Popular Mechanics

Veterinary Guide
for Farmers

Completely Revised Edition
By G.W. Stamm

Edited by R.C. Klussendorf, D.V.M., Veterinary Consultant

Dr. Klussendorf is well known as a former
successful veterinary practitioner and, later
in his career, as Editor of the *Journal of
the American Veterinary Medical Association*.
He received his Bachelor of Science degree
with honors at the University of Wisconsin,
and his Doctorate at Cornell.

Book Division, The Hearst Corporation,
New York, N.Y. 10019

ISBN 0-910990-61-1

Library of Congress Catalog Number: 75-18653

Foreword

THE SHORTAGE of veterinarians in farm animal practice is greater today in many areas than ever before. Thus, the publication of this completely revised edition of the *Veterinary Guide for Farmers* is most opportune.

The book fulfills a need in several important respects. It helps a man engaged in the care of farm animals to recognize with greater accuracy the early symptoms of a disease and thereby get veterinary assistance more quickly. The book also enables an individual to carry out with greater efficiency the routine treatments as directed by a veterinarian.

A large portion of the book is devoted to basic knowledge of the animal body, the function of its organs, and the bacteria, viruses and parasites that interfere with these functions. Thus, the over-worked veterinarian will find the book invaluable in teaching the elements of veterinary medicine to a non-professional assistant.

No book related to biology is ever completely up-to-date. New findings come so fast that a book is hardly off the press before parts of it are obsolete. Also, in the same manner that a drug for arthritis may relieve one person but be detrimental to another, so the delicate relationship between a drug and an animal patient often leads to conflicting conclusions in evaluating a pharmaceutical. In the confusion arising from such a situation it is probable that some valuable drugs may have been omitted from the text.

Contents

The causes of disease

ALL LIVING THINGS are made up of cells, bits of living matter so small that they can be seen only with the aid of a microscope.

These cells are specialists in the work they do. Muscle cells can change their shapes—become shorter or longer—so that your muscles can shorten up and lift things. Nerve cells carry messages between the brain and other parts of the body—tell us when a toe is injured, how food tastes, enable us to enjoy the sound of music. The cells of the inner eye are sensitive to light and can pick up images that are sent to the brain.

An animal is sick whenever something interferes with the life and work of its cells. And this happens most often when microbes invade the body and overcome the natural defenses.

Microbes, also called *microorganisms*, are found everywhere in almost unbelievably large numbers. It has been estimated that those in the top eight inches of an acre of soil weigh nine tons. There may be more of them in a handful of rich topsoil than there are people on earth. Most of them are not only completely harmless but are helpful to plants, animals and people. Some enter into the making of cheese and vinegar. Others have the ability to take nitrogen from the air and soil and put it in such a form that it serves as food for plants.

Those microbes that cause disease are said to be *pathogenic*. They are called *pathogens* although this word includes other things that cause illness, such as hay fever pollen.

How microbes destroy

Some people may wonder why things so small can bring on such violent illness. When pathogenic microbes gain a foothold in the body, they start breaking down the cells and body fluids. In doing so they create poisons called *toxins*. This is done in the same manner that yeast cells consume sugar and make alcohol.

The toxins produced by a few thousand or a few million microbes won't always make an animal sick. But unless they are stopped, microbes multiply until there are billions of them.

Sometimes they multiply so fast that the animal is sick—shows *disease symptoms*—in a few days. In other cases, it may take months from the time the microbes enter the body until the symptoms appear.

The period from the time infection occurs until symptoms are present is called the *period of incubation*. This varies in length with the kind of disease, the *virulence*, or strength, of the organism and the resistance of the infected animal. To be *resistant* means that an animal can fight off invading germs, at least to some extent. *Susceptible* is a word that means just the opposite.

What is metabolism?

Besides their ability to multiply and make toxins, there is another reason why microbes can do so much damage. This is their *rate of metabolism,* or metabolic rate.

Metabolism is the over-all process whereby the body of an animal or plant takes in food and changes it into energy or tissue, or stores it. Animals store it in the form of fat or protein.

The metabolic rate of a microorganism is about 50 times as great as that of a man. This is as though a 150-pound man sat down to breakfast on Sunday morning and ate five dozen eggs, 30 waffles, six loaves of bread, a kettle of oatmeal, and drank 80 cups of coffee. Then for fear of getting hungry at church, he topped this off with a small snack consisting of a boiled ham and five custard cream pies.

Microbes vs body forces

But microbes entering the body don't remain unchallenged. A conflict at once arises between the invaders and the body forces. These forces are of several kinds, chiefly certain white blood corpuscles called *phagocytes* and substances in the blood known as *antibodies.* The latter act like chemicals and kill the invaders or so weaken them that they fall easy prey to the phagocytes. The phagocytes also produce substances that neutralize toxins, fittingly called *antitoxins.*

All animals are born with natural resistance to some diseases. Cattle, for example, won't get glanders, a disease of horses, nor will horses come down with hog cholera. When an animal is not susceptible to a disease it is said to be *immune* to that disease.

There is a great difference in immunity among animals. This difference applies not only to animals of different kinds but to individual animals of the same kind.

When hog cholera strikes a susceptible herd, many animals die in a few days; some after a week or more. Others will be sick and recover, while a very few will go blithely about their business and won't be sick at all. Why this should be, no one knows. Inheritance seems to play an important part.

Antibodies, the mysterious substances that spell death to microbes, are made by the cells in the blood and tissues. With some diseases, when the animal recovers, the cells seem to keep on making antibodies as long as the animal lives. It remains immune to that disease.

Toxins and other substances that cause cells to make antibodies are called *antigens.* An antigen is specific in its action. For example one that will bring on protection against hog cholera will not protect against erysipelas.

And now we come to one of the greatest discoveries in all human history.

Pasteur's great discovery

If antibodies protect animals against disease, why not inject some from another animal? Or why not cause them to be made in the body? Herein lies the idea that has saved the lives of untold millions of animals, not to mention human beings. It is sometimes termed *artificially induced immunity*.

The principal products used to induce such immunity are vaccines, bacterins and serums. These and similar products are called *biological products, biologicals,* or simply *biologics*.

Vaccines are made of living germs that have been weakened or changed so as to lose much of their original virulence or power. When an animal is vaccinated, it is given a mild attack of the disease. This produces antibodies and often results in permanent immunity. When antibodies, also called *immune bodies,* are produced by an animal in this way, its resistance against the disease is called *active immunity*.

Animals susceptible to a disease should be immunized while they are healthy, not after they are sick. Usually it takes a few weeks for the body to build up a supply of antibodies. And during that time the animal is more susceptible to the disease than if it had not been vaccinated at all.

The formation of antibodies is influenced by the age of the animal. Neither the very young nor the old respond as well as those between these two extremes.

Bacterins are similar to vaccines, but the microbes in them have been killed. The dead organisms are placed in oil or in water that contains the same amount of salt as the body fluids.

Like vaccines, bacterins cause cells to make antibodies. In theory they could be used to advantage in the treatment of all diseases where the microbes are known. In practice this doesn't work out.

Serums, properly called *immune blood serums* or *antiserums,* contain no organisms, either dead or alive. When the corpuscles are removed from blood, plasma is what remains. Plasma contains *fibrinogen,* a substance that makes blood clot and so stops the bleeding when the skin is cut. Remove the fibrinogen from plasma and you have serum.

To make immune blood serum, a healthy animal is purposely infected with the disease for which the serum is wanted. In due time the antibodies are formed in the lymphocytes and pass into the blood. This blood is withdrawn in proper amounts and the immune serum is recovered.

The injection of immune blood serum supplies antibodies, but does not cause cells to make antibodies. For this reason it is called passive immunity, and gives only the temporary protection.

Immune blood serums are used to protect animals temporarily against disease epidemics. They are also used to advantage in combination with vaccines. In such cases they permit the use of much larger doses of vaccine than would otherwise be possible and so hasten the production of immune bodies. Also, since vaccines are living microbes, they will sometimes kill animals unless used with immune serums.

Microorganisms are sometimes said to be simple one-celled animals. Actually, they are by no means simple.

Small as they are, microbes contain within themselves manufacturing units that change many substances into heat and energy and living matter. Within themselves, the microbes use vitamins and enzymes. They have what amounts to well-equipped machine shops that make repairs when needed. And they do these things, and many more, automatically.

Most microbes multiply by what is called simple division. This means that when they grow to a certain size, they simply divide in half and then there are two of them instead of one. In this way their blood lines have been carried on through the ages. Outlines of the remains of their colonies are found in rocks that were formed long before man came upon this earth.

Some microbes live only in the presence of air. These are termed *aerobic*. Others can live only without air and so are called *anaerobic*. They have many shapes and sizes.

Certain germs make powerful toxins that are dissolved in the blood. Others carry the toxins in their bodies until they die and these are released when the organisms are broken up.

Some microbes form spores

Under certain conditions, some microbes form *spores*. When in this form, they have shell-like coverings which enable them to resist destruction. Spores can live several years without food. They can withstand poisons that would kill them without spore casings. They can live through bitter cold winters, and some of them can endure a 16-hour bath in boiling water.

Diseases, such as anthrax, that occur year after year in certain areas are perpetuated by spores. Animals eat them with their food, they are spread by insects, or enter the animal bodies through open cuts.

Let conditions be right and spores again become their former selves. Shortly they are back in fighting trim.

Animal flesh and blood must be considered quite a delicacy among the lower forms of life. Otherwise why should animals have so many enemies? And why should these enemies have so many different methods of attack?

Let's take up some of the worst offenders:

Bacteria comprise a large portion of all microscopic life. Their bodies are made up of just one cell. According to their shapes, there are three kinds.

Bacilli are rod-shaped bacteria that cause such diseases as tuberculosis and tetanus.

Cocci are round or oval-shaped. They cause pneumonia, the well-known streptococcus infections, and many other diseases.

Spirilla are bacteria that are thread-shaped or corkscrew-shaped. One form may cause abortion among cows and ewes.

Viruses are so small that 500 to 1,000 of them will fit into a bacteria cell. Since they cannot be seen with an ordinary microscope, they are studied by means of an electron microscope. Viruses always live and multiply within living cells. Consequently they cannot be killed by means of chemicals or antibiotics such as the sulfa drugs and penicillin which circulate only in body fluids.

Viruses cause foot-and-mouth disease, hog cholera, rabies, fowl pox and numerous other diseases of animals.

Some virus diseases bring on *secondary infections*. These are caused by bacteria normally present in animals without harm, but which flare up with disastrous results after viruses have broken down the natural body resistance. This often occurs in distemper of dogs and horses, and in swine influenza.

Protozoa are like bacteria in that they are composed of only one cell. However they are 50 to 100 times as large as bacteria. Most protozoa are *motile*, that is, they have ways of propelling themselves.

One kind, called *amoeba*, moves by letting body substances flow out in the direction it is moving. Then the rest of the body fills in this extended portion until the whole animal occupies a new position. Another kind of protozoa moves by means of whip-like lashes, called *flagella*. A third uses hair-like vibrating projections, called *cilia*, to propel itself.

A few kinds of protozoa prey upon animals and produce serious and fatal diseases. Among the animal diseases are coccidiosis of poultry, cattle and sheep, and anaplasmosis of cattle.

Other causes of disease

Although bacteria, protozoa and viruses are the principal causes of disease, there are other important ones. Among them are:

Parasites, which may be internal or external. Internal parasites are technically called helminths, and commonly called worms; but they may also be flukes. They infest the stomach, intestines, liver, lungs, and other parts of the body.

The external parasites are lice, flies, mites, and ticks. These not only cause direct injury to the health of animals but often do a great deal of indirect damage by harboring pathogenic microbes. Parasites often have these microbes inside their bodies and carry them from sick animals to healthy ones in the same way that malaria is spread by mosquitoes.

Poisonous plants and chemicals.

Lack of certain foods, vitamins or minerals, collectively called deficiency diseases.

How to tell what's wrong

FARM ANIMALS, like people, generally show by their actions and appearance when something is the matter with them. Successful livestock men form the habit of watching their animals closely for early signs of disease. In this way, they come to recognize the symptoms of many of the more common ailments.

With a few diseases, of course, there are at first no observable symptoms. In cases of tuberculosis, for example, the presence of the disease can be determined only by means of special tests.

Diagnosis—how to tell what ails a sick animal—should be based on evidence. Mere guesswork won't do.

When a cow that has recently calved goes off her feed, has a faltering gait, develops a listless expression about her eyes or becomes wildeyed, she probably has milk fever or acetonemia, or both. Further tests will determine the truth. A sheep that spends an unusual amount of time lying down, but seems otherwise in good health may have foot rot. The appearance of its feet and the characteristic foul odor make it almost certain that this disease is present.

Some ailments usually appear only at certain times of the year; some attack only the young animals; others affect only the old. The presence of a particular disease in the locality, and whether or not new animals have recently been added to a herd, must also be considered.

Usually the first signs of a disease are very slight. But to notice these early symptoms before more serious ones appear helps greatly in the control of disease. Animals recover more quickly when given care and treatment at the onset of sickness. What's more, the spread of a disease can often be stopped if a sick animal is at once separated from the rest of the group.

Symptoms and what they mean

Symptoms of many diseases vary somewhat in different animals of the same kind. And a particular ailment may bring on different symptoms in different kinds of animals. A horse with colic will paw the ground with its forefeet. It may break out in a sweat, lie down, roll and groan. A cow with a similar digestive disturbance may also groan but she will be dull and inactive.

When one or more symptoms of sickness are noticed, a more thorough examination of the affected animal should be made. In most cases it is unwise to arrive at a definite conclusion until all symptoms and all conditions that might influence the animal's health have been considered.

Only a few symptoms point to disease of particular parts of the body. Most symptoms are general. When one part of the body is diseased, symptoms appear in other parts as well. This is like an upset stomach that brings on a headache and makes a person feel sick all over.

Symptoms, considered singly, are often misleading. They merely indicate that a disease is present. The task in diagnosis is to find out what causes the symptoms. Many ailments have some symptoms in common, and symptoms considered alone are often misleading. Even a sudden change of feed may cause symptoms like those of an infectious disease.

In making an examination it is advisable to do the simple things first. In this way you may learn at once what ails a sick animal. You can then check your findings by looking for other symptoms that will make certain the presence or absence of a particular disease.

Noting the general behavior

When an animal acts in a manner that is contrary to its nature, it is often showing the first signs of disease. For this reason a good diagnostician must know how healthy animals appear and behave. Only in this way can he recognize behavior that is unnatural.

An animal may show signs of sickness by keeping away from the rest of the herd, by droopiness, lack of normal energy and loss of appetite.

It is natural for cattle to lie down part of the day, especially after feeding. They usually do not get up when someone approaches them. Cattle seldom lie on their sides but rest on their breastbones with legs folded under them.

A cow with milk fever will rest on her breastbone, but her head will fall limply to the side. If not attended to, she will soon fall into a stupor and roll over on her side. In this position she may bloat and her legs will stick out straight and stiff.

Animals that are very sick usually hold their heads down. Their ears droop and they seem to move only with great effort. A cow that extends her head stiffly may have tetanus, muscular rheumatism, a throat ailment, catarrh or a disease of the nervous system.

In diseases where there is a rapid loss of condition, animals get a

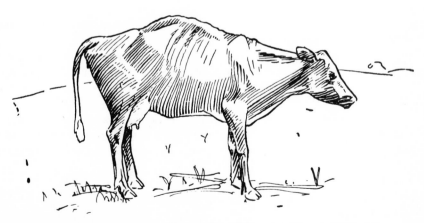

Although an arched back occurs with a number of diseases, it is nonetheless a valuable clue in diagnosis when considered together with other symptoms

dejected, woebegone look. Eyes become sunken; the face gets a blank expression.

The way an animal stands is often a clue to its ailment. An arched back occurs with a number of diseases but is nonetheless a valuable clue when considered with other symptoms. For example, it occurs with severe vaginitis—inflammation of the vagina—but a cow with this disease, in addition, will hold her tail high and spread her legs apart. She doesn't like to be forced to "move over," and she'll stop often to urinate when driven. A cow with a piece of metal puncturing her heart wall—traumatic pericarditis—will often stand with arched back but in such cases she'll keep her body stiff when turning to go in another direction.

In severe cases of grass tetany, a disease that often occurs when cows are first turned out into lush pastures, a cow has a stumbling gait and may fall forward, almost turning a somersault. Fever often causes a labored, wobbly gait.

Loss of condition

When an animal loses weight, the manner in which it is lost and the circumstances surrounding the loss often indicate the cause.

It is usually easy to tell the differences between loss of weight caused by not enough feed and that due to sickness. The behavior of the animal reveals this even to one who does not know that the animal was underfed.

Emaciation—extreme loss of weight—occurs commonly with Johne's disease and tuberculosis, although in some cases a tuberculous animal may seem to be in the best of health. Lack of certain minerals and the presence of internal parasites—the so-called helminths, or worms—are common causes of emaciation.

When a disease seriously affects the digestive tract, an animal always loses condition. This is true whether the disease affects the digestion directly or whether the digestive disturbance is brought on indirectly by an ailment in another part of the body. When an animal loses condition gradually and continuously even though it eats enough good feed, it probably has a chronic disease.

Sometimes an animal loses weight because a sore mouth or an infected tooth makes eating painful or an injured foot keeps it from moving around for feed. If a cow in good condition suddenly gets a painful infection in a hind foot, it may lose a lot of weight within a few days.

Appearance of skin and hair

The appearance of the skin not only reveals local disease conditions but often indicates maladies of a general nature involving the internal organs.

Local skin diseases or external parasites are usually present when an animal frequently scratches itself and its hair falls out in large amounts, sometimes leaving the skin completely denuded. When an infected spot has been found, a complete inspection of the skin should be made.

The location and extent of a skin infection are sometimes clues to its nature. When parasites cannot be found with the unaided eye, skin scrapings from infected spots should be examined with a magnifying glass or under a microscope.

Rashes, widespread swellings and discoloration of the skin often occur with diseases seated in other parts of the body. Some diseases cause skin reactions that appear on certain parts of the body only or are most evident in certain places. For example, cowpox sores seldom appear other than on the teats and udders of cows. In blackleg, swellings appear mainly on the upper parts of the legs—never on the tail or on the lower parts of the legs.

The skin of healthy animals is soft and pliable. It tends to become hard and leather-like when an animal loses condition either from under-nourishment or from a wasting disease. The skins of healthy animals, when clean, have a faint odor that is not unpleasant.

The appearance of hair changes with disease. It loses luster and sometimes tufts appear. When an animal suffers a chill, whether from fever or from cold air or water, hair will stand on end.

Unusual odors

Each kind of animal has an odor peculiar to itself. In disease these odors change, but only in a few cases do offensive odors have diagnostic value. Odors may indicate that an animal is sick but seldom point to the nature of the malady.

Unpleasant odors of the breath sometimes have definite diagnostic value. These may come from the mouth, the lungs, the stomach or the intestines. The smell of acetone is present in acetonemia. A sour smell with a sticky feeling in the mouth parts accompanies chronic indigestion. Mouth ulcers always have an offensive odor.

The mouth and eyes

Too much saliva in the mouth may indicate that more is being secreted than usual or that the animal cannot swallow the amount that

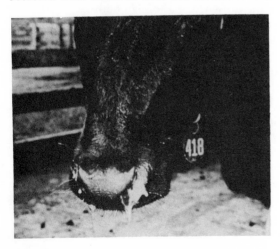

A nasal discharge such as exhibited by this heifer is often seen with the respiratory form of infectious bovine rhinotracheitis

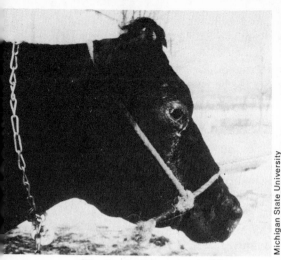
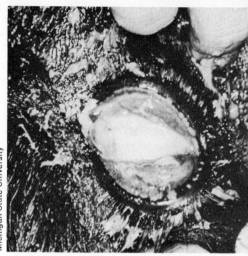

The eye discharge seen in this photograph was caused by the conjunctivitis form of IBR (the conjunctiva are the pink tissues which surround the eyes)

Note the severe inflammation and swelling of the mucous membranes which surround the eye in this case of the eye form of IBR (conjunctivitis). ["-itis" on the end of a word means inflammation of that tissue.]

normally flows from the gland. Excessive saliva is usually caused by irritation brought on by an infection of the tongue, cheeks or jaws, or by an injury in the mouth as from bad teeth. Wood splinters, thorns or other foreign objects that penetrate the soft tissues or become lodged between the teeth are common causes. Lumpy jaw and wooden tongue are fairly common mouth and jaw infections that cause driveling.

The flow of saliva is decreased in most acute diseases accompanied with fever, in severe ailments of the intestines, and generally with colic. When the mouth of an animal remains open, the condition may be due to swelling of the tongue or to the presence of a foreign body.

In sickness, the eyes lose their normal moist, clear appearance. Diseases of the eye, such as pinkeye, are fairly easy to recognize because of the extent of the discharge. But the eyes are also affected in diseases of a general nature such as hog cholera and gray eye in fowl paralysis.

When the pupils of the eyes fail to become smaller upon shining a strong light into them, it may be due to a local ailment or to a disease of the nervous system. Both eyes should always be examined.

Fever as a symptom

The temperature of an animal's body rises above normal when more heat is produced than is given off. This happens naturally under a number of conditions, such as during exercise, after eating, in very hot weather and among cows in the later stages of pregnancy.

When the temperature of an animal rises without apparent reason, it is generally caused by illness or injury. That is why the presence of fever is of great importance in the diagnosis of disease, especially those that affect the internal organs.

An increase in temperature is not the only symptom of fever. Sometimes after the temperature goes up rapidly, chills may occur, and these in turn are accompanied by trembling muscles, cold skin, erect hair coat and arched back.

Chills do not occur with all fevers but with disease where microbes or toxins are in the blood stream. Among them are anthrax, shipping fever and maladies accompanied by pus formation. Once the body becomes used to a higher temperature, chills cease. But they will come back if the animal is taken to a colder place.

Fever brings with it a more rapid breathing and heart beat. At the same time the pulse becomes weaker. The more rapid the pulse, the higher the fever.

A strange thing about fever is that the legs, ears, nose and base of the horns in cattle and sheep become alternately hot and cold even though the internal temperature of the animals remains uniform. One ear may be hot while the other is cold. Later these conditions may be reversed, or both ears may be hot or both cold. The same thing hold true of legs and other extremities.

Other signs of fever are dry muzzles and snouts, loss of appetite, indigestion, constipation, increased thirst, decreased urination and mental depression.

Differential diagnosis

The symptoms of several diseases are sometimes so much alike that it's hard to tell the ailments apart. Even veterinarians with years of experience have this difficulty now and then. The differences in the symptoms are there all right, but they are so slight that they cannot easily be found.

Such situations call for what is known as a "differential diagnosis." This merely means that you use greater care and often more technical methods to find more symptoms and to find any differences among symptoms already found. You "differentiate" between the diseases that might be present.

A very slight difference in symptoms may be a clue to the nature of the disease. The symptoms of swine erysipelas and hog cholera are very much alike, but in hog cholera eyelids become glued together while in erysipelas they do not. The red blotches that appear in hog cholera remain red when pressed. Similar areas in swine erysipelas disappear or turn white under pressure.

The rapidity of the onset of a disease, the number of animals affected and the death rate are valuable aids to diagnosis. If many animals suddenly take sick, the cause is probably an infectious disease or poison. Other symptoms make it easy to tell whether or not animals have been poisoned.

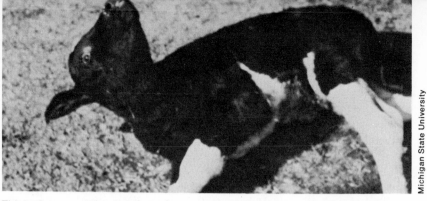

This calf was unable to stand or walk normally. It was born with a condition called cerebellar hypoplasia (defective development of a part of the brain) as a result of its mother being infected with bovine virus diarrhea during the middle of pregnancy

Symptoms of a disease sometimes change or new ones are added as a malady progresses. For this reason it is helpful to know when the first signs of the malady appeared and how long it took for later symptoms to develop. The speed with which a disease reaches a climax is often a clue to its nature.

Performing an autopsy

Whenever there is any doubt about the presence of a serious disease, post-mortem examinations should be made and affected body organs should be sent to the laboratory for examination.

When a suspected disease is dangerous to man, such as anthrax, special care should be taken to guard against infection. In such cases it is better to leave the examination to someone with veterinary or medical training. In any event, don't open the carcass of an anthrax victim or you may contaminate your premises. Instead, cut off an ear and send it to the laboratory. Never try to salvage pelts of animals where anthrax is suspected. Such bodies should be burned or deeply buried in quick lime.

Autopsies should be made as soon as possible after death. Decomposition of a carcass starts early, especially in warm weather. If you wait, the changes in a body organ caused by decomposition may be mistaken for disease symptoms.

An autopsy should be complete. After thorough examination of the outside of the carcass, start work on the interior—lungs, liver, spleen, stomach, intestines and bladder.

How to take the temperature

TAKING THE TEMPERATURE of animals is of great value during outbreaks of infectious diseases. Fever is often the first noticeable sign of an infection. By taking daily temperatures, preferably in the evening, you can detect infected animals much sooner than otherwise.

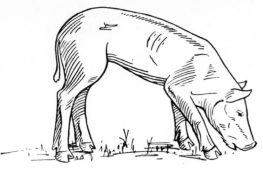

Fever is accompanied by loss of appetite and loss of moisture from the body. This results in rapid loss of condition

Taking daily temperatures is especially valuable in combating pneumonia, swine plague, hog cholera and influenza. It is useful, both in diagnosing a disease and in observing its course. With important diseases and especially with valuable animals, temperatures are often taken twice a day, preferably at 8 a.m. and 5 p.m.

The instrument used for taking body temperatures is known as the maximum thermometer. When its bulb is warmed, the mercury rises in the column and remains at its highest point after the warmth is no longer present. This makes the thermometer easy to read, but it has one disadvantage. After the instrument has been used, the mercury must always be shaken back into the bullb before the instrument is used again. A cattle thermometer is generally five inches long, and the one for smaller animals is four inches long.

The temperature of domestic animals is usually taken by inserting the thermometer into the rectum. In special cases, the vagina is used.

After you have shaken down the instrument, grease it with some harmless grease or oil before inserting it into the rectum. Push it in its full length, bulb first, and allow it to remain in position for three minutes or longer. Large animals should be restrained since they are apt to kick. Use care not to break the thermometer and injure the animal. Always clean the thermometer thoroughly after each use.

The normal body temperature of animals varies much more than that of people. The normal range of rectum temperatures of principal farm animals is given in the chart on the next page.

Rectum temperatures are higher than those of the mouth and much higher than those of the skin. If the temperature of animals rises 2 degrees or more above the highest figures given, fever is present.

Taking the pulse and what it tells

THE PULSE TELLS how the heart is beating. Fever, inflammations and local diseases of the heart increase the heart beat and consequently the pulse rate. So do exercise, excitement, hot weather, pain and the digestion of food.

The blood vessels that lead away from the heart—the arteries—have a pulse. With a few exceptions, those that lead toward the heart—the veins—do not have one. Most arteries are more deeply embedded in the tissues than the corresponding veins. This makes the arteries a little harder to find.

In cattle, the artery used most often for taking the pulse is called the submaxillary. This can be felt where it winds around the lower edge of the jawbone at the lower part of the flat muscle on the side of the cheek. If a cow or a horse is lying down, the metacarpal artery may be more convenient. This can be felt on the back part of the fetlock of a front leg.

In sheep the femoral artery is the most convenient at the point where it comes out of the groin and runs down the inner surface of the upper part of the hind leg.

To take the pulse, place the tips of the first three fingers over the artery. The best spot can be found by rolling the artery a little under the fingers. Make sure that all beats are plainly felt before starting the actual count. The thumb cannot be used for taking the pulse because the thumb has a pulse of its own that might be mistaken for that of the animal.

Interpreting the pulse

There is a big variation in the normal pulse rate of animals. This applies not only to animals of a different kind but also to individual animals of the same kind. In general, large animals have slower pulse rates than small ones. Also, the older the animal the slower the pulse. The pulse of females is faster than that of males. Purebred or blooded animals often have a slower pulse than others of the same kind.

When the pulse rate of a cow approaches 110, it has an ailment from which it probably will not recover.

Other variations of the pulse

In addition to the pulse rate, the pulse has other variations that may indicate the presence of a disease, especially ailments of the heart or blood vessels.

A slow or infrequent pulse means that the number of beats per minute is less than normal. An irregular pulse is one in which the beats do not occur at regular intervals although there may be a normal number per minute. To say a pulse is strong or feeble means that it is stronger or weaker than normal. A pulse is said to be hard or soft when the artery feels harder or softer than normal—is more, or less, compressible.

An intermittent pulse is one in which beats are skipped. But this does not always means that there is something the matter with the animal. When a horse, used to hard work, is rested for a while, its pulse will often skip a beat at regular intervals—usually one beat out of every five. When this horse is back at work, the missing beat will reappear.

Farm animals—names and useful facts about them

	Cattle	Swine	Sheep	Horses
Adult male	Bull	Boar	Ram	Stallion
Adult female	Cow	Sow	Ewe	Mare
Young male	Bull calf	Shote[1]	Ram lamb	Colt
Young female	Heifer	Gilt	Ewe lamb	Filly
Newly born	Calf	Pig	Lamb	Foal
Castrated male	Steer	Barrow[2]	Wether	Gelding
Normal body temperature (degrees F.)[3]	98.0 to 102.8	101.6 to 103.6	100.9 to 103.8	99.0 to 100.6
Pulse rate per minute	40-70	60-80	70-80	32-44
Respiration per minute	10-30	8-18	12-20	8-16
Age of puberty (female)	4-8 months	3-5 months	First fall	One year
Length of pregnancy (average)	283 days	113 days	150 days	336 days
Length of cycle (time between heat periods)	21 days	21 days	17 days	22 days

[1] The word shote applies to a pig of either sex under one year old.

[2] To be considered a barrow, a pig must be castrated when young, before sex characteristics have developed. If castrated when mature, he is called a stag.

[3] Temperatures of animals vary in accordance with such things as the time of day, season of the year, the part of the body and whether or not the animal has recently eaten or had exercise.

To determine whether an animal has fever, temperatures are usually taken in animal's rectum. It may be necessary to take two or three readings at intervals of an hour, or compare readings with those of healthy members of a herd. A rapid rise in temperature of six or eight degrees that soon returns to normal is less dangerous than a slow rise of three or four degrees that does not subside.

Diagnosis chart of the more common animal diseases

Disease	Kinds of animals affected	Age at which animals are most susceptible	Principal symptoms
Anaplasmosis	Cattle	Seldom attacks animals under one year old	Anemia, jaundice, frequent urination, rough coat, depression. In severe form death occurs in few days. Mild form occurs mostly in calves, with quick recovery
Anthrax (splenic fever, charbon)	Nearly all warm-blooded animals, including man. Cattle, horses, sheep, and goats are most often affected	All ages, but mature animals are most often affected	In peracute (highly acute) form, animals seemingly in good health suddenly die. In acute and sub-acute forms, victims are excited and later depressed. Thirst increases; appetite fails. Breathing is rapid and labored. Bloody discharges come from natural body openings. Soft swellings that pit upon pressure appear on various parts of the body
Atrophic rhinitis	Hogs	Young pigs. Symptoms seldom noticeable until pigs are three weeks old	Sneezing. Discharge from the eyes. Failure to make satisfactory gains. Extreme irritation of nose. Pigs rub snouts in corners and against legs. Nasal hemorrhage. Distortion of face. Marked wrinkling
Black disease (infectious necrotic hepatitis)	Sheep	Adults	No definite symptoms. Death comes suddenly. Animals look as though they had died in their sleep. Sometimes bloody foam runs from nose
Blackleg (black quarter, quarter ill)	Cattle, sheep, goats	Usually occurs between six months and two years of age	First symptoms are high fever, loss of appetite, followed by depression. Swellings appear under skin of shoulders, hip, beneath breast, on flanks and thighs. At first, small and painful, but rapidly become larger. When pressed, swellings make crackling sound.
Bluetongue	Sheep	May occur at any age	Starts with lack of appetite and depression. Within few days inside of mouth and nose become inflamed. There is frothing and labored breathing. Inflamed parts may become blue. Bloody spots with ulcers and bleeding may appear. There is often a discharge from the nose which changes to catarrh in a few days with formation of crusts on upper lip

Geographic distribution and seasons of greatest occurrence	Fever, in degrees Fahrenheit	Death rate (mortality)	Internal conditions (post-mortem findings)
Mostly in Far West, South and Southwest, but cases have occurred in 29 states. Summer and fall	Sometimes as high as 106	From 25 to 60 percent of older animals die. Recovered animals are carriers throughout life	Skin, teats, mouth parts are yellow. Gall bladder contents are dark green and resemble gelatin. Liver enlarged and yellow. Spleen soft, large and resembles blackberry jam. Blood thin and watery.
Occurs all over the world in certain areas or districts. Summer and fall: occasional cases at other times	105-108	90 to 100 percent of affected animals die	In peracute cases, changes are slight. In other cases, spleen is enlarged and dark red to blackish in color. There are bloating and tarry blood. Hemorrhages beneath skin are common. In hogs, changes are most noticeable in the throat—hemorrhages in the glands, enlarged dark-colored tonsils. Use extreme care in handling carcasses. The disease is deadly.
Europe, North America, probably elsewhere. May occur at any time of year	No fever	Death rate around 20 to 30 percent of pigs affected	Bones of snout and face often completely wasted away
Swampy, poorly drained land where liver flukes are present, especially California, Montana, Oregon and Idaho. Late summer and fall	Not known	90 to 100 percent	Hemorrhages under skin on back and sides. Clear fluid present under heart covering. Yellowish spots on liver, some as large as a walnut
Occurs in nearly every state but most widespread in Mississippi Valley states. Spring and fall; but may occur at other times. Stable cattle may get it in the winter	105 to 107	Usually nearly 100 percent. Milder form with recovery sometimes affects older animals	Extreme bloat appears shortly after death. Bloody froth comes out of mouth, nostrils and rectum. Bloody serum is found under skin and between muscles. It has a sweetish-sour odor like that of rancid butter
Appears in California and has been suspected in Western States. Is known in South Africa, Cyprus and Israel	Temperature 106 to 107	Death rate among affected animals usually under 10 percent but may rise to 30 or 40 percent	In addition to outward symptoms there is often muscular degeneration. About half the victims have blood and fluids in their lungs

Diagnosis chart of the more common animal diseases

Disease	Kinds of animals affected	Age at which animals are most susceptible	Principal symptoms
Brucellosis (Bang's disease, contagious abortion)	Cattle, hogs, goats, man (when the disease attacks people it is called undulant fever)	Any time after animals are sexually mature	In cattle: abortion, retention of afterbirth, reduced milk production. In hogs: abortion, arthritis, inflammation of the testicles
Calf diphtheria (necrotic stomatitis, gangrenous stomatitis, necrotic laryngitis, malignant stomatitis, sore mouth)	Young suckling calves	As early as three days old. Mature animals infected only in severe outbreaks	Animals are depressed. Even suckling calves refuse feed. Drooling of saliva occurs; swelling may appear at side of throat; there are wheezing and coughing. Sticky yellowish to greenish-yellow discharge may come from nostrils. Tongue sometimes sticks out and mouth has offensive odor
Calf scours (See White Scours)			
Circling disease (listerellosis, encephalitis in sheep)	Sheep Goats Cattle Hogs, to small extent	May occur at any age	In sheep, goats and cattle: dullness, staggering, pushing head into fences, walking in circles, paralysis. In hogs: trembling, dragging hind feet, stilted movements of forelegs, paralysis.
Coccidiosis (red dysentery)	Cattle Hogs Sheep Goats Poultry	Any age. Young calves and young pigs are susceptible to serious attacks	Bloody diarrhea, anemia, weakness and emaciation. In young pigs, principal symptom is usually pronounced unthriftiness
Hog cholera	Hogs	All ages	In highly acute form, animals die suddenly without showing any symptoms. In acute form, symptoms are loss of appetite, great depression, high fever, head held down and tail straight, often purple patches on ears and abdomen, discharge that often makes eyelids stick together. Weakness, especially in hind legs, gives animals peculiar wobbly gait
Johne's disease (paratuberculosis, chronic specific enteritis of cattle)	Principally cattle but also horses, sheep, goats and deer	Young animals become infected most easily but symptoms may not appear until animals are three or four years old	Loss of condition while appetite remains good, thirst, diarrhea without straining, rough coat, dry skin and no fever. Animals seem to recover but symptoms later appear again. Toward the end, animals refuse to eat

Geographic distribution and seasons of greatest occurrence	Fever, in degrees Fahrenheit	Death rate (mortality)	Internal conditions (post-mortem findings)
Occurs the world over in all seasons of the year	None of diagnostic value	Very low among mature animals. High in interrupted pregnancies—fetuses mostly dead	None of diagnostic value
Any part of country but most often in cold climates, though only occasionally in eastern states. Winter	105	Very high	Cheesy, crumbly grayish-yellow mass present in upper windpipe and on base of tongue. In severe cases lungs, stomach, intestines and liver also contain this mass
Worldwide. Fall, winter and spring	104 to 106 in cattle	Nearly 100 percent among affected animals	None that can be seen without the aid of a microscope
May occur anywhere and in any season, though largely in fall and winter	Temperature normal or below normal	Death rate low except in severe outbreaks among very young calves	Intestines and rectum tissues are thickened and bloody. Rectum wall is often two or three times as thick as normal. Contents of large intestines and rectum may consist largely of blood
In Middle West occurs most often in late summer and fall, with only occasional light outbreaks at other times. In the South, where winters are mild, severe outbreaks may occur at any time	104 to 107	Nearly 100 percent	Diagnosis difficult to make from appearance of internal organs because symptoms vary greatly in degree and resemble those of some other diseases. Spleen, or milt, is soft and easily torn and is full of blood that is darker than ordinary. Kidneys have hemorrhages the size of a pinhead or smaller. Bladder and intestines have similar hemorrhages. Raised ulcers may occur in large intestines. These are called "button ulcers"
Worldwide. Occurs at any time of year though somewhat more often in summer	Practically none	Practically all animals that show symptoms die within a period of one month to two years	In young calves, redness and swelling of small intestines occurs, but sometimes only a small area is affected. In mature animals, the ileum, cecum, large intestines and rectum are thickened and often have red patches. In severe cases, infected portions are sometimes two to five times their normal thickness.

Diagnosis chart of the more common animal diseases

Disease	Kinds of animals affected	Age at which animals are most susceptible	Principal symptoms
Ketosis (acetonemia, hypoglycemia)	Dairy cows, especially heavy milkers	May occur during any lactation period but most often from third calving on	Disease occurs in three forms: (1) indigestion, constipation, listlessness, loss of appetite; (2) indigestion, trembling, weakness, collapse; (3) extreme nervousness, bellowing, insane actions. In all three forms there are rapid loss of condition, large reduction in milk flow, a sweetish, offensive odor of the breath and off-flavored milk
Leptospirosis	Cattle Hogs Horses	Any age	In calves, typical symptoms include fever, prostration, labored breathing, anemia, jaundice and red urine. In older cattle anemia and red urine may occur but disease is usually much milder. There is a sharp drop in milk production. Milk is thick, yellow, blood-tinged though udder shows no inflammation. Abortions occur in any stage of pregnancy. Hogs show common signs of sickness plus meningitis and circling
Malignant edema (gas phlegmon, braxy in sheep)	Horses Hogs Sheep Cattle	Any age	Sudden onset within few hours to a few days following an injury caused by such things as splinters, nails, castration, docking or shearing. Symptoms are high fever, loss of appetite, and swelling that may appear on any part of body; in horses, they usually start on the head and legs. The swellings make a crackling sound when touched and a thin, dirty, reddish fluid flows from them
Milk fever (parturient paresis)	Dairy cows, principally, though female sheep, goats and hogs may be affected	Occurs only after calving and seldom until after second calving	Symptoms are of two kinds: (1) great depression, refusal to eat or move about; (2) excitement, trembling, wild look in eyes, staggering, weakness. In either case, loss of consciousness follows, with head turned to one side
Navel ill (joint ill)	Horses Sheep Cattle Hogs	Newborn foals. Lambs from one to three weeks old. Newborn calves and pigs	Usually hot swollen joints, lack of appetite, listlessness, fever and lameness. In some cases disease does not cause swollen joints or lameness but the other symptoms are present

Geographic distribution and seasons of greatest occurrence	Fever, in degrees Fahrenheit	Death rate (mortality)	Internal conditions (post-mortem findings)
May occur in any locality and at any time of year	Temperature usually normal but has been known to reach 107 in exceptional cases	Very low	Liver and kidneys contain large amounts of fat
Probably world wide. Any time of year	104 to 107	In cattle, 25 percent of young animals, 5 percent of older ones. Mortality in hogs not known	Anemia, jaundice. Urine in bladder color of port wine. Kidneys show reddish-brown or white spots after capsule is stripped
Worldwide. Spring, summer and fall	106 to 108	Nearly 100 percent	Thin, dirty, reddish fluid mixed with gas flows from swellings when they are cut open. Swellings may appear in lungs or throughout body as in blackleg
Worldwide. Occurs at any time of year	Temperature usually below normal	Animals that are not treated usually die within a few hours to several days	Internal organs apparently normal
Worldwide. May occur at any time of year	Up to 105 in foals	When disease occurs a few hours after birth, death rate is between 90 and 100 percent. Average death rate 30 to 75 percent	One or more joints may contain pus, especially stifle and hock joints. Abscesses may occur in spleen, liver or lungs. Usually navel is inflamed and abscesses are present in surrounding veins

Diagnosis chart of the more common animal diseases

Disease	Kinds of animals affected	Age at which animals are most susceptible	Principal symptoms
Pig typhus (infectious necrotic enteritis, often called "necro")	Hogs	Two to four months old	Usually starts with fever, loss of appetite, diarrhea and dullness. Animals that recover are generally unthrifty. Disease may be mistaken for hog cholera. If animals sick with pig typhus are vaccinated with anti-hog-cholera virus and hog-cholera serum, many deaths will follow
Pink eye (infectious keratitis, infectious conjunctivitis)	Cattle Sheep	Any age	Onset is sudden. There is a watery discharge from one or both eyes, eyelids become red and swollen, are painful and remain closed. When forced open, a yellow deposit is found over eyes. In severe attacks, eyeballs may become infected with loss of sight. Course of disease is two or three weeks with high percentage of recovery. In dairy cows, milk flow may be reduced as much as 50 percent
Pneumonia (inflammation of the lungs)	All warm-blooded animals	Any age	Dullness, high temperature, rapid breathing, dilated nostrils, loss of appetite, strong, hard pulse, hot, dry muzzle. Discharge often flows from nostrils that may be a clear fluid or sticky and pale yellow. Victims may stand with forefeet spread apart or lie on breastbone for easier breathing. Wheezing, splashing or gurgling sounds may be heard in chest. Pulse is rapid. In cattle there is open-mouth breathing and extension of tongue
Pregnancy disease (acidosis, acute hepatitis, ketonuria)	Sheep	Among ewes before lambing, especially when carrying twins or triplets. Ewes between three and six years old are most susceptible	Animals lag behind the flock or stand by themselves, nearly always grind their teeth, become dull and weak, urinate often, tremble when exercised. Later they refuse to eat, drink hardly any water, becomes stupid or excited and may appear blind. Finally they become too weak to move, lie on their breastbones, heads to one side

Geographic distribution and seasons of greatest occurrence	Fever, in degrees Fahrenheit	Death rate (mortality)	Internal conditions (post-mortem findings)
Worldwide where hogs are raised under crowded conditions. Occurs at all seasons	104 to 107	Moderately high	Walls of large intestines much thicker than normal, with patches of dead tissue of various sizes. These may be small circular spots or may involve several feet of the bowel. Lymph glands of stomach and intestines may be enlarged and reddened and look like gelatin. Spleen is dark and swollen and dark irregular hemorrhages appear on kidneys
Worldwide. May occur at any time of year	Fever is rare and never high	Death rate is low and indirect as a result of occasional blindness. Animals so blinded may die, especially on the range, from hunger, thirst and exposure	No changes take place in internal organs
Worldwide. Occurs most often in fall and winter, particularly when quarters are damp, cold and drafty or animals are exposed to cold winds and rain	In cattle, fever is between 103 to 107	Severity of disease varies greatly. This, coupled with fact that pneumonia often occurs with other diseases, makes it impossible to predict percentage of deaths	Surface of lung covering has reddish or grayish-red patches. The small air tubes in the lungs contain yellowish or grayish pus. In severe cases, serum is present in the chest cavity and the lungs contain pus
Worldwide. Occurs only before lambing	Temperature normal	Over 90 percent	Liver is yellow, crumbles easily and contains a great deal of fat. The kidneys are usually pale and softened. Victims nearly always carry more than one fetus

Diagnosis chart of the more common animal diseases

Disease	Kinds of animals affected	Age at which animals are most susceptible	Principal symptoms
Red-water disease (bacillary hemoglobinuria)	Cattle Sheep	Any age	Sudden onset, high fever that soon falls, depression, loss of appetite, bowel movements at first scanty followed by bloody diarrhea. The pronounced symptom is foamy urine the color of port wine. Death occurs in 24 to 36 hours after first symptoms appear
Scrapie	Sheep	Most common among sheep two years old but may occur in older ones. Seldom seen in sheep less than 18 months old	At onset, animal becomes excitable, fine tremors extend over head and neck and produce slight nodding movements. Intense itching starts on rump, then extends over entire body. Emaciation and weakness become worse and worse. There is a high stepping action of forelegs in trotting. Disease lasts six weeks to six months
Shipping fever (hemorrhagic septicemia stockyards pneumonia)	Cattle, principally. Sometimes sheep and hogs	The young are most susceptible but the disease attacks animals of all ages	High fever, loss of appetite, discharge from nose, hacking cough, swollen watery eyes, stiffened gait, sometimes swollen tongue that causes animals to drool and slobber
Sleeping sickness (equine encephalomyelitis)	Horses Mules Man	Any age	First symptom is fever, followed by sleepiness, grinding of teeth, wobbly gait and difficulty in chewing and swallowing. Most animals become dejected, a few become wild and unmanageable. The mouth is usually foul smelling and a watery discharge flows from the nostrils. Eyes become infected and muddy or dull yellowish in color. Lips, tongue or cheeks may be paralyzed
Sore mouth (contagious ecthyma, contagious pustular dermatitis)	Sheep Goats	Young lamps and kids	Reddening and swelling of lips, gums or tongue, with small blisters on these parts. In a few days these become filled with pus and finally break, leaving raw sores that bleed easily. Thick grayish-brown scabs form on raw spots. The scabs fall off in three or four weeks leaving no scars

Geographic distribution and seasons of greatest occurrence	Fever, in degrees Fahrenheit	Death rate (mortality)	Internal conditions (post-mortem findings)
Occurs principally in poorly drained mountain valleys of Nevada, California and Oregon. Has also occurred in Idaho, Montana, Louisiana, Utah and Texas. Usually occurs from June to November	May reach 106 but soon falls	95 percent of untreated animals	Most important change is in the liver, which always has a pale area of dead tissue. Other symptoms are severe anemia and jaundice
Probably worldwide. Occurs any time of year	No fever	Nearly 100 percent	No internal symptoms observable without use of microscope
Principally in the Middle West in the fall and early winter	104 to 107	Usually 1 to 4 percent, but may reach 10 percent	Principal post-mortem changes are in throat and lungs. Lymph glands of throat are swollen, windpipe and its larger branches in the lungs are coated with phlegm, while smaller branches may be tinged with blood. Cavities in lungs contain reddish serum
Worldwide. Occurs principally in spring, summer and fall	May reach 110	Very high	Disease causes no noticeable internal changes. Secondary infections of pneumonia, gangrene or edema may cause changes in lungs
Worldwide. In the United States greatest number of cases are reported in sheep-raising states west of the Mississippi from the Dakotas to Mexico. Occurs most often in spring and summer and dies out with cold weather	None	Very low from disease itself but secondary infections may cause loss as high as 50 percent	None that are not observable in living animals

Diagnosis chart of the more common animal diseases

Disease	Kinds of animals affected	Age at which animals are most susceptible	Principal symptoms
Strangles (equine distemper)	Horses Mules	Colts older than six months and horses between two and five years old. The disease is rare among animals either younger or older than this	Sudden onset, depression, reduced appetite, discharge from nostrils which is at first watery but after one to three days becomes thick. It is expelled in large amounts by snorting and coughing. Usually swellings appear under the jaw and in the throat. These become filled with a thick yellow pus and interfere with breathing
Swine erysipelas (diamond skin disease)	Hogs Man Sometimes sheep, turkeys and other animals	Three to 12 months, in hogs, but the disease affects animals of all ages	Acute type resembles hog cholera. Onset is rapid. Sometimes first signs of disease are death of one or more animals that seemed to be in good health shortly before. Other symptoms are fever, reduced appetite, stilted gait, depression, red patches on belly, arched back, vomiting, constipation at first and later diarrhea. Sometimes diamond-shaped patches appear on lighter portions of skin. In chronic type, joints become stiff, animals are usually unthrifty
Swine influenza (hog flu)	Hogs	All ages	Onset sudden, often affecting every animal in a herd. Symptoms: loss of appetite, listlessness, coughing, discharge from nose, eyes red and swollen, breathing labored and jerky, high fever. Victims squeal when handled
Tetanus (lockjaw)	All warm-blooded animals, including man. Animals most often affected are horses, mules and sheep	Any age	Nearly always can be traced to cuts, wounds or punctures. First symptoms usually appear around head. Chewing and swallowing become difficult. One group of muscles after another becomes rigid, animal stands with legs stiff and spread apart, ears rigidly erect, tail raised

Geographic distribution and seasons of greatest occurrence	Fever, in degrees Fahrenheit	Death rate (mortality)	Internal conditions (post-mortem findings)
Worldwide. Occurs most often in the spring but may occur at any time of year	104 to 106	Very low; usually less than 5 percent	Changes other than those noted under "Symptoms" are abscesses that often appear in other parts of the body
Occurs principally in the Corn Belt but has been reported in more than half the states. Occurs at any time of the year, but mostly in summer and fall	105 to 110	Very high in acute form	Swollen lymph glands and spleen, hemorrhages in stomach, intestines and kidneys. In chronic and subacute forms, joints may contain fluid and parts of the joint bones may be wasted away
Worldwide. Greatest losses occur in the late fall and winter	104 to 107	Very high when animals are not treated. Percentage figures not available	Hemorrhages in one or more organs of body. Swellings, tinged with blood, may be found under skin. Lymph glands may contain blood. Hemorrhages occur in fatty tissue around kidneys and in intestines and heart wall. Body cavities and lungs often contain fluids
The eastern type is found on the Atlantic seaboard and in the Gulf States; the western type prevails elsewhere. Symptoms of the two types are the same	102 to 107	One of every four or five with the western type die; nine of every 10 with eastern type die	No changes of definite diagnostic value observable without aid of microscope

Diagnosis chart of the more common animal diseases

Disease	Kinds of animals affected	Age at which animals are most susceptible	Principal symptoms
Trichomoniasis (bovine)	Cattle	Sexually mature animals	Abortion is principal symptom among cows. This differs from that caused by brucellosis in that the dead fetus remains in the womb for some time. Abortions usually take place in eight to 16 weeks after service. In bulls, symptoms are inflammation of the prepuce and pus formation
Vesicular exanthema	Hogs	Any age	Blisters form on snout, in mouth, between toes, the soles, and dew claws. Appear as blanched flat areas and are filled with clear fluid. Blristers break in 24 to 48 hours, leaving raw areas. These may become infected, otherwise heal in two to three weeks
White scours (calf scours, infectious diarrhea, acute dysentery)	Calves	Up to five days old	Yellowish-white, foul-smelling diarrhea. Calves become dull, weak, eyes become sunken, breathing hurried, temperature may go below normal
X disease (bovine hyperkeratosis)	Cattle	All ages, though calves and young cattle are more susceptible	Skin is dry, thickened, wrinkled and hair is lost in these areas. Raised rounded bumps appear in and around mouth. Watery discharge comes from eyes and nose. There is depression, loss of appetite and diarrhea

Geographic distribution and seasons of greatest occurrence	Fever, in degrees Fahrenheit	Death rate (mortality)	Internal conditions (post-mortem findings)
May occur anywhere and at any time following sexual activity	None	Does not cause death in adult animals but kills many fetuses	None that cannot be observed in living animals
Has been found in nearly all states. Occurs at any time of year	Fever 104 to 107	In old pigs death rate is negligible. Losses high in young pigs	No internal abnormalities
Nation-wide among stabled animals. Occurs most often in fall, winter and spring	Little or none. Temperature may drop below normal	90 to 100 percent of seriously affected animals die	Reddish serum present in body cavities. Liver, kidneys and spleen often partly wasted away. Digestive tract inflamed. Carcass thin and has foul odor
May occur anywhere and at any time of year	There is no fever	Death rate up to 80 percent in calves less than six months old; older calves 60 percent; adults up to 25 percent	Gall bladder, liver, pancreas and kidneys are affected. There may be abortion and severe mastitis in cows

How to inject drugs and biologicals

THE INJECTION of drugs and other products through skins of animals has several advantages over giving them by way of the mouth. Action is quicker. Substances are not changed by the digestive juices before entering the blood. Smaller doses are required because substances are not thinned out by being mixed with food and water.

Absolute cleanliness—the certainty that no unwanted microbes are forced into the body—is of extreme importance in making injection. Before use, instruments should be cleaned and then sterilized by boiling them in water for 10 minutes. If it is not convenient to boil the instruments, they can be disinfected by filling them with ethyl alcohol or ether and squirting out the contents several times. If alcohol is used, a 70 percent solution is best. All of it should be forced out before the instrument is used. Needles should not be allowed to touch anything before insertion. Syringes and needles should be disinfected between injections so as not to introduce infection into the herd.

The fluids to be injected and the syringes should generally be at body temperature or a little lower—never higher. Serums may be given at body temperature although they can also be given cold or even when chilled. Needles should be sharp and of the proper size. The place where injection is to be made should be cleaned and treated with a suitable antiseptic such as alcohol and, if the site is covered with hair, clipping and shaving are advisable.

There are a number of different ways to make injections. The kind used depends upon the purpose for which it is intended and the amount and the kind of solution to be used. Biological products and solutions of drugs to be injected are usually measured in cubic centimeters, written "cc." for short.

Subcutaneous, or hypodermic injection

The subcutaneous injection is made so that the fluid is deposited directly beneath the skin—not in the flesh or in a blood vessel. The words subcutaneous and hypodermic mean the same thing.

It is easiest to make the injection where the skin lies in loose folds. Favorite places are: the flat side of the neck of cattle, just behind the ear of swine, and the inner surface of the upper hind leg of sheep.

Injection is made by gently pinching up the skin with thumb and forefinger, then thrusting the needle quickly and firmly through all layers of the skin. The point of the needle can be moved sideways when it is in the right position.

Serious results may follow if certain fluids are injected into a vein. To make sure that the point of the needle is not lodged in a vein, the plunger of the syringe should be pulled out a trifle before injection is made. If blood appears, another site should be used. Care should also be taken

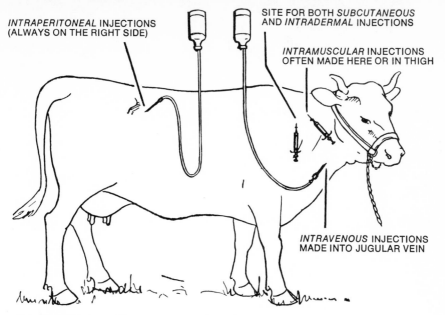

INTRAPERITONEAL INJECTIONS (ALWAYS ON THE RIGHT SIDE)

SITE FOR BOTH *SUBCUTANEOUS* AND *INTRADERMAL* INJECTIONS

INTRAMUSCULAR INJECTIONS OFTEN MADE HERE OR IN THIGH

INTRAVENOUS INJECTIONS MADE INTO JUGULAR VEIN

Common sites for making various injections. Other sites are sometimes used

not to inject fluid into a muscle, otherwise a large swelling and abscesses may later result.

After injection has been made, the point of injection should be massaged gently. This hastens absorption.

Intradermal injection

The intradermal injection differs from the hypodermic injection in that it is made into the skin instead of beneath it. After insertion, the needle is so close to the surface that it can usually be seen through the outer layers of skin. Unless this is done very carefully, and with a very fine needle, it is likely to become subcutaneous rather than intradermal injection.

Common sites for intradermal injections are the same as those used hypodermically, although in cattle, horses and mules, the flank, areas around the sternum (breastbone), and caudal (tail) fold are also used.

A very fine needle is used, commonly 19 gauge or smaller and $^3/_4$ of an inch long. Injection is made by pinching up the skin between the thumb and forefinger so as to form a ridge two or three inches long. The needle is held almost parallel to the skin and inserted its full length. The dose should be injected slowly while the needle is drawn out, distributing the dose along the needle's course.

To keep the fluid from leaking out, press a finger firmly over the puncture after withdrawing the needle. If the injection is properly made the fluid will raise a small elongated lump. In cases of vaccination, this lump will become enlarged in a few days.

Intravenous injection

The intravenous injection is used with certain fluids that are too irritating when given hypodermically or when the prescribed dose is so large that it cannot be absorbed after hypodermic injection. But some substances should never be given intravenously because they bring on dangerous reactions. Be sure the product you intend to use is labelled "For intravenous use."

In cattle, sheep and horses the injection is usually made into the left jugular vein. This can be felt in what is called the jugular furrow that runs along the side of the gullet. Jugular veins carry blood from the head to the heart.

In swine the injection is made into the veins on the outer surface of the ears; in poultry, into the large vein at the inner surface of the wing at the elbow.

How to make an intradermal injection

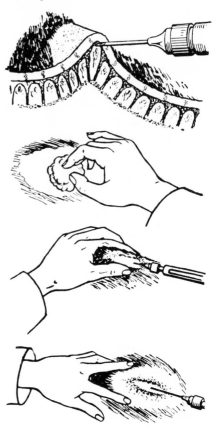

Enlarged cross section of skin shows how needle should be inserted between the layers

Clean the site. Then treat it with 70-percent alcohol or some other good antiseptic. Practitioners often remove hair before applying antiseptic

Pinch up the skin between the thumb and forefinger, making a ridge a few inches long. Hold the needle almost parallel to the skin and insert it the full length

Inject the dose slowly, at the same time withdrawing the needle. This distributes the dose along the needle's course. After the needle is withdrawn, press a finger over the puncture to keep dose from flowing out

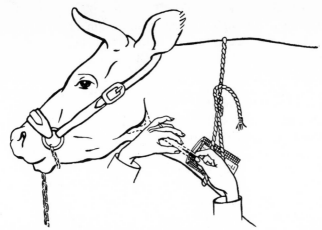

Some operators use a tourniquet to compress the jugular vein in making an intravenous injection. A rope, twisted tight, presses a pad of burlap or other material against the vein. This stops the flow of blood

The ordinary large hypodermic syringe is good for doses up to 40 cc. When larger doses are required, it is necessary to use an injecting outfit. This consists of a container attached to a needle with a rubber tube. Pressure for injection of the fluid is supplied either by gravity—holding the bottle considerably above the point of injection—or by pressing an attached rubber bulb. A 16-gauge needle two or three inches long is generally used for large animals such as cattle and horses. Smaller needles are of course used for smaller animals.

Remove the needle from the syringe or hose before making the insertion. This makes it easier to manipulate the needle and makes less likely the injection of fluid into the skin or muscles.

After the spot for injection has been prepared, the vein is compressed at a point towards the heart. This enlarges the vein at the right place and makes it easier to insert the needle. If the jugular vein is used, the proper place to apply pressure is below the injection site.

A vein can be compressed by hand by an assistant, by the operator himself or by use of a tourniquet. A tourniquet can be made with a piece

In hogs, a vein on the outside surface of an ear is used to make an intravenous injection. Here the operator is making an injection while an assistant shuts off the flow of blood with his thumb

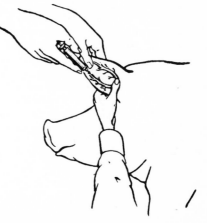

of rope and a small thick pad of burlap. The pad is placed in the jugular furrow. The rope is put around the neck of the animal so that it passes over the pad. When the rope is twisted tight with a stick, the pad shuts off the flow of blood and makes the vein swell up for easy insertion of the needle.

There is less danger of getting air into the vein if the insertion is made against the blood stream. Hold the needle parallel to the vein and nearly parallel to the skin. Push the needle quickly through the skin with the bevel outward. After the point of the needle is through the skin, hold it a little more upright before pushing it through the wall of the vein. This makes it easier to push through. When the point is in the so-called lumen, or hollow of the vein, push the needle in its full length to keep it from slipping out.

Blood should come out of the needle if it is in the right place. If no blood appears, it may be because the needle is clogged or the bevel rests too firmly against the inside of the vein wall. If by chance the needle has become embedded in the flesh, pull it out and start over at another site.

The rubber tube should be completely filled with fluid—so that a few drops escape—before attaching it to the needle. When a syringe is attached, care should be taken that no air is forced into the vein with the fluid. Air bubbles reaching the heart may cause death.

The pressure applied to the vein must be released before starting the flow of fluid into it. The flow should be very slow, particularly at first. In the treatment of large animals, 10 to 15 cc. the first minute is enough, with less for smaller animals, depending upon their weight. Allow at least 10 minutes for injecting 250 to 300 cc. of calcium gluconate and similar products. Some practitioners use a 20-gauge needle or smaller so that too rapid a flow of fluid is almost impossible.

How to fill a syringe

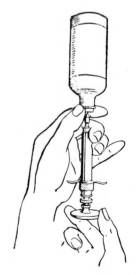

Before using a syringe, make sure it is clean. Then boil it for 10 minutes. To fill a syringe, first shake the bottle, then force the needle through the stopper and fill the syringe while holding the bottle upside down. Replace the needle with another sterilized one before making the injection. Always protect biological products from heat and sunlight. After using a syringe, take it apart, clean it and put it where it will stay clean until you need it again. Another way to fill a syringe is as follows: Proceed as above except fill the barrel of the syringe with air by pulling the plunger outward before pushing the needle through the stopper. Hold the bottle up and force a little air into it. Then pull the plunger down and suck in some fluid. Continue to pump in this manner until the syringe is full. This method is quicker than the first because it creates pressure instead of a vacuum inside of the bottle

If injections are made too rapidly, shock follows. Symptoms of this are short breath, rapid and irregular heart beat, frothing at the mouth and final collapse. Animals should be watched closely during the injections. If signs of shock appear, injection should be halted until the animal recovers.

Before pulling out the needle following an injection with a fluid that might be dangerous, it is good practice to compress the vein again until blood appears in the needle. In this way, any fluid that may remain will not drip out into the tissues while the needle is being withdrawn.

Intramuscular injections

Fluids injected intramuscularly are not absorbed so fast as those given in the veins but are absorbed faster than those injected under or into the skin.

Injections of this kind are made deeply into the larger muscles. Favorite sites are muscles of the neck or thighs. Special care must be used to avoid infections because deep-seated sores that may follow are painful and difficult to treat.

The needle should be thrust quickly through the skin at right angles to it and into the muscle without stopping. To make sure that the needle has not penetrated a blood vessel, pull the plunger of the syringe out a little before starting the injection. If blood is sucked into the syringe, choose another site.

How temperatures affect biologicals

37° — Living vaccines are no longer any good if kept at this temperature for more than a few days. Other biologicals may lose strength so that they are not dependable at their stated expiration dates — 98.6°

21° — For dependable service, no biological should be kept at temperatures higher than this — 70°

10° — Living viruses, rabies vaccine and tissue vaccine should not be kept at temperatures higher than this — 50°

0° — At this temperature, all biologicals keep their strength for a long time and are dependable long after reaching their expiration dates. *Caution:* Biological products freeze at a few degrees below the freezing point of water and may become useless when frozen — 32°

Centigrade   *Fahrenheit*

Intraperitoneal injections

The peritoneum is the membrane which lines the abdominal cavity. It is penetrated most easily in the cow from the right side and between the hip bone and the last rib.

An intraperitoneal injection is one in which the needle is pushed through the skin, muscles, and body wall, then squirting the contents of the syringe into the abdominal cavity. Since as inner fold of peritoneum also covers the intestines and other organs, one must use care not to penetrate these before making the injection.

Drugs and biologicals injected in this way are absorbed quickly though not so fast as when injected into the veins.

The preferred site for intraperitoneal injections is the middle of the hollow of the right flank—never the left one—otherwise the needle might penetrate the wall of the rumen. After preparation of the site, the needle should be pushed straight through the skin and peritoneum. The operator can tell by the feel when the point of the needle has pierced the peritoneum and is in the right place.

This type of injection is beset with greater dangers than the others and should be learned under the guidance of an experienced person.

The care of biologicals

Most biological products lose their strength when they are warmed up or left in the light. Some lose strength when too old. And there's no easy way to tell when a biological is no longer any good.

Research men have determined just how these products should be handled for best results and just how big the doses should be. Official regulations require licensed manufacturers to put this information on the labels or supply it to buyers of the products in leaflets or folders. The proper way to determine whether a biological is still potent is to observe The "Expiration Date" with which most are marked.

What you should know about antibiotics

SERUMS, VACCINES and related biological products have certain limitations in the treatment of animal diseases. They are effective against a comparatively small number of disease-producing viruses and bacteria. None have been found successful against the protozoa and various other injurious parasites.

Chemical poisons like lye or carbolic acid have been used for a long time to kill microbes or to stop their growth. But the trouble with nearly all such strong poisons is that they can't be used inside of the body because they destroy living tissue. They kill disease germs but they also kill the patients.

In the treatment of farm animals three groups of drugs are used to overcome this difficulty. They are the sulfonamides, or so called sulfa drugs, the nitrofurans, and the antibiotics.

The sulfa drugs and nitrofurans are man-made chemicals. The antibiotics, such as penicillin and streptomycin, are produced by molds and bacteria.

In proper doses, these drugs can be used within the body to kill certain microbes—usually with little or no bad side effects on the patient. The drugs act in a different manner than the common germ-killers. They don't destroy protoplasm, the living substance of cells, but interfere with the life processes of microbes. The latter do not grow and increase in numbers and so fall easy prey to the germ-fighting forces of the blood.

Like most drugs, the sulfas, nitrofurans and antibiotics are selective in their action. One that will help cure a specific disease will not necessarily be of any use in a similar disease. This is often true even when the organisms that cause the maladies are almost identical. The drugs are also selective in another way. One that will cure a disease in one kind of animal will not always cure the same disease in another kind of animal.

Drugs of all kinds should always be given in the doses recommended by the manufacturers for each purpose. If doses are too small they will not be effective; if too large, the animals may be injured and may even die.

The first step in the treatment of sick animals should be proper diagnosis—finding out what makes them sick. The next step is to find out whether the disease can be cured at a reasonable cost. If treatment with drugs or biological products is practicable, then these should be employed in accordance with methods that have proven effective.

How to drench an animal

WHEN IT IS NECESSARY to have animals swallow a medicine, the simplest way is to mix it in feed or drinking water. This won't always work, especially if the medicine has a disagreeable taste. In such cases the medicine can be poured into the animal's stomach by means of a rubber tube or into its mouth from a long-necked bottle. The latter method is called drenching.

Care must be taken when drenching animals. There is danger that the medicine will enter the lungs instead of the stomach. This often causes pneumonia.

The entrance to the gullet (esophagus) of a cow is closed by a "valve" except when the animal is in the act of swallowing. The entrance to the windpipe is of course open while an animal is breathing. It closes when the animal swallows. When medicine is poured into an animal's throat and the animal does not swallow it voluntarily, the medicine will go down the windpipe instead of the gullet.

To drench an animal, its head should be raised slightly—just enough so that medicine in the mouth will flow towards the throat. If the head is raised too high, the danger of strangling the animal is greatly increased. The head can be held in the right position by grasping the nostrils between the thumb and forefinger.

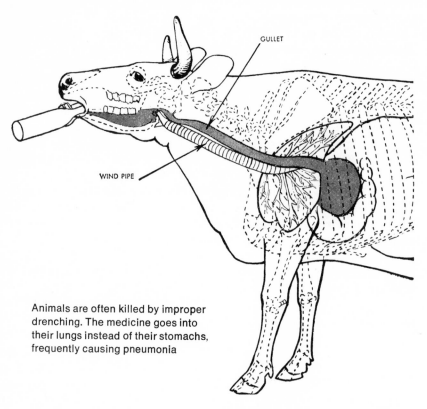

GULLET

WIND PIPE

Animals are often killed by improper drenching. The medicine goes into their lungs instead of their stomachs, frequently causing pneumonia

The neck of a long-neck bottle should be put into the side of a cow's mouth so that the mouth of the bottle rests on the middle of her tongue. Care should be taken to avoid getting the bottle between the teeth, otherwise the bottle may be broken. Better still, by a rubber drenching bottle. The medicine should be poured slowly while the mouth is closed, stopping often to giving the animal time to swallow. If the cow coughs, the head should be lowered at once to permit the fluid to escape.

Sheep are more difficult to drench than cows. In general never drench sheep unless they are standing firmly on all four feet, and never raise their noses any higher than their eyes during drenching. Sheep are often given medicines with a syringe, or through a piece of rubber tubing with a funnel attached to one end and a metal tube to the other end. The metal tube is inserted into the sheep's gullet and the medicine is poured into the funnel. This is a delicate operation, because the tube will slide into the trachea very easily, and the medicine will enter the lungs.

How to treat wounds and abscesses

MOST WOUNDS AND CUTS are not serious. Treat small, shallow injuries just as you would a cut on your finger. Wash them thoroughly and then apply tincture of iodine or some other good mild antiseptic. If dirt has been ground into a wound, an application of hydrogen peroxide has the advantage of "boiling out" the germ-laden particles.

If a cut or a wound is in a place where dirt may get into it after treatment, cover it with a bandage that has been dipped in an antiseptic solution, or apply a piece of sterile cotton and hold it in place with adhesive tape.

If you don't find a wound until after a scab has formed, just leave it alone. It will probably heal without causing any trouble.

The more serious wounds

The more serious wounds are those through which harmful microbes may enter the blood stream or muscles, where an internal organ has been punctured, or where a blood vessel has been severed.

Deep puncture wounds—those made by sharp-pointed objects—are the most dangerous and the most difficult to treat. It is often hard to tell how deep they are. Yet the innermost part of such a wound should be disinfected, otherwise a deep-seated dangerous pus pocket may develop.

A puncture wound should be searched with a sterile probe. If you do not have a probe specially made for this purpose, use a knitting needle or make one by smoothing a small stick or by doubling over a piece of slender wire so that the flattened loop end has no sharp edges.

After you have determined the depth of the wound, pull out the probe and wrap absorbent cotton around the end of it. Dip the cotton end into a mild antiseptic solution and insert it into the wound as far as it will go. After this is done, pour antiseptic into the opening and around the outside of the wound. Avoid the use of strong, irritating antiseptic solutions. Such wounds should not be sewed.

On premises where tetanus (lockjaw) has occurred, wounds made by nails and glass lying in the soil are especially dangerous. Because the tetanus germ grows only in the absence of air, such wounds should at once be enlarged and treated with an antiseptic. Where valuable animals are concerned, especially horses, injections of tetanus antitoxin should be made.

When blood merely oozes from a wound, a clot usually forms in a short time and bleeding stops. If bleeding fails to stop of its own accord, you can sometimes stop it by applying pressure over the spot with a pad of sterile gauze or a clean cloth. Or you can apply cold water, or a styptic pencil—the kind used by barbers. Don't use cobwebs, flour or similar home remedies to stop bleeding. Such substances may be laden with harmful microbes.

How to stop a hemorrhage

When a blood vessel is cut, bleeding is sometimes so heavy that an affected animal will die unless the hemorrhage is stopped. In all cases bleeding should be stopped before a wound is treated and bandaged. This is a surgical procedure and surgical cleanliness must be observed.

Here's the way many surgeons tie a knot

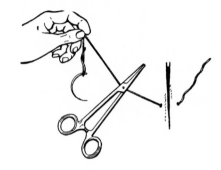

Right: This is a good way to tie a knot, especially when suture material is short or slippery. Instead of using forceps, as shown, the operator can use a pair of long-nose pliers

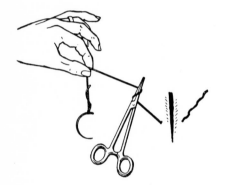

Left: The suture is wound around the forceps, taking care not to disturb the stitch

Rigt Right: The end of the suture is pulled through the loop

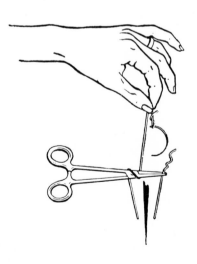

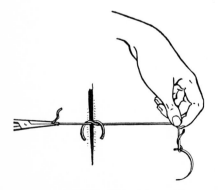

Left: After tightening the first part of the knot, make the second loop by winding the suture around the forceps in the opposite direction. Then complete the knot by winding the third loop like the first

Some operators press a white-hot iron against a bleeding vessel for a few seconds to stop the flow of blood. The iron should not be applied longer, otherwise the tissue will char and stick to the iron when it is pulled away, and the bleeding won't stop.

When an artery is badly mashed or cut through, simple methods for stopping the hemorrhage may not work. To save an animal's life, a ligature may be necessary. Such a ligature is nothing more than a piece of string or thread tied around the end of a blood vessel to stop the blood from flowing out.

Veins are seldom ligated—large ones never. The reason is that tying off a vein often results in gangrene.

You can easily tell whether an artery or a vein has been cut. The blood from an artery is bright red and flows in spurts corresponding to the pulse. Blood from a vein is dark red and flows in an even stream. Among farm animals, the only vein at the surface of the body that sometimes has a pulse is a jugular vein of an ox.

To find the end of a bleeding artery, gently clear the wound of blood with a piece of cotton dipped in cold water. You can then see where the blood comes from. A blood vessel is slippery. For this reason, use a forceps, tweezers or a small pair of pliers to pull it out so you can tie it off, that is, ligate it.

When an artery is cut through, it often contracts and its ends become hidden in the flesh. In such cases, a sharp-pointed hook, called a tenaculum, is sometimes used to draw it clear of the surrounding tissues.

After pulling a vessel out of a wound so you can work on it, tie the cord or thread tightly once around it with a firm knot and cut off the ends. Sometimes you may tie up a little flesh with the artery but make sure you do not also include a nerve.

Another way to stop a hemorrhage is by means of torsion. This consists of twisting the vessel around a few times with forceps so that the inside becomes mangled and thus stops the flow of blood. Torsion is used with small vessels and has the advantage over ligating in that no string or thread is left in the wound. Small veins may often stop bleeding if grasped firmly with a pair of forceps.

After an artery is tied off, the wound should be thoroughly cleaned, disinfected and bandaged or otherwise protected from dirt.

Hemorrhage of a wound on a leg can be reduced or stopped by using a tourniquet, which should not be too tight. Even then, the pressure should be released at intervals of about 20 minutes. A tourniquet is only for temporary use—to stop the flow of blood until it clots. The flow of blood beyond the injured tissues should not be cut entirely.

An artery carries blood away from the heart, so should be compressed between the wound and the heart. A vein carries blood to the heart, so should be compressed on the side of the wound farthest away from the heart.

When a wound should be sewed

A small gaping wound will often heal properly if the skin is pulled back in place and held there with a piece of adhesive tape, or by the application of collodion. But a large gaping wound may require suturing, that is, it has to be sewed up.

Suturing is generally done with catgut, silk, nylon or stainless steel wire. Straight needles are convenient where only the skin is sutured, but when suturing flesh it is necessary to use a curved surgical needle.

When curved needles are inserted with the fingers, they tend to turn while their points are in the flesh and then they don't come out where they should. To make them come out at the right place they should be held with forceps or pliers.

As nearly as possible, stitches should be the same length, same depth, and the same distance apart. The purpose of this is to distribute the strain equally over all the stitches. Knots should be made at the side of a wound, not over it.

Some of the more common sutures

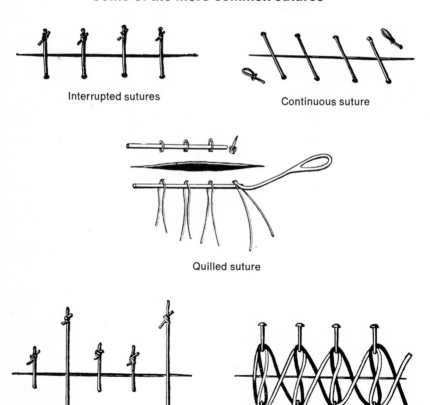

Interrupted sutures

Continuous suture

Quilled suture

Interrupted sutures for deep wounds

Figure-of-eight, or pin, suture

An opening should be left at the bottom of a wound so that any discharge can run out. Deep wounds often require drainage, that is, a rubber tube or a piece of gauze should be kept in it to drain out pus and serum until healing starts from the inside.

When a wound is shallow, the lips (edges) can be brought together by making independent stitches through the skin only. These should be about one-half to three-quarters of an inch apart and about three-quarters of an inch long—three-eighths of an inch on each side of the lips. The opposite edges of the skin should *not* be brought together tightly—just tight enough to touch each other. There will be sufficient swelling to hold the edges together. When the stitches are not connected with one another, the suture is called an interrupted suture.

When a wound is deep, the needle should be pushed straight through the skin and some of the flesh. The needle should be inserted at a distance far enough from the lips and deep enough to insure strength. Sometimes two sets of stitches are used: deep ones to hold together the deeper tissues and others to hold the skin in place.

When a deep wound cuts a muscle crosswise, such as a leg muscle, a very strong suture is necessary. The best one for this purpose is called a quilled suture. It requires a double thread and a needle with an eye in the point.

Start the stitch at least an inch back from the lip, making a stitch at least two inches long. When the needle comes through, seize the thread and hold it, at the same time withdrawing the needle. This leaves a loop at one end of the stitch and two loose ends of thread at the other.

After all the stitches have been made, run a stick about the size of a lead pencil through the loops. Then tighten and tie the loose ends of thread around a similar stick at the opposite side of the wound. Pieces of small rubber tubing may be used instead of sticks.

Dressing and aftertreatment of wounds

Before suturing or dressing a wound, bleeding should be stopped. The hands of the operator and all instruments and dressings used must be kept clean and treated with an antiseptic before coming in contact with a wound. While healing, wounds should be protected from contamination by the use of dressings. Dressings should be changed when they become smeared with pus or get out of place.

When swelling appears at the outside of a bandage, it's a sign that the bandage is too tight. When a wound is in a place on the body where movement keeps the wound from healing, the affected animal should, if possible, be kept quiet until the wound heals sufficiently.

Taking care of abcesses

An abscess is a swelling filled with pus, commonly called a boil. In nearly all cases, an abscess should not be opened until it is nearly ready to break. When this point is reached, the swelling usually softens somewhat, though there is an outer ring around it. The skin often becomes whitish where a head is about to form.

If you open an abscess too soon, you may cause some of the microbes to get into the blood and spread the infection to other parts of the body. Or you may not be able to drain out all the pus, in which case a new abscess may form near by, even after the first one has healed.

When an abscess first starts, it does not have a sharply outlined shape. But by the time it is ready to come to a head, a "wall" has formed around the infected area. The abscess has become a sac filled with pus.

Hot moist applications help bring an abscess to a head so it may be

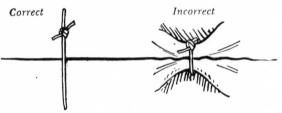

Correct *Incorrect*

Above: A common mistake is to pull sutures too tight. This may retard healing and always leaves a bad scar

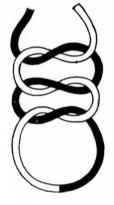

Right: A few suturing materials—especially nylon—are so smooth that they won't hold with an ordinary knot. The double reef knot shown at the right will keep such materials from slipping

How to treat an abscess

Right: Put the end of a long round stick into the center of a piece of sterile cotton

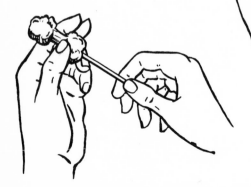

Left: Twist the stick until the cotton becomes packed at the center and firmly attached to the stick. The cotton will remain fluffy at both ends. Such a cotton plug is called a "tampon"

Right: With a sharp knife or razor blade, cut through the skin covering abscess

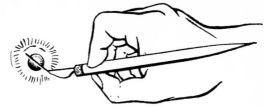

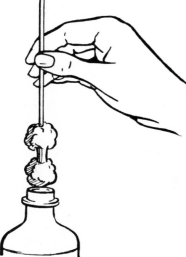

Left: Dip the tampon into a good antiseptic solution such as tincture of iodine. The tampon should be wet but not dripping

Right: Gently squeeze out the pus and remove it with a piece of cotton or cloth

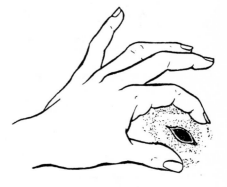

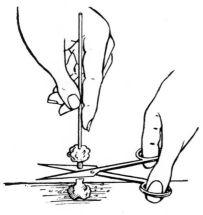

Left: Insert the tampon into the wound and cut it off below the end of the stick. The lower part, which remains in the wound, can be held in place with adhesive tape if necessary

Parts of a dairy cow

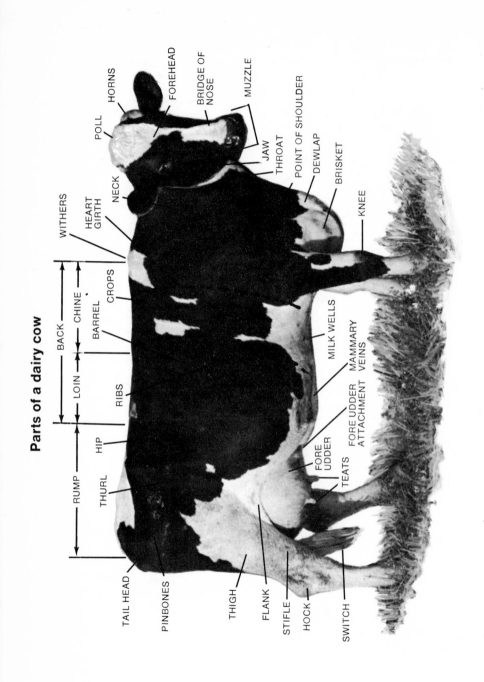

POLL
HORNS
FOREHEAD
BRIDGE OF NOSE
MUZZLE
JAW
THROAT
POINT OF SHOULDER
DEWLAP
BRISKET
KNEE
NECK
HEART GIRTH
WITHERS
BACK
CROPS
CHINE
BARREL
LOIN
RIBS
RUMP
HIP
THURL
MILK WELLS
MAMMARY VEINS
FORE UDDER ATTACHMENT
FORE UDDER
TEATS
TAIL HEAD
PINBONES
THIGH
FLANK
STIFLE
HOCK
SWITCH

opened. The only time an abscess should be opened before a sac has formed is when delay might have serious consequences. This is the case when an abscess is on a joint or adjoins a ligament, a tendon, or a bone. The danger is that the pus might drain inwards and infect these parts.

To treat an abscess, cut it open with a sharp knife or razor blade, gently squeeze out the pus, and drench the wound with a good antiseptic. Do not cut *through* the abscess; merely cut it open. Keep the wound open with a piece of sterile gauze until the pus has drained out. It can also be kept open with a cotton plug, called a "tampon." The wound should not be allowed to heal over, but should heal from the inside out.

What happens when a cow becomes pregnant

THE LIFE OF an animal starts when one of the spermatozoa, or sperm, of the male combines with an ovum, or egg, of the female. With the exception of birds, the testicles of domestic animals are enclosed in the scrotum, or bag, suspended outside of the body. The reason for this is that a temperature somewhat lower than that of the body is necessary for the formation of sperm. The testicles are thus "air-cooled." Should they be inside the body, as in the case of a ridgling, sperm are rarely formed and the animal generally is sterile.

A sperm is composed of a head that contains the substance that fertilizes the ovum, a small body, and a tail which enables it to swim. Sperm are too small to be seen without the aid of a microscope. In fact, they are the smallest cells in the body.

While in the testicles, sperm are motionless but by the time they reach the penis they have become mixed with several fluids which make them active. The glands that supply these fluids are the prostate that lies at the base of the bladder and the two seminal vesicles which lie close to the prostate. The mixture of these fluids together with the sperm comprises the semen.

A single ejaculate of semen may contain a billion or more sperm.

Sperm cells go through the periods of youth, middle age and old age. If a male is serviced too often, immature cells that are infertile are released into the semen. On the other hand, if a male does not ejaculate often enough, many of the sperm cells become inactive or die because of old age. While in the female tract of cows, sperm generally live between 36 and 48 hours.

The female reproductive organs

The principal reproductive organs of the female are the ovaries, oviducts, uterus, vagina and vulva.

The ovaries lie within the body cavity below the kidneys, one on

The reproductive organs of a cow

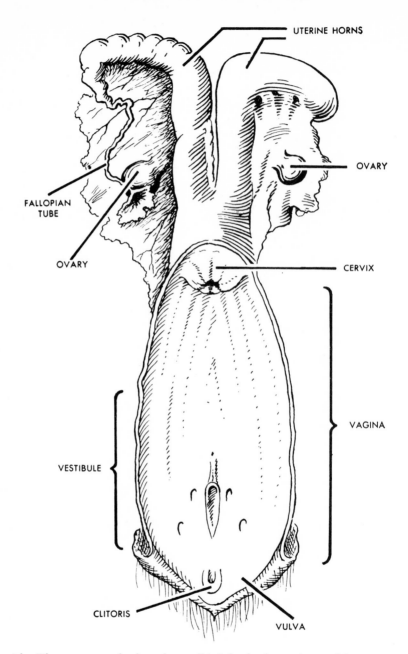

each side. They are attached to the wall of the body cavity and in a cow are about the size of pigeon eggs.

The normal ovary contains thousands of eggs. These eggs look like the yolks of birds' eggs but each one is only about 1/130 of an inch in diameter. They can be seen without the aid of microscope or magnifying glass by a person with good eyes.

It was formerly believed that a female was born with a full life-supply of eggs but we now know that this is not the case. New eggs are now known to form in a number of mammals up to the age when the change of life occurs.

How eggs are shed from ovaries

Each egg is lodged in a small sac, an enclosure known as a Graafian follicle. When an animal comes in heat, one or sometimes more than one of these follicles begins to grow rapidly until it bulges from the surface of the ovary. Finally, the follicle bursts and the egg is released or "shed," as it is called.

When an egg is shed from an ovary, it drops into the funnel-shaped membrane that partly surrounds the ovary. Thus the egg is guided into a slender tube, called an oviduct or Fallopian tube. Under normal conditions, if a female has been bred, the egg is fertilized in the oviduct by a sperm that has come to meet it.

Only one sperm cell merges with an egg. After the two have merged, the egg in some mysterious way rejects all further suitors. Upon fertilization, the egg proceeds on its trip in the oviduct to the uterus. A fertilized egg starts growing at once. The single cell becomes two, two become four, and so on.

Each of the two oviducts merges into a horn of the uterus. These horns open into the body of the uterus—a muscular bag with a spongy wall. The uterus opens into the vagina or female passage, by way of the cervix. The cervix is usually sealed with mucus except when the animal is in heat. This helps prevent the uterus from becoming infected.

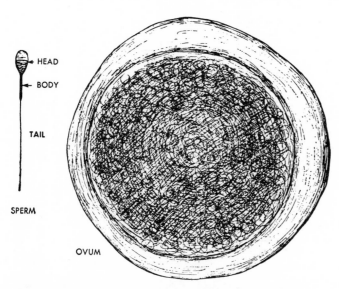

HEAD

BODY

TAIL

SPERM

OVUM

Sperm of a bull and egg of a cow magnified 500 times. Sperm move by means of whip-like movements of their tails in a manner similar to that of tadpoles

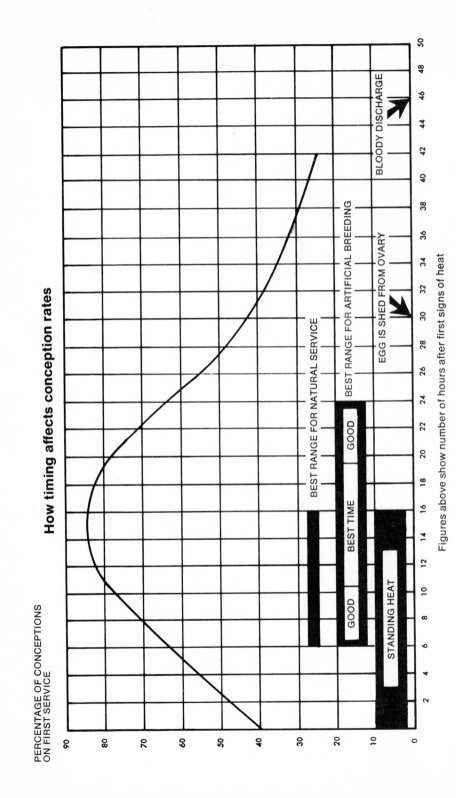

How timing affects conception rates

Figures above show number of hours after first signs of heat

A fertilized egg develops within the uterus where it sends out membranes that become attached to the spongy wall. The fetus is nourished through these membranes. The lining of the uterus of a cow is provided with knob-like elevations called cotyledons through which blood is supplied.

The corpus luteum or "yellow body"

When a follicle bursts, the cavity left almost immediately starts to fill up with a yellow, fat-like substance called the yellow body, or corpus luteum. It forms a brightly colored dome-like elevation, somewhat smaller than the follicle that it replaced.

The corpus luteum remains during pregnancy. It gives forth a hormone which prevents follicles from ripening. In this way, no more eggs can be fertilized nor are there normally any heat periods while an animal is pregnant.

The corpus luteum helps to maintain pregnancy. If it is removed during pregnancy, abortion usually occurs, particularly if it is removed during the early part of a pregnancy period.

Normally, if pregnancy does not occur at a heat period, the yellow body gradually disappears. It is gone before the next heat period is due.

Heat periods vary in length between six and 27 hours, with an average of about 16 hours for heifers and 20 hours for cows. About 70 percent of cows show the first signs of heat in the forenoon and the others show it in the afternoon.

Shedding of egg or eggs from the ovary usually occurs about 14 hours after signs of heat have stopped. This time varies greatly, however. Research indicates that eggs may be shed anywhere from two hours before the end of heat to 26 hours after it.

Eggs die between six and 10 hours after they are shed from the ovaries unless they are fertilized during this period. Sperm will live about 24 hours or more in a cow. It takes six hours for an egg to travel one-third of the way down an oviduct. Living sperm must be present in the upper third of the oviduct if fertilization is to occur.

Taking all these facts into consideration, the best time to breed a cow is just before the end of the standing heat period or just after that time. With artificial breeding, a good conception rate can be obtained as late as eight hours after the end of standing heat. For cows that do not become pregnant at the first or second heat periods, it often helps to give them two services, one early in the heat period, the other 12 to 18 hours later.

On an average twins are born once in 80 births among animals which usually produce one offspring at a time. Triplets are born once in about every 6400 births.

Twins can be produced in two ways: two eggs can be shed at the same time, either from one follicle or from two follicles. When such eggs are fertilized, each by a sperm, they become unlike twins upon birth. Two eggs and two sperm are involved.

The other way twins are produced is when one egg is fertilized and thereafter separates into two individuals. In such cases only one sperm and one egg are involved. The twins have the same inheritance and are identical in nearly every respect. They are always either both male or both female.

Triplets are formed by any of three ways: a single egg which divides into two and one of the halves again divides into two; by two eggs, one of which divides into two; or by three separate eggs.

How to detect pregnancy

USUALLY A COW is pregnant if she fails to show signs of heat three to four weeks after service. But this is not absolute proof. She may skip one or more heat periods because there is something the matter with her.

On the other hand, a cow may show signs of heat and accept service, even though she's in calf. This occurs in about $3^{1}/_{2}$ percent of cows. Such heat periods may happen from one to four times in a gestation period.

A cow that is in calf usually becomes quiet and docile and puts on flesh, especially in the first four months of gestation. After the fifth month, the movements of the calf can often be seen when the cow drinks cold water. This stimulates the calf into activity, causing a sudden outward jerking movement in the right flank of the cow, nearly in front of the stifle.

In the latter months of pregnancy, the common way to tell whether a cow is in calf is to press the hand strongly and several times in succession against the right flank, about eight inches in front of the stifle and a little below it. Upon holding the pressure, you can usually feel the movements of the calf.

Diagnosis early in pregnancy

To determine pregnancy early in a gestation period it is necessary to reach into the rectum and feel the fetus in a horn of the uterus.

This procedure is called rectal palpation and it enables an experienced veterinarian or technician to detect pregnancy as early as 30 days after service. But the method requires great care, much practice, and a well-developed sense of touch. These can only be acquired with practice, and kept dependable by much use. Very few persons can reliably determine pregnancy under 60 days.

Before starting the examination, trim the fingernails closely, oil the hand and lubricate with soap and water. With the palm down, insert the hand into the rectum slowly, waiting for it to relax to let the hand advance freely. For easy entrance, let the fingers overlap to form sort of a cone, remembering that the intestine is a delicate membrance which is easily punctured. This would lead to peritonitis and death of the cow.

It is sometimes necessary to remove manure from the rectum. If the rectum is "ballooned" with air, examination of the uterus is difficult or

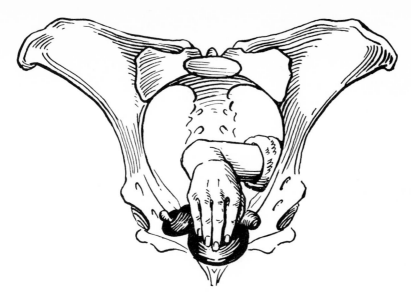

When a cow is pregnant, the fetus can be felt by reaching into
the rectum and feeling the enlarged horn of the uterus

impossible. In such cases hold the hand still until the rectum is relaxed.

Run the fingers along the center of the floor of the rectum. The pear-shaped outline of the bladder can easily be felt. It will be more or less rounded depending on the amount of urine it contains.

The uterus usually lies between the bladder and the floor of the rectum. But if the bladder is full, it may push the uterus to one side or upward so that it cannot immediately be found. Do not mistake the bladder for the uterus. The body of the uterus of an open (non-pregnant) cow is from $1^1/_2$ to 2 inches thick.

When you have located the uterus, pick it up and hold it in the hollow of your hand with your middle finger extended. This finger will lie over the place where the horns of the uterus come together. Push the finger down between the horns until you hook it under the web of tissue that connects them.

If you lift upward and pull gently backward, you will uncoil the horns. Each one can then be felt its entire length so you can find whether a fetus is present. A horn is about 15 inches long and tapers off gradually in thickness from the place where it joins the body of the uterus until it merges with the slender Fallopian tubes. (See drawing in the preceding chapter.)

The fetus itself cannot be felt in early pregnancy. But it lies in a sac, or bag, surrounded by a fluid. The sac is called an amnionic vesicle. This in turn is enclosed in the fluid-filled chorionic vesicle. To determine early pregnancy, a search is made for the latter.

A fetus, if present, will be found in one of the horns. In case of twins there may be one in each horn or two in one of them.

Thirty days after conception, the fetus of a heifer is less than a half inch long and the vesicle containing it is a sphere about ³/₄ of an inch in diameter.

At five weeks, the vesicle is balloon-like and about 1¹/₄ inches in diameter. It can be be felt if the horn of the uterus is allowed to slide between the thumb and the first two fingers. It has a characteristic slippery feeling—unlike anything else that might be in the horn. The reason for this slippery feeling is that the larger vesicle contains its fluid rather loosely—its covering is not taut—while the inner vesicle is firm to the touch.

The slipperiness is usually present up to the seventh week of pregnancy after which it rapidly disappears. At the same time the pressure within the vesicle decreases.

The vesicle grows rapidly in size between the 35th and 49th day of gestation. Also it changes from spherical to egg-shaped. These changes are uniform so that during this period an experienced operator can tell the age of a fetus within a week or two. He does this by working out a set of standards whereby he compares the length of the fetus at various ages with that of his fingers. Also, through practice he develops a fine sense of size.

Pregnancy during third and fourth months

At the end of 60 days, the fetus is about 2¹/₄ inches long. The vesicle is about the shape and size of a fairly large hen's egg. At the spot where the fetus lies, the horn is about 2¹/₂ inches thick as compared with a thickness of about one inch in a non-pregnant heifer or young cow.

The reproductive organs of a cow. The uterus is tilted so as to show the two horns

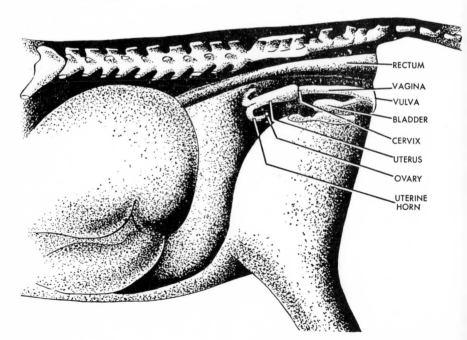

RECTUM

VAGINA

VULVA

BLADDER

CERVIX

UTERUS

OVARY

UTERINE HORN

By this time, the membranes that cover the fetus can be felt the full length of the pregnant horn. As the fetus grows, the non-pregnant horn also usually grows somewhat in thickness. This is because the membranes that cover the fetus become larger and extend into the non-pregnant horn.

At 80 days, the fetus is about four inches long and the horn is about three inches in diameter at its thickest part. The pregnant horn is now noticeably longer than the other one.

At three months the fetus is about six inches long. The thickest part of the horn measures about $3^{1}/_{2}$ inches. In most cases the uterus lies at the brim of the pelvis and can easily be felt. But in some older cows it falls down and lies in the abdomen. In such cases veterinarians often use a special forceps to grasp the cervix and pull the uterus up where it can be examined.

It is sometimes possible to feel the fetus itself at 90 days of pregnancy. By tapping the horn with the fingers, the fetus can be felt floating in the fluid. With gentle manipulation it may be picked up without injury.

At the end of the third month it is sometimes possible to detect the cotyledons, or "buttons" that stud the fetal membrane adjoining the trunk of the fetus. At this time the large ones are about the size of walnuts.

As gestation continues, cotyledons grow larger until at birth of the calf some of them may be 4 inches in diameter or even larger. Cotyledons also appear in the non-pregnant horn but these are small as compared with the others.

Pregnancy from the fifth month on

By the beginning of the fifth month of pregnancy, the uterus has sunk below the pelvic brim. Yet from then until the middle of the sixth month,

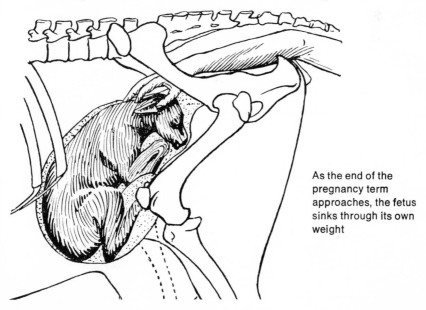

As the end of the pregnancy term approaches, the fetus sinks through its own weight

Gestation table of farm animals

Date of Service	Date Animal is Expected to Give Birth			
	Mare	Cow*	Ewe	Sow
Jan. 1	Dec. 6	Oct. 10	May 30	Apr. 22
Jan. 6	Dec. 11	Oct. 15	June 4	Apr. 27
Jan. 11	Dec. 16	Oct. 20	June 9	May 2
Jan. 16	Dec. 21	Oct. 25	June 14	May 7
Jan. 21	Dec. 26	Oct. 30	June 19	May 12
Jan. 26	Dec. 31	Nov. 4	June 24	May 17
Jan. 31	Jan. 5	Nov. 9	June 29	May 22
Feb. 5	Jan. 10	Nov. 14	July 4	May 27
Feb. 10	Jan. 15	Nov. 19	July 9	June 1
Feb. 15	Jan. 20	Nov. 24	July 14	June 6
Feb. 20	Jan. 25	Nov. 29	July 19	June 11
Feb. 25	Jan. 30	Dec. 4	July 24	June 16
Mar. 2	Feb. 4	Dec. 9	July 29	June 21
Mar. 7	Feb. 9	Dec. 14	Aug. 3	June 26
Mar. 12	Feb. 14	Dec. 19	Aug. 8	July 1
Mar. 17	Feb. 19	Dec. 24	Aug. 13	July 6
Mar. 22	Feb. 24	Dec. 29	Aug. 18	July 11
Mar. 27	Mar. 1	Jan. 3	Aug. 23	July 16
Apr. 1	Mar. 6	Jan. 8	Aug. 28	July 21
Apr. 6	Mar. 11	Jan. 13	Sept. 2	July 26
Apr. 11	Mar. 16	Jan. 18	Sept. 7	July 31
Apr. 16	Mar. 21	Jan. 23	Sept. 12	Aug. 5
Apr. 21	Mar. 26	Jan. 28	Sept. 17	Aug. 10
Apr. 26	Mar. 31	Feb. 2	Sept. 22	Aug. 15
May 1	Apr. 5	Feb. 7	Sept. 27	Aug. 20
May 6	Apr. 10	Feb. 12	Oct. 2	Aug. 25
May 11	Apr. 15	Feb. 17	Oct. 7	Aug. 30
May 16	Apr. 20	Feb. 22	Oct. 12	Sept. 4
May 21	Apr. 25	Feb. 27	Oct. 17	Sept. 9
May 26	Apr. 30	Mar. 4	Oct. 22	Sept. 14
May 31	May 5	Mar. 9	Oct. 27	Sept. 19
June 5	May 10	Mar. 14	Nov. 1	Sept. 24
June 10	May 15	Mar. 19	Nov. 6	Sept. 29
June 15	May 20	Mar. 24	Nov. 11	Oct. 4
June 20	May 25	Mar. 29	Nov. 16	Oct. 9
June 25	May 30	Apr. 3	Nov. 21	Oct. 14
June 30	June 4	Apr. 8	Nov. 26	Oct. 19
July 5	June 9	Apr. 13	Dec. 1	Oct. 24
July 10	June 14	Apr. 18	Dec. 6	Oct. 29
July 15	June 19	Apr. 23	Dec. 11	Nov. 3
July 20	June 24	Apr. 28	Dec. 16	Nov. 8
July 25	June 29	May 3	Dec. 21	Nov. 13
July 30	July 4	May 8	Dec. 26	Nov. 18
Aug. 4	July 9	May 13	Dec. 31	Nov. 23
Aug. 9	July 14	May 18	Jan. 5	Nov. 28
Aug. 14	July 19	May 23	Jan. 10	Dec. 3
Aug. 19	July 24	May 28	Jan. 15	Dec. 8
Aug. 24	July 29	June 2	Jan. 20	Dec. 13
Aug. 29	Aug. 3	June 7	Jan. 25	Dec. 18
Sept. 3	Aug. 8	June 12	Jan. 30	Dec. 23
Sept. 8	Aug. 13	June 17	Feb. 4	Dec. 28
Sept. 13	Aug. 18	June 22	Feb. 9	Jan. 2
Sept. 18	Aug. 23	June 27	Feb. 14	Jan. 7
Sept. 23	Aug. 28	July 2	Feb. 19	Jan. 12
Sept. 28	Sept. 2	July 7	Feb. 24	Jan. 17
Oct. 3	Sept. 7	July 12	Mar. 1	Jan. 22
Oct. 8	Sept. 12	July 17	Mar. 6	Jan. 27
Oct. 13	Sept. 17	July 22	Mar. 11	Feb. 1
Oct. 18	Sept. 22	July 27	Mar. 16	Feb. 6
Oct. 23	Sept. 27	Aug. 1	Mar. 21	Feb. 11
Oct. 28	Oct. 2	Aug. 6	Mar. 26	Feb. 16
Nov. 2	Oct. 7	Aug. 11	Mar. 31	Feb. 21
Nov. 7	Oct. 12	Aug. 16	Apr. 5	Feb. 26
Nov. 12	Oct. 17	Aug. 21	Apr. 10	Mar. 3
Nov. 17	Oct. 22	Aug. 26	Apr. 15	Mar. 8
Nov. 22	Oct. 27	Aug. 31	Apr. 20	Mar. 13
Nov. 27	Nov. 1	Sept. 5	Apr. 25	Mar. 18
Dec. 2	Nov. 6	Sept. 10	Apr. 30	Mar. 23
Dec. 7	Nov. 11	Sept. 15	May 5	Mar. 28
Dec. 12	Nov. 16	Sept. 20	May 10	Apr. 2
Dec. 17	Nov. 21	Sept. 25	May 15	Apr. 7
Dec. 22	Nov. 26	Sept. 30	May 20	Apr. 12
Dec. 27	Dec. 1	Oct. 5	May 25	Apr. 17

*The average gestation period of all cows has long been given as 283 days. However the American Dairy Science Association recommends a new table for dairy breeds under which the number of days of gestation are as follows: Ayrshire, 287.7; Brown Swiss, 290.8; Guernsey, 284.0; Holstein-Friesian, 278.9; Jersey, 279.3. In first calf heifers gestation is usually about two days shorter than with adult cows.

the fetus can be touched without much difficulty in more than half the cases. When it is within reach, it lies below the pelvic brim and slightly in front of it.

When it cannot be reached, it is because it has sunk to the bottom of the uterus which in turn rests on the pelvic floor. Sometimes it can be reached at the beginning of an examination but promptly slips away. It may be out of reach on one day but within reach the next.

From the middle of the sixth to the middle of the seventh month of gestation, pregnancy can best be determined by the condition of the uterus —its blood vessels, the uterine "buttons" and the tension on the cervix.

The arteries of a pregnant horn are larger and the pulsations are stronger than those of its mate. The increase in the flow of blood causes the pulse to become tremor-like in its beats. This can be best felt by applying only light pressure when taking the pulse. Some of the arteries of the uterus become as large as lead pencils and assume more winding paths during the last weeks of pregnancy.

Why some cows don't settle

MANY otherwise good animals are sold for slaughter because they fail to come in heat.

Pregnancy is the most common cause of heat failure and is the first thing to look for when an animal does not "come around." Sometimes an animal is bred without the owner's knowledge. Now and then a male, believed to be too young to breed, is responsible for a pregnancy.

Watch out for "silent heats"

The onset of heat in cows is sometimes hard to recognize because symptoms are not always pronounced. Heat is easier to recognize among heifers than in older cows, more apparent in summer than in winter and when a cow is warm rather than cold. Signs are more noticeable when cows are in a pasture or barnyard than when they are stanchioned. Every cattle owner knows the usual signs.

A cow in heat will often bellow, twitch her tail and raise it. She will remain standing while being mounted by another animal or will attempt to "ride" other animals. She will put her head on the back or rump of another animal throwing her head as if to mount. She will nose and smell other animals, snort and work her rump and tail like a bull.

But how about the cow with "silent" heats—those that are not noticeable?

Most cows bleed from the vulva about two days after their heat period although sometimes the amount of blood is so small that it is hardly noticeable. Some stockmen believe that the absence of such blood indicates that a service has been successful, but this is not true.

If a bloody discharge is noticed even if other signs of heat were not present, it is almost certain that the cow has been in heat and that she will probably be in heat again in 16 to 22 days. A good way to be sure of observing even mild symptoms of heat is to make a note of all heat periods, and begin to watch for the next one from about the 17th day after.

A bull calf is an excellent heat detector when running with a herd. A good way to find cows that are in heat in a barn is to lead a bull calf through each morning. He will show interest in cows in heat by sniffing at their hind quarters.

Research workers have found that 44 percent of the cows have silent heats during the first 60 days after calving. Among cows that have been fresh more than 60 days, silent heats occur about 11 percent of the time.

Persistent "yellow body"

As pointed out in the chapter "When a cow becomes pregnant," after an egg is discharged from an ovary, a small yellow body, known as a corpus luteum, immediately starts to form in the hole that had been occupied by the egg.

If an animal becomes pregnant, the yellow body remains during pregnancy. If conception does not take place, it is normal for the yellow body to increase in size for a short time and then gradually to disappear. It is gone before the next heat period.

Sometimes, for reasons that are not completely understood, the yellow body persists. It remains for an indefinite period of time even though the animal is not pregnant. In such cases the affected animal does not come in heat and conception does not occur.

Two methods are used to remove the yellow body. One consists in giving the animal the synthetic hormone, diethylstilbestrol. A cow should not be bred in the heat following the use of this drug. The use of hormone products is always accompanied by the danger of overdosing and unbalancing the entire system of endocrine glands.

The second method for removing a persistent yellow body consists in pinching it out of the ovary or removing it from the surface by reaching through the rectum. This requires experience. With unpracticed hands there is danger of causing a hemorrhage that may result in the death of a cow.

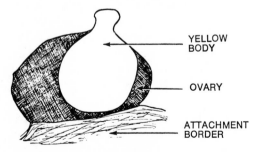

Cross section of a cow's ovary showing relative size of a yellow body. If the yellow body in a pregnant cow is removed, abortion follows

The ovary containing the yellow body is usually quite a bit larger and more egg-shaped than the other one. Before attempting to remove the body, the operator should be certain the cow is not pregnant. If the cow is pregnant, an abortion will follow.

The ovary should be picked up through the wall of the rectum and the yellow body pressed between the thumb and fingers. Pressure should be gentle but firm.

Usually the body is removed without much trouble and heat follows in one to five days. Removal of the yellow body is difficult when it has been present for some time and scar tissue holds it in place.

Mummified calf in uterus

Sometimes a pregnant cow has all the signs of dropping a calf, then labor pains stop and nothing happens. The unborn calf, or fetus, dies and remains in the uterus. Such a calf loses its water content and becomes hard and leathery like a mummy.

No heat periods occur while the mummified calf is in the uterus. Unless something is done about it, the calf may remain in the uterus for years.

The presence of a mummified calf can be determined by feeling it. This is done by reaching through the rectum. The firmness as compared with a living fetus is unmistakable.

Treatment consists in expelling the mummified calf, either through the injection of diethylstilbestrol or by removing the yellow body as explained above.

Sickness may cause lack of heat

Sickness and improper feeding may keep animals from coming in heat. Sickness of any kind will often disturb an animal's regular heat cycle. Even lice, worms or mange mites will sometimes keep cows from coming in heat. The presence of pus or abnormal growths has the same effect.

A fairly common cause of lack of heat in heifers is failure of the ovaries to develop eggs. This condition is accompanied by a small uterus and vagina. It is more often found in under-developed heifers than in those of normal size. The injection of gonadotropic hormone sometimes causes the ovaries to become normal.

Other causes of failure to come in heat are: Milk production of a cow so heavy that it saps all surplus energy. Animal has passed the breeding age. Lessening of sexual urge due to extremely cold weather. A decided change of climate has a temporary effect.

Freemartins

A freemartin is a female born twin to a bull calf. About nine out of 10 times such heifers are sterile and nothing can be done to make them otherwise.

The reason for the sterility is that the blood of the twins becomes intermingled. This blood carries the hormones produced by both the testicles and the ovaries. But it so happens that the testicles develop first. The hormones they give off stop the ovaries and other female organs from developing. This mingling of blood does no harm if both twins are either male or female.

Outwardly a freemartin may look normal while young but her sex organs never reach full development. As she grows older she will usually develop a tuft of hair near her vulva and she will take on some of the appearance of a steer.

Veterinarians usually diagnose freemartinism by examining the vagina by means of a speculum. This is inserted and a light is shown into it so that the inside of the vagina can be observed. With experience, a man can also detect abnormal female sex organs by feeling of them through the rectum, a method known as "rectal palpation." By testing the blood of a pair of twins, a male and a female, it can now be determined even at birth whether the heifer is a freemartin.

Chronic bullers

Some cows are in heat all the time or come in heat much more often than the usual 21-day interval. This ailment is called "nymphomania." Such cows will accept service but do not become pregnant.

When an egg is ripe and ready to be shed from an ovary, the fluid in which the egg lies give off a hormone that enters the blood stream and causes the cow to become sexually excited. The fluid and egg are contained in a sac, called a Graafian follicle or ovisac.

Ordinarily this follicle ruptures about 14 hours after the end of heat and releases the egg and the fluid. But sometimes for some unknown reason this rupture does not occur. The hormone continues to be developed and the cow is permanently or frequently in heat. The ailment is often referred to as a "cystic ovary."

The best way to treat a cystic ovary is to give the animal an intravenous injection of pituitary gonadotrophin or an intramuscular injection of chorionic gonadotrophin. These hormones are generally available only to veterinarians and physicians. Breeding should be delayed until the second heat period following use of the drugs.

The method of treatment used for many years consists in breaking the cysts by pinching them through the rectum, again using great care.

Feeding and sterility

Generally, if an animal is in good physical condition, sterility or other breeding disorders are seldom due to improper or insufficient feed. The organs of reproduction do not require special food elements, minerals or vitamins that are not required by the rest of the body.

Well-fed heifers have their first heat periods earlier than poorly fed ones but they also mature earlier in other ways. Lack of certain minerals may affect breeding efficiency before other signs of the deficiency appear but such cases are believed to be rare.

Hermaphrodites

Now and then animals are born with the characteristics of both sexes. Such animals are known as hermaphrodites. Since there is no way to correct this defect in dairy herds, the animals are usually sold for slaughter when it is found that they are unable to reproduce. In beef herds they are often allowed to attain full growth before being sold.

Many cases of so-called hermaphroditism are cause by incomplete development of the sex organs during gestation. In other words, the defect is like the hare-lip or cleft palate that often occurs among human beings. Most of these animals are really males whose development is imperfect. In extreme cases these are sterile but in mild cases they are capable of reproduction.

The tendency to give birth to hermaphrodites is to some extent inherited. Evidence of this has been noted particularly among sheep and goats where the defect occurs more often in certain families than in others.

White heifer disease

So-called white heifer disease is limited primarily to Shorthorn cattle, and is not a disease but a genetic defect in which the genital organs do not develop. The vagina grows to only half its normal length, and the ovaries and uterus are underdeveloped. The defect occurs only in animals that are entirely white, and only in a small percentage of those.

The tendency to the defect is inherited, usually occurs in beef cattle (notably Shorthorns), and in inbred animals or families. The heifers come in heat regularly, but the bull cannot penetrate to the usual depth, and thus the sperm cannot enter the oviducts. There is no cure nor treatment, the defect being inherited.

Vitamins

Cows under range conditions do not get enough vitamin A when they are kept for long periods on dry grass. Another cause of vitamin A deficiency is the feeding of a large amount of cotton-seed meal without sufficient green feed. Young animals are more apt to suffer from the deficiency than older ones.

Vitamin A deficiency may cause birth of dead or weak calves and frequent retention of afterbirth. Heat periods are also disturbed. Other symptoms of the deficiency are eye inflammation, night blindness and diarrhea.

To ward off vitamin A deficiency, animals should be fed green and yellow plants. These contain carotene which converted into the vitamin. Green legume hays are a good source of carotene. The feeding of synthetic vitamin supplements is the easiest and surest way to correct the deficiency.

Inheritance and fertility

Fertility is an inherited characteristic just like milk production, color of coat or body conformation. History records that certain breeds and families of livestock have passed out of existence because of their failure to reproduce.

It has been demonstrated that hormone activity and a tendency to cystic ovaries are inheritable. Both of these influence the efficiency of reproduction.

Granular venereal disease

Vaginitis means inflammation of the vagina. Some such inflammations do not interfere greatly with conception, but one kind definitely does when it occurs in severe form. This is known as granular venereal disease or nodular vaginitis.

Symptoms of the disease are bilsters or nodules in the vagina, especially just inside the vulva. These vary in size from that of a pinhead to a rice kernel and can easily be seen. In the acute state the nodules are red and bleed easily. A flaky, sticky discharge from the vulva is often present.

The troublesome time of the disease is when the vulva and vagina are reddened and a pus discharge dries to a crust on the tail. This may happen to virgin heifers even at the age of six weeks. When the granules form, the disease is apparently on the way out.

Granular vaginitis is spread through contact, especially by bulls. Its cause is not known but is suspected of being a virus. The disease runs it's course, sometimes through a herd, and then dies out. A common treatment for females is a sexual rest for 60 days. The disease is most severe among heifers.

Most cases of granular vaginitis will recover within a few weeks of their own accord. Medicines, though, will often hasten recovery.

In heifers, swabbing the infected vagina with acriflavine ointment, or douching with 5 percent silver nitrate solution, Lugol's solution or gentian violet is common practice. The acute signs disappear quickly in cows but the granules often persist for a month or more. In bulls the disease is often stubborn and may last for many months. Sexual rest, the use of tranquilizers to reduce sexual excitement, and douching the sheath with acriflavine or 5 percent silver nitrate solution is often helpful.

Problem cows

A small percentage of cows fail to breed for no apparent reason. They come in heat regularly, tests fail to indicate the presence of the common breeding diseases or ailments, yet repeated service fails to bring them with calf. Research indicates that 80 percent of these non-breeders have a mild infection of the uterus which cannot be detected by ordinary means.

Samples taken from the uterus during successive heat periods show that these microbes may remain for months. The injection of penicillin and the sulfa drugs has no effect on them.

It is believed that the microbes destroy the fertilized eggs or young embryos since they seem to have no effect on sperm. The fact that such barren cows often skip one or two heat periods indicates that they have been temporarily pregnant.

Many of these repeat breeders will recover of their own accord if given a long rest period—three months or more. Apparently, cows become immune to the infection with time and the infection disappears.

Suggestions on cattle breeding troubles

1. Keep records of heat dates, dates of breeding and unusual occurrences such as abortions and vaginal discharges. If a heat period is missed and you later notice bleeding from the vulva, watch for the heat period about 19 days later. Sometimes ovaries operate normally but cows do not show sexual excitement. Such cows can be bred successfully with proper timing.

2. Before you sell a cow for sterility, make sure she is not in calf. A large number of cows butchered for sterility have been found to be pregnant.

3. Do not breed cows until they have been fresh at least 60 days. A cow needs a rest period for a good conception rate.

4. Do not breed a cow with an unnatural discharge—one that is flaky or discolored.

5. If a cow has had a retained placenta (afterbirth), make sure that she is clean before breeding her.

6. Be sure of proper timing. For best conception rate, breed just before or just after the end of the heat period.

7. If a cow does not conceive with three services, she should be examined by a veterinarian before being bred again.

8. Never allow other cows or other livestock to come in contact with the discharge or bedding of a cow that has aborted. Such contaminated material should be burned or buried. Keep the cow that has aborted away from other animals until you are sure that the abortion was not caused by a contagious disease.

9. Cows should have plenty of sunlight and exercise in winter as well as in the summer.

10. Since cows breed better when they are gaining weight, reduce the weight of fat cows and let them be gaining in weight at the time they are to be bred.

11. Let the cows stand dry for 60 days before calving.

12. Raise your own replacements so far as practicable. If you buy them, you may expose your herd to disease or may be buying someone else's breeding problems.

13. Make sure that the bull is not at fault. If he settles most cows but not all of them he's presumably all right.

What to do in difficult calving

THE FIRST SIGN of calving is enlargement of the udder. It becomes firm with more or less swelling in front. The vulva becomes enlarged and discharges a stringy mucus. The belly droops.

When the muscles at the sides of the root of the tail fall in, so as to leave deep hollows, calving will normally occur in from one to three days.

Signs of labor

Just before labor pains begin, the pregnant cow becomes uneasy, stops eating, separates from the herd, lies down and rises again as though in pain, shifts upon her hind feet, moves her tail and may bellow or moan. With contractions of the womb and labor pains, the back becomes arched, the rump drops, the belly is drawn up and straining starts. At the same time, blood may appear on the vulva and tail. Soon "water bags" protrude between the lips of the vulva.

These bags increase rapidly in size. They hang down towards the hocks. In normal births the fore or hind feet of the calf can be seen within them. They finally break. When the water runs out, more violent contractions of the womb occur and normally the calf is shortly born.

The water bags should not be broken. They provide a soft cushion and uniform pressure within the womb while the solid body of the calf passes through it.

A cow often calves while standing, in which case the navel string is broken as the calf falls to the ground. If the calf is delivered while the cow is lying down, the cord is torn when the cow rises. Afterpains normally come three or four hours later and expel the afterbirth.

As soon as the calf is born, clip the navel cord about one inch from its belly and squeeze out the few drops of blood. Then apply tincture of iodine.

Usually a cow will calf without help. One cause of difficult calving is an unnatural position (a malpresentation) of the fetus. The front feet and nose should appear first as shown in Fig. 1.

With twins, the second one should be delivered hind feet first. In this case, or when a single calf is born hind feet first, someone should be on hand to see that delivery is hastened when the blood supply to the calf through the navel cord is shut off. If the calf is unable to start breathing at that time, it will smother.

Make sure of proper delivery

Before labor has progressed to any great extent, it is well to make sure that the fetus lies in the proper position for easy delivery. Sometimes the position of the fetus makes calving without assistance difficult or impossible.

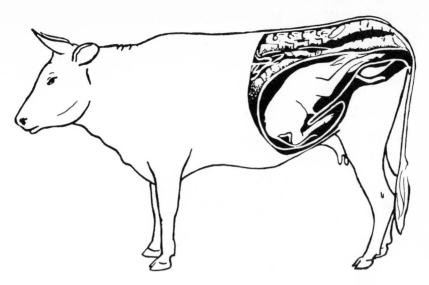

This is the normal position of a calf as it is lodged in the uterus shortly before birth

A calf should be delivered on its belly, with front feet and head first. In this way its curved body follows the natural curvature of the canal through which it must pass.

Unless a person is skilled in the work, he should call a veterinarian when difficulties in calving arise, that is, if two hours have elapsed without delivery, or if the water bag has broken leaving the calf dry. A bungled job may mean serious injury to the uterus or vagina or death of the cow or calf. Sometimes assistance is needed even when presentation of the calf is normal. This is especially true with heifers.

No help should be given a cow in labor unless it is necessary. Time must be allowed for the relaxation of the openings of the uterus and vagina. Generally, labor should continue for an hour or two before help is given, if an examination shows that the calf is being presented in a normal position, although the condition of the cow must be taken into consideration. If there is no mechanical obstruction, or malpresentation, the unaided efforts of the cow will nearly always expel the calf.

When assistance is needed, the operator should prepare himself for the work. He should trim his fingernails and scrub his hands and arms thoroughly. The whole arm should be bare. The arm and hand should be smeared with sterile oil, grease, unsalted lard or vaseline, before inserting the hand into the womb.

The use of a mild antiseptic will protect the cow against the introduction of infection into the passage and the operator against possible disease. The membranes of the vagina and uterus are delicate, so strong antiseptics must be avoided and all movements of the hand must be slow and gentle.

An examination should be made with the hand when any of the following situations arise:

71

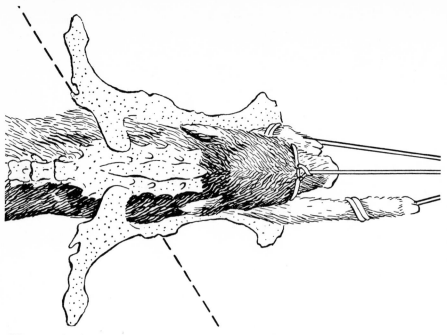

When a calf is too broad through the shoulders for delivery, pulling out one leg ahead of the other helps to offset the difficulty. Dotted line shows position of shoulders as they pass through the pelvis

Labor pains have lasted for some several hours without the appearance of water bags or other signs of calving.

The head and only one forefoot appear.

Both forefeet but not the head appear.

The head appears without the forefeet.

One hind foot appears without the other.

When some but not all the parts appear, do not at once attempt to manipulate the fetus into proper position. Wait until after you have secured with a rope or chain and running noose the parts that are within reach. (Fig. 2) This is done so that these parts can easily be pulled back into the vagina if it should be necessary temporarily to push them back into the womb.

In the search for a missing part, it is easier to work if the cow is lying on an incline with her head lower than the hind end. In this way the fetus and internal organs tend to be pulled forward by their own weight and leave more room in which to bring up a missing part.

In cases of difficult labor, a block and tackle are often used to raise the hind end of a cow or raise her completely off the floor. The block is hung from the rafters of a barn.

Do not attempt to bring a missing leg into its proper place during labor pains. Wait until the pains stop and straighten the leg out before the next pain begins. If the pains are violent and continuous, they may be checked by pinching the back or by putting a tight surcingle around the body in front of the udder. These failing, 1 ounce or 1¹/₂ ounces of chloral hydrate in a quart of water may be given to check the pains.

If the passages have dried up or lost their natural, lubricating liquid, smear the interior of the passages and womb and the surface of the calf, as far as it can be reached, with pure fresh lard; or pure sweet oil or mineral oil may be run into the womb through a rubber tube (fountain syringe).

In dragging out the fetus apply strong traction only while the mother is straining and drag downward toward the hocks as well as backwards. The natural curvature of both fetus and passages is thus followed and the extraction made easier. A number of good calf pullers are available at agricultural supply companies. (Fig. 3)

Labor pains that precede abortion

Any of the causes of abortion may bring on labor pains before it is time for the calf to be born. Straining may occur days or even weeks before time. In such cases there are not the usual enlargement, swelling, and mucus discharge from the vulva. There is little or no falling in by the sides of the root of the tail. The abdomen has not dropped to the usual extent. When abortion occurs early in pregnancy, early advance symptoms are, of course, often lacking entirely.

In spite of the pains, sometimes no water bags appear. If the hand is cautiously introduced into the vagina, the neck will be found to be firmly sealed. If it is definitely known that the cow has not reached her proper time for calving, examination of the vagina should be omitted. The animal should be placed in a dark quiet place by herself.

In some cases the external parts are relaxed and duly prepared, but the neck of the womb remains rigidly closed. In such case the solid extract of belladonna should be smeared around the constricted opening and the animal left quiet until it relaxes.

Oversized calf from prolonged gestation

Some cows repeatedly carry their calves past the normal calving date. The calf continues to grow and when delivery is finally attempted,

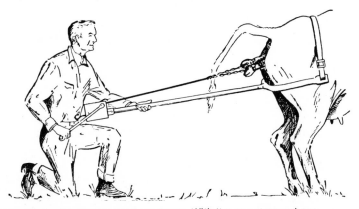

Various kinds of calf extractors are in use. With the one shown above, great pulling power is obtained with comparatively little effort

the calf is too large and must be taken by cesarean operation to save the cow.

This type of calf seldom lives. The trouble can usually be traced back to the cow's sire, many of whose daughters have had the same trouble.

Twisting of the neck of the womb

Quite often the neck of the womb becomes twisted in such a way that the cervix cannot open, or at least cannot open completely. In such cases the calf cannot be expelled. Veterinarians call such twisting *torsion of the uterus*.

The twist is usually a partial one, that is, the uterus rotates less than half way around. Rarely does it make a complete rotation, although cases have been known where several complete rotations were made.

Torsion of the uterus occurs both among heifers having their first calf and among cows that have calved several times. The twist may be in either direction.

When such a womb is untwisted, the cervix is usually found completely open. In view of this, some authorities believe that twisting takes place during the latter stages of labor, and is caused by the movements of of an unusually active fetus.

Even though the womb is twisted, the onset of labor is normal. But when labor pains continue for some time without any signs of water bags, if possible, the vagina should be examined with the oiled hand.

A womb may be twisted without the vagina or the vagina may be included in the twist. When the vagina is included in the twist, the folds run forward in a spiral manner and can usually be felt. It is then easy to tell whether the twist is to the right—like the threads in a righthanded screw—or to the left.

Sometimes it is not possible to tell through the vagina whether the twist is to the right or to the left. Examination may then be made by reaching into the rectum and feeling of the uterus. Ridges indicate the direction of the twist.

If the twist is to the right, the cow should be laid on her right side with her head downhill. The operator should put his hand in the cow's vagina. If possible, he should then insert his hand through the cervix and seize one or both legs of the calf. This should be done carefully so as not to injure the delicate tissues.

If the hand cannot be passed through the cervix, it is advisable to call your veterinarian, because the longer the cow labors unsuccessfully the more difficult delivery becomes. If cesarean section becomes necessary, early operation affords the best prospects for a living cow and a living calf. This operation is now successful in most cases that are performed early.

If the hand can pass through the cervix and grasp a foot, two or three assistants should then roll the cow quickly over on her left side. While doing so, the foot which can be grasped should be doubled back at the fetlock to provide a more secure hold and better leverage to prevent the calf from rolling when the cow rolls. The object of this is to hold the

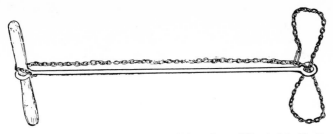

This is what is known as a detorsion rod. When the calf lies twisted in the uterus, the loops of the chain are put around two of the animal's legs. Turning the rod by means of the wooden handle helps bring the calf into proper position for delivery

womb and calf still while the body of the cow rolls over. If the procedure is successful, the womb becomes untwisted. The cervix opens and the water bags and calf slip through the opening.

If the first attempt is not successful, the process should be repeated —several times if necessary. If the womb is twisted to the left, the cow should be laid on her left side and rolled over to her right side.

This method of treatment for a twisted womb will not bring relief in all cases. Sometimes the fetus has dried and its decomposition has set in. Inflammation of the womb and pus in the twisted neck of the womb may hinder the rotation of this organ.

In difficult cases, instruments are sometimes used. One of these, called a detorsion rod. (Fig. 4) In rare cases a cesarian operation must be performed to save the cow's life.

Wrong presentations

When a calf lies in a womb in a position other than the natural one, the calf is said to have malpresentation. The most common wrong presentations together with methods for their relief are as follows:

Back turned to one side

A calf is thicker from breastbone to spine than from side to side. (Fig. 5) The pelvis of a cow—the large bone through which the calf must pass on delivery—is shaped so as to allow for this difference in dimensions. If a calf lies on its side in a womb, delivery is difficult if not impossible.

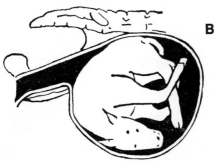

Back turned to one side

The remedy for this is, of course, to rotate the body of the calf until its spine turns toward the spine of the cow. The operation is easy unless the calf has become wedged sideways in the passage. Simply twist the legs over each other in the direction wanted, until the head and spine of the calf are in the proper position for delivery or double a leg at the fetlock, as described previously, to provide more leverage for rolling the calf. If it is possible to repel the calf back into the uterus for a few inches between labor pains, the turning is made easier.

If the body is firmly wedged in the pelvic canal, the problem of delivering the calf becomes more difficult. First, freely lubricate the calf where it is in contact with the obstructing bone. Then proceed with twisting the feet as set forth in the paragraph above.

Often it is necessary to engage the legs with a rope to be pulled by an assistant, while the operator rotates the head. Sometimes quite a bit of manipulation is needed to bring the calf into proper position. This is called a breech presentation, and is very difficult to correct. If it is possible, it will be difficult, and can only be done by repelling the calf far enough to straighten the legs—first at the hock, then at the fetlock. When an attempt is made, care should be taken that the feet do not break through the roof of the vagina.

If early attempts to get a normal presentation are unsuccessful, cesarean section is the preferred procedure.

Calf upside down and backwards

It is possible but sometimes difficult to extract a calf in this position. (Fig. 6) If an attempt is made, care should be taken that the feet do not break through the roof of the vagina.

Other ways to handle such cases are to rotate the body of the calf so the spine will run in the same direction as the spine of the cow, or push the rump and hind legs back so that the calf rotates in the womb, end to end. In the latter case the calf will be presented head and forelegs first.

Twins jammed in passage

Twins are usually born one at a time but in rare cases they both move into the vagina at the same time. (Fig. 7) In such cases the forelegs of one and the hind legs of the other move together. Since the pas-

Calf upside down and backwards

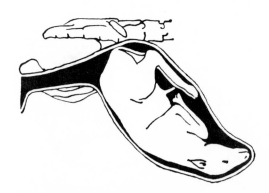

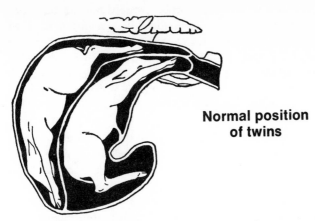

**Normal position
of twins**

sage is not big enough for both calves, they become jammed, or impacted, in the pelvis. The difficulty can be recognized by the fact that two of the feet extending into the vagina are in the normal position (soles down) and the other two are reversed (soles up). It is also possible to differentiate by following the leg up until reaching the knee or else the hock.

If the front feet and head are being presented, it is usually easiest to repel the hind legs, and deliver the other calf first. This can usually be done by having an assistant pull the front feet while you repel the rear legs of the twin. Place a running noose around each of its legs just above the hoof or fetlock. The operator or an assistant should pull on these ropes while the feet of the other calf are pushed back. As soon as one calf has been brought forward so as to occupy the pelvis, the other twin will be crowded back and will then no longer obstruct the passage.

Forelegs bent at knees

When the forelegs are bent at the knees, the shoulders are pushed backward. (Fig. 8) This adds the thickness of the shoulder blades and muscles to that of the chest, greatly increasing the bulk of that already bulky part. The forearm from the elbow to the knee further increases the bulk in the chest area and makes it difficult or impossible for the calf to pass through the pelvis.

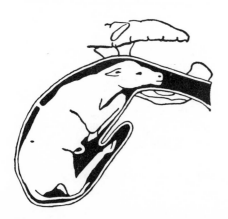

Forelegs bent at knees

For delivery of the calf, the forelegs can be brought into proper position by repelling the shoulders with one hand while straightening a leg with the other—being careful, as always, to avoid puncturing the uterus or the vagina. The ease with which this can be done depends upon how far the calf has advanced into the pelvic cavity. If it has advanced only a short distance, the legs can be brought into their proper position by means of the hands. It is easier to use the right hand to straighten the left leg and the left hand for the right one.

The easiest way to straighten a leg is to grasp the foot, bend it forcibly on the fetlock, and lift it over the brim of the pelvis. In doing this, the knee of the calf will be pressed upwards. As soon as the foot has been raised into the passage, the leg can be straightened out with ease.

When the calf has advanced to the extent that the shoulders have entered the pelvis, delivery of the calf becomes much more difficult. The calf must be pushed back into the womb. A repeller can be used for this purpose.

Use of a repeller

A repeller is an instrument with a long straight stem and several branches, two or three inches long, attached to the end. The end with the branches is introduced into the womb and placed against the breast of the calf. When the operator pushes on the stem of the instrument, the calf is repelled back into the womb. This makes it possible to manipulate the legs into their proper position for delivery.

If a repeller is not at hand, a round smooth staff, such as the handle of a pitchfork, can be used, or an assistant can strip his arm to the shoulder and push back the calf while the operator brings out the legs.

Pressure against the calf's breast should be forward or slightly upward. This carries the shoulders of the calf upward and makes room for bringing out the missing feet.

When repelling a calf into the womb, it is good policy to put a halter on the head or a noose around the lower jaw, and a rope around each knee. This guards against loss when any of the parts are pushed back into the womb. If the cow is lying down, the operator should first secure the foot on the upper side and if necessary turn the cow over to secure the one on the other side.

Foreleg bent back from shoulder

This may happen with one leg, as shown in Fig. 9, or with both legs. In either event, the remedy is more difficult than when legs are bent at the knees.

One of the symptoms of the condition is that the head is presented at the passage and may even protrude from the vulva during active labor pains, but draws back quickly when straining stops. This is a very difficult malpresentation to correct, and every hour of delay will make it more difficult for your veterinarian.

The missing leg or legs usually cannot be found when you insert

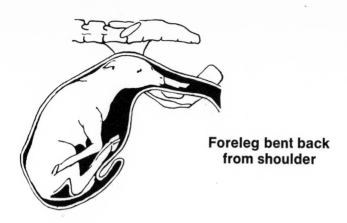

**Foreleg bent back
from shoulder**

the oiled hand into the womb between labor pains. However, if you introduce the hand during a pain it may be possible to reach the elbow or upper foreleg.

In the absence of pain, you can put a halter or noose on the head and move the body towards you so as to grasp a foreleg just below the elbow. If you hold this firmly and at the same time push the head and body back into the womb, you will have room to bring up the knee. From then on, continue to bring out the leg as explained in the preceding section, "Forelegs bent at knees."

Head bent down beneath breast

In this case the nose of the advancing calf has struck the lower brim of the pelvis and the head was bent downward as shown in Fig. 10. On examination, the neck can be felt between the forelegs. As a rule the head is out of reach since it is lodged against the breastbone.

If you keep your hand on the neck and drag the feet with the aid of ropes you may reach an ear or better still be able to put your fingers into the sockets of the eyes. If you then push on the legs, you may be able to slip your hand down and grab hold of the nose. A repeller may be used to push the body back instead of pushing on the legs.

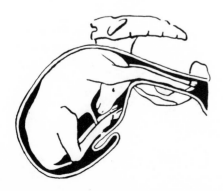

**Head bent down
beneath breast**

If it is impossible to deliver the calf with the hand alone, veterinarians use blunt hooks that are placed in one or both eyes. Sometimes a noose around the calf's upper jaw or around the muzzle is used in combination with the eye hooks.

Calf upside down

This position is unnatural and highly unusual. Moreover, delivery is difficult for two particular reasons: First, the natural curvature of the calf and that of the passage are in opposite directions; second, the thickest part of the calf—the upper part—must pass through the lower, or smaller, part of the pelvis. Despite this, in most cases delivery will occur naturally with little or no assistance. (Fig. 11)

If the calf is unusually large or the pelvis of the cow abnormally narrow, calving is sometimes difficult. In such cases, either the body of the calf may be rotated as in cases where the calf lies on its side or the operator can push back the head and forelegs and reach for the hind legs, pulling them through the pelvic opening. The calf will then be delivered hind feet first.

All four legs presented

In this position all four legs extend into the passage. The calf lies across the womb with its back arched. The head may be felt to the right or the left and indicates the position of the calf. (Fig. 12)

The remedy is to push back into the womb the pair of legs that are least advanced or the two which will leave the fetus in the position for easiest delivery. Where the calf can be so turned that its back runs along the spine of the dam, the calf should be turned in this manner, even though the hind legs will be presented first.

Before attempting to turn the body of the calf, it is best to put a noose on each of the four feet, marking the ropes that lead to the forelegs so you can identify them. If the forelegs are to be brought into the passage, a noose should be placed on the lower jaw. Run the ropes attached to the legs that are to be pushed back through the ring of a cord carrier and pass the rings down to the feet.

With the aid of the carrier, push the feet well back into the womb and hold them there. In the meantime pull on the ropes attached to the other two feet and bring the feet into the passage. If the forefeet are

All four legs presented

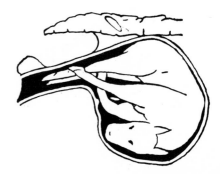

coming out first, at the same time pull on the rope attached to the lower jaw.

The feet that are to come out last should be pushed back in the womb until the body of the calf has entered the passages. In this way they cannot again enter the pelvis until the rest of the body has emerged.

In all cases where it is necessary to push the calf back into the womb before bringing it out, the cow's head should be kept lower than the rear end. In cases of long standing, it is often advisable to give the cow a full 2-ounce dose of chloral hydrate, but it would be safer to call your veterinarian before the cow is greatly weakened.

Epidural anasthesia

Difficulties attending wrong presentations are due largely to straining on the part of the cow. This can be completely overcome through injection of an anesthetic into the base of the cow's tail. This procedure is explained in the latter part of the chapter "Eversion, or prolapse, of the uterus".

When a cow fails to clean

THE AFTERBIRTH, or placenta, of a cow is usually expelled within a few hours after a calf is born. If it is not expelled naturally within 36 to 48 hours, opinions differ as to what should be done.

Some veterinarians say the afterbirth should be removed by hand if it is possible to do so without using force. Others recommend immediate treatment with antiseptics, antibiotics or hormones. A few say just leave the afterbirths alone; after a certain length of time they will come out of their own accord with no harm done.

When an afterbirth is retained, part of it usually hangs from the vulva and develops an offensive odor in a few days. For hygienic reasons, dairymen do not want this to occur. Moreover, infection of the uterus usually follows a retained afterbirth, with general symptoms of illness.

Sometimes a gallon or more of fluid and pus accumulates because of the infection. Such an infection is known as metritis or endometritis.

Retained afterbirth is often caused by an infection. Trichomoniasis, and vibrionic abortion are the principal diseases involved though it may also be caused by other infections. Retained afterbirth often happens among animals without any symptoms of disease. Cases occur more frequently when calves are born before or after the expected time. They often accompany the birth of twins and painful or slow delivery of young.

Treatment

The placenta is attached to the uterus by cotyledons, sometimes called "buttons." These are often swollen in cases of retained afterbirth. In any event they stick tight instead of letting go when the calf is born.

Therein lies the danger of removing the afterbirth by hand. If the cotyledons are injured, or the cervix is forced open, the cow may thereafter be barren.

It takes experience to remove an afterbirth properly. If it does not detach readily from the cotyledons, further attempts should not be made at the time, as there is danger of tearing the cotyledon from the wall of the uterus. Sometimes several trials at intervals of a few days will be successful. Only gentle pulling should be done. Care must be taken not to infect the uterus with unclean hands or a contaminated irrigating tool.

The external genitals of a cow should be thoroughly cleaned before the work is begun. A straining cow should not be cleaned. The operation increases straining and may result in prolapse, or eversion of the uterus.

The injection of what is known as "posterior pituitary hormone" immediately after delivery of the calf greatly reduces the chance of a retained afterbirth, but this should become routine practice only after a series have been retained, and the preventive injection is recommended by your veterinarian.

Whether a retained afterbirth is removed by hand or allowed to come out of its own accord, the uterus should immediately be treated with drugs to avoid infection. The antibiotics generally recommended are a combination of penicillin and Streptomycin, chlortetracycline (Aureomycin), or oxytetracycline (Terramycin). Nitrofurazone (Furacin) suppositories are also used. The afterbirth comes away in about a week with no odor or discharge.

The use of sulfa drugs in the treatment of the disease is no longer recommended since they delay the healing process.

It is not believed that drugs hasten the expulsion of an afterbirth. They keep the womb from becoming infected and the afterbirth is expelled through natural causes.

Prolapse of the uterus

Prolapse or eversion of the uterus sometimes follows calving. When this occurs, the uterus is partly or wholly turned inside out and hangs from the vulva. Between 50 and 100 mushroomlike bodies (cotyledons) are on its surface, each two to three inches in diameter and attached by a narrow neck.

When fully everted, the two horns of the uterus hang down toward the hocks. In cases of long standing the organ becomes inflamed and engorged with blood until it is as large as a bushel basket.

Treatment

Before proceeding with treatment, the hands and arms should be thoroughly washed and when there is a possibility that brucellosis is present they should also be oiled.

In partial eversion, with the cow standing, an assistant should pinch the cow's back to prevent straining while the operator pushes his closed fist into the center of the mass and carries it back through the vagina.

In the meantime he should use his other hand to return the surrounding parts that overlap the lips of the vulva.

These directions sound simple, but following them will present difficulties. One is, that a finger may be pushed through the wall of the uterus in trying to return it to the inside of the cow. This occurs especially when attempting to cover a wider area by spreading the fingers instead of keeping the fist closed.

In more complete eversion, with the cow standing, a sheet is used by two men to lift the womb to the height of the vulva. It should be sponged with clean cool water and then with a mild antiseptic solution. Allow a little time for as much blood as possible to drain out of the swollen organ. A closed fist should then be planted in the largest horn to push it back within itself and into place through the vagina. The uterus should be pushed completely through the cervical ring and into the abdomen—an arm-length procedure. Great care must be taken not to damage the "buttons" or any other part of the organ.

In case the above procedure fails, take a long linen or cotton bandage, five or six inches wide, and wind it around the protruding womb as tightly as it can be drawn. Begin at the free end and gradually cover the entire mass up to the vulva. This forces the greater part of the blood out of the organ and greatly reduces its bulk. After this is done, proceed with the first as described above.

As the womb is turned within itself the wrapping bandage gradually loosens. Once the great mass has entered the passages it is easy to compel the rest to follow. When the womb is completely replaced, the bandage is left inside and can easily be taken out. It is well to move the hand from side to side to make sure that the two horns are fully extended and on about the same level.

If a womb is everted and the cow is lying down, she should be brought to her feet. This is usually done by means of a block and tackle if other methods fail.

Treatment with a spinal anesthetic

Bringing a cow to her feet and replacing an everted womb can be done much more easily with the aid of what is called *spidural anesthesia,* This consists of injecting an anesthetic into the spinal column.

With an everted uterus, the site for injection is the depression between the first and second caudal vertebrae or tail bones. To find the site, hold the tail of a standing cow straight back and move it up and down. It is then easy to feel, by the movement of the bones, which ones are the first and second of the tail.

The anesthetic used is generally procaine hydrochloride, sold under the trade name of novocaine. The size of the dose is 8 to 12 cc of a 2 percent solution depending on the weight of the animal. If too much is used, the animal will not be able to retain a standing position. Use a strong hypodermic syringe, preferably glass, with a needle 2 to 3 inches long.

Stand at the right side of the animal. After proper preparation of the

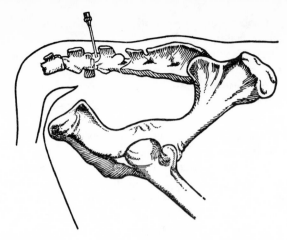

This shows the place and the approximate angle at which to insert the needle when making an epidural injection

site—clipping, shaving and disinfecting the skin—push the needle into the center of the depression, slanting it slightly as indicated in the accompanying sketch. The needle should be pushed in to a depth of $3/4$ to $1^1/2$ inches.

When you think you have reached the proper depth, attach the syringe and try to inject a little of the fluid. If it flows easily, as in the open air, the point of the needle is in the right place. But if pressure is necessary to make the injection, the needle should be pulled out and inserted in a slightly different spot or at a little different angle, but always in line with the exact center of the tail.

If the needle penetrates too deeply and the point goes into the cartilage beneath the canal, a slight withdrawal of the needle will generally bring the point to the right place. Sometimes the needle will puncture a small blood vessel but this does no harm.

The fluid should be injected slowly with occasional short pauses, taking one or two minutes. With rapid injection there is danger of death from shock. The drug starts to take effect in a few minutes and reaches maximum effectiveness in ten to 15 minutes. Its effects last one-half to two hours.

When a cow is lying down, epidural anesthesia will often bring her to her feet immediately. If not, she can nearly always be made to stand with a little stimulation. The anesthetic overcomes completely the straining on the part of a cow that comes on when her genital organs are handled. Hence putting a womb back where it belongs, as per instructions set forth above, becomes comparatively easy following epidural anesthesia.

Eversion of the uterus seldom recurs, once the organ is put back in place. But to guard against possible recurrence, a rope harness is often applied around the vulva for a few days. Sometimes the upper part of the vulva is stitched shut to keep the organ in place. Stitches are removed at the end of a week, when straining has stopped completely.

Eversion, or prolapse, of the vagina

DURING PREGNANCY eversion, or prolapse, of the vagina is common. This protrusion of the vagina comes from relaxation of the vaginal walls and occurs most often when cows lie in stalls that are lower behind than in front, or when stalls are so short that the rear quarters extend over the edge and into the gutter.

The protrusion is rounded and smooth and if it embraces both sides of the urinary canal it is double with a passage between. It occurs most often in a cow or ewe after the third or fourth month of pregnancy. It rarely happens in animals bearing young for the first time.

In some cases, the protruding part disappears of its own accord after the calf is dropped. While it is present a truss may be applied. If the everted vagina does not disappear after calving, the condition can sometimes be remedied by raising the hind part of the stall higher than the front. Raise it about four inches at first and a little higher later if this does not work. In severe cases, treatment should proceed as in case of eversion of the uterus.

Removing extra teats

OFTEN DAIRY HEIFERS have one or more extra or so-called supernumerary teats. Although these teats do a heifer no harm, often they don't look well and sometimes they interfere with milking. In some cases an extra teat may secrete milk and cause a lot of bother by leaking at milking time.

Extra teats can easily be removed up to one year of age. Simply stretch out the extra teats and cut them off close to the udder with a sharp pair of scissors. Apply tincture of iodine or some other good disinfectant both before and after the operation. In some cases in older animals it may be necessary to cut out a teat and its accompanying gland. This should be done by someone skilled in this work and only during the dry period.

Bull castration

THE PRINCIPAL REASON for castrating bull calves is to make the animal more valuable for beef purposes. Steers have a better quality of meat than bulls and have more flesh on the most valuable portions of their dressed carcasses. Castration also aids in growth and fattening.

Still another reason for castrating some bull calves is to keep scrub or inferior males from mating with purebred or superior cows. Bulls are sometimes castrated when they become dangerous. This is done so they can be sent to market in better condition and with less hazard.

Bull calves are usually castrated when about two or three months old but they may be castrated as early as a few days after birth. The younger the animal, the easier the work and the less the danger.

There is a growing tendency to not castrate dairy bull calves, but to market them when not more than a year old. Sometimes the testicles are forced back up and into body, and held there by an elastrator band (as described later), thus creating what is known as a "short scrotum."

Early spring is the best time for castration although fall is also a good time for it. Castration may be done in the winter but, except for the bloodless type (discussed later), it should not be done when flies are troublesome. Otherwise there is danger of fly-borne infections.

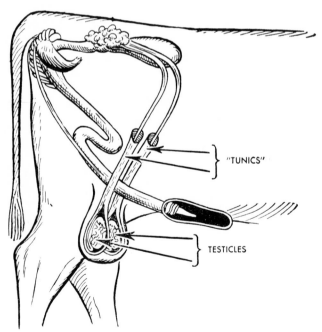

Sex organs of a bull, showing the testicles and how the *tunica vaginalis* surrounds them and the spermatic cord

Methods in use

There are two main ways to unsex bovine males: remove the testicles from the scrotum (bag); or crush the blood vessels that lead to the testicles so that the testicles waste away.

Testicles can be removed by a number of methods. However, only two of these methods are in common use. These are the lateral (side) incision method and the end-incision method.

The Lateral-Incision Method—Grasp the scrotum with the thumb and forefinger of the left hand so as to stretch the skin tight over the right side of the right testicle. Then with a sharp sterilized knife cut a slit down the right side of the scrotum, starting a few inches above the top of the testicle and ending a little below it. This incision should be deep enough to cut through layers of skin and tissue and expose the testicle.

Grasp the testicle with one hand and with the other hand strip the cord of its loose surrounding tissue so that the cord is exposed well up to the top of the scrotum. Pull the testicle down with the left hand, using a force of about two pounds. Apply an *emasculator* to the cord with the right hand, forcing it up so that the jaws surround the cord high up in the scrotum. Press the handles of the emasculator together to cut the cord.

The emasculator has a dull or crushing edge and a sharp or cutting

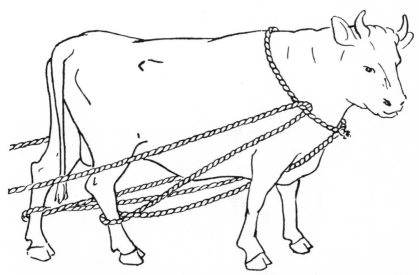

Proper restraint of animals is a necessary precaution when castrating animals. Bulls are especially treacherous

edge; and it must always be applied so that the crushed end of the cord remains with the animal.

An emasculator, as shown on this page, is used to cut off the cord because it crushes before it cuts. This mangles the blood vessels and wards off serious hemorrhages.

After the removal of one testicle, the other one can be removed in the same manner.

End-Incision Method—To perform this operation, grasp the buttom of the scrotum with the left hand and squeeze it so as to force the testicles upwards. Then start cutting the scrotum crosswise, about one third of the way up. Completely encircle the scrotum so as to remove the buttom third.

This should leave the testicles dangling uninjured, encased in a sac called the *tunica vaginalis*—"tunic," for short. Nick the tunic with the knife and a testicle will be exposed. Grasp the testicle, strip the cord of its surrounding tissue and proceed as in the lateral-incision method.

As in all operations, the greatest care must be used to avoid infection. To do a professional job, you should first wash the site for cutting with 70-percent alcohol and then treat it with tincture of iodine. The iodine solution should be allowed to dry before you make an incision. All instruments should be thoroughly cleaned and sterilized before they are used.

Bloodless castration

Bull castration by surgical means is rapidly being supplanted by a method popularly called "bloodless castration." It is done by crushing the cords and blood vessels that lead to the testicles without injuring the scrotum. By this method the testicles wither away. Danger of infection and screwworm infestation are avoided. The operation can be performed safely at any time of the year.

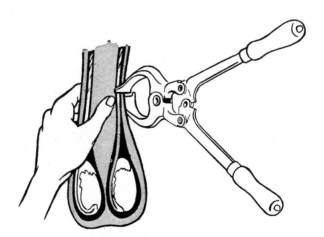

Before applying the emasculatome, squeeze the cord as far over to the outside edge of the scrotum as it will conveniently go. In this way only a small part of the scrotum is injured

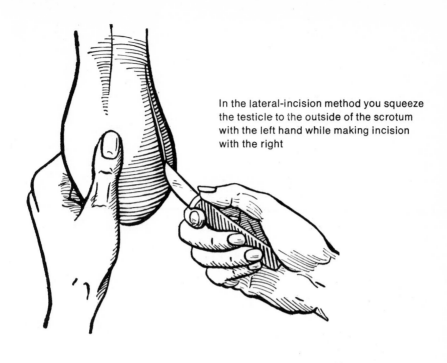

In the lateral-incision method you squeeze
the testicle to the outside of the scrotum
with the left hand while making incision
with the right

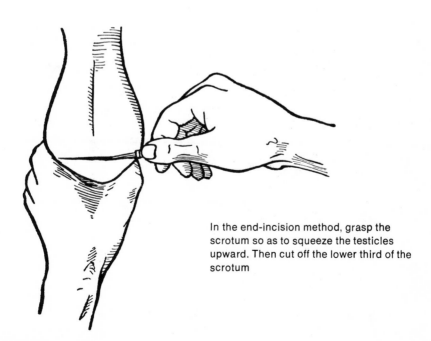

In the end-incision method, grasp the
scrotum so as to squeeze the testicles
upward. Then cut off the lower third of the
scrotum

The instrument used for bloodless castration is called the *emasculatome*. It is a special pincers whose jaws do not quite come together regardless of how much pressure is put on the handles.

To apply the emasculatome, first open the jaws far enough to slip over the edge of the scrotum, an inch-and-a-half or more above one of the testicles. Then crowd the cord of this testicle over to the outer side of the scrotum as far as it will conveniently go. Next, bring the jaws of the instrument together so that the jaws crush the cord, yet cover as little of the scrotum as possible.

By crowding the cord over to the side and pinching only a small section of the scrotum, very little damage is done to blood vessels other than those that serve the testicles. Make sure, however, that the cord is thoroughly crushed, otherwise the operation will not be successful.

The more recent emasculatomes have metal protrusions on one of the jaws, or one protrusion on each jaw, called "cord stops." These make it much easier to apply the instrument in just the right place.

It takes about five seconds effectively to crush a cord. After crushing one cord, apply the instrument to the other. Never try to crush both cords at the same time. Testicles become completely wasted away in a month to six weeks.

With slight variation in method, the emasculatome can be used in castrating many kinds of males other than bulls. However, the method is more difficult with animals having a less pendulous scrotum, such as pigs and dogs.

Elastration

Elastration is a method of castration in which a rubber band is placed around the base of the scrotum and left there. This cuts off the supply of blood to the parts below the band, causing the testicles and affected tissues to shrivel up and fall off. The process takes a few weeks. Specially made rubber bands and a device for attaching them, called an "elastrator," are sold by breeders' supply houses.

The method is "bloodless" but soreness and swelling occur during the first few days that the band is attached. It is claimed that the testicles are made useless as soon as the band is put on. Opinions among stockment differ as to the merits of elastration as compared with other methods of castration.

How to tell the weight of a dairy cow

THE HEAVIER the animal, the bigger should be the dose of a medicine or biological. Instructions that come with such products nearly always tell what size, dose to give farm animals at various weights.

The table below is for livestock owners who do not have scales large enough to weigh cattle. The table is based on work done by H. P. Davis and R. F. Morgan at the University of Nebraska. With few exceptions it has proved to be correct within 7 percent of total weight.

To tell the approximate weight of a dairy cow, draw an ordinary household tape measure snugly around the animal's chest, just back of the shoulders, as shown in the sketch. Then check with the table.

If your cattle are of a breed not included in the table, pick the breed closest to yours and weigh a few members of your herd to find out how the weights of the two breeds compare. Then by perhaps making a small percentage adjustment, you can apply the figures in the table to your own herd.

Chest girth Inches	Live weights in pounds				
	Holstein	Jersey	Guernsey	Ayrshire	Average
21	....	32	....	....	....
22	....	37	....	....	....
23	46	42	38	38	41
24	51	47	43	43	46
25	57	52	48	49	52
26	64	59	54	54	58
27	71	65	61	61	64
28	78	72	67	67	71
29	86	80	74	74	78
30	95	88	82	82	87
31	104	97	90	90	95
32	113	106	99	99	104
33	123	115	108	108	114
34	134	125	118	118	124
35	145	136	129	128	135
36	156	147	140	139	146
37	169	159	151	150	157
38	181	172	163	162	170
39	195	185	176	175	183
40	209	199	190	188	196
41	224	213	204	202	211
42	239	228	219	216	226
43	255	244	234	231	241
44	272	260	250	247	257
45	289	277	267	264	274
46	307	295	285	281	292
47	326	314	304	299	311
48	345	333	323	317	330
49	365	353	343	337	350
50	386	373	364	357	370
51	408	395	385	378	392
52	430	417	407	400	414
53	453	440	431	422	436
54	477	464	455	446	460
55	502	489	480	470	485
56	527	515	506	495	511
57	553	541	532	521	537
58	580	568	560	548	564
59	608	597	589	575	592
60	637	626	618	604	621
61	667	655	648	633	651
62	697	686	680	664	682
63	728	718	712	695	713

Chest girth Inches	Live weights in pounds				
	Holstein	Jersey	Guernsey	Ayrshire	Average
64	761	751	746	727	746
65	794	784	780	760	780
66	828	819	815	794	814
67	863	855	852	830	850
68	899	891	889	866	886
69	935	929	928	903	924
70	973	967	968	941	962
71	1012	1007	1009	981	1002
72	1052	1048	1050	1021	1043
73	1092	1089	1093	1062	1084
74	1134	1132	1137	1104	1127
75	1177	1176	1183	1148	1171
76	1220	1221	1229	1193	1216
77	1265	1267	1277	1239	1262
78	1311	1314	1326	1285	1309
79	1357	1362	1376	1333	1357
80	1405	1412	1427	1383	1407
81	1454	1463	1480	1433	1458
82	1504	1514	1534	1484	1509
83	1555	....	1589	1538	....
84	1607	....	....	1592	....
85	1660	....	....	1647	....
86	1715	....	....	1703	....
87	1760	....	....	....	....
88	1827	....	....	....	....
89	1884	....	....	....	....
90	1942	....	....	....	....
91	2002	....	....	....	....
92	2064	....	....	....	....
93	2127	....	....	....	....
94	2190	....	....	....	....
95	2254	....	....	....	....

Dehorning cattle

CATTLE WITH HORNS often injure one another and sometimes cause deaths. Bruises from horns lower the value of hides and meat. For this reason polled or hornless breeds have become popular, while a percentage of cattle owners continues to dehorn their animals. On the other hand, many owners of valuable purebred animals do not dehorn them because they feel that removal of horns detracts from the appearance of the stock.

The easiest way to keep animals from having horns is to apply caustic potash or a similar substance to the horn buttons when the calves are from four to 10 days old—the earlier the better. Growing horns can also be treated successfully with caustic up to the age of two or three months. But horns of older calves require more caustic and treatment is more troublesome.

Caustic potash is available at drug stores. It comes in the form of a stick about the size of a lead pencil. Operators should wear gloves when handling it, or wrap it in paper, leaving one end of the stick uncovered.

To treat horn buttons, first remove the hair from them with a pair of scissors or clippers. Then apply petroleum jelly to the area surrounding

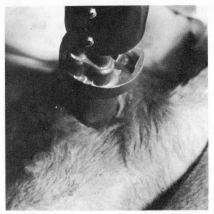
Be sure the dehorner is hot and place it directly over the horn button

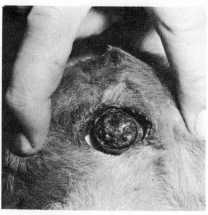
Rotate the dehorner to form a ring around the base of the horn

Michigan State University

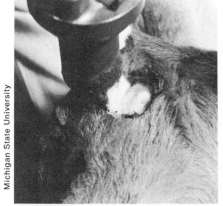
The "Cap" is easily flipped off when properly done

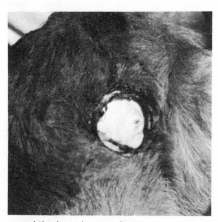
—and the horn is gone forever

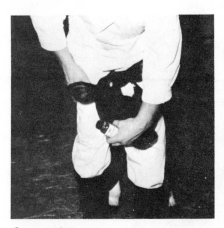

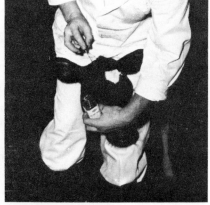

Commercially prepared dehorning liquids or caustic potash can do a neat job of dehorning

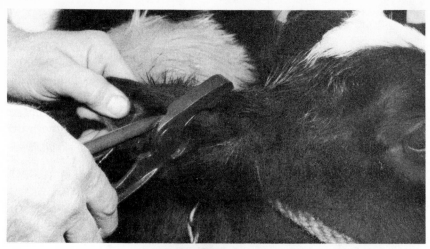

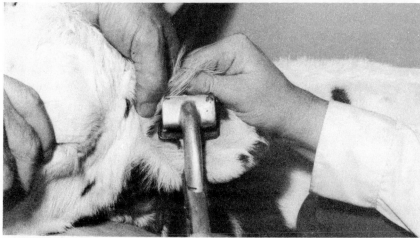

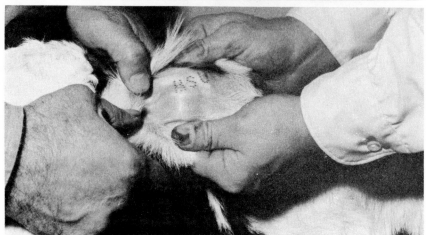

Identify calves temporarily by number. Ear tag or tattoo for permanent identification.
Record the identification with birth date, sex, sire, and dam in the herd record
system. A tattoo is permanent identification

the buttons to prevent the caustic from coming in contact with the skin, causing hide-damaging burns and pain.

To apply the caustic, slightly moisten the end with water and rub each horn button. Cover an area about the size of a nickel. Do not continue rubbing until the spots bleed; merely remove the outer skin from the horn buttons.

When treating growing horn, rub the caustic completely around the base of the horns where they join the skin. Development of the horn stops when this tissue is destroyed. Use only a minimum of water, otherwise the caustic may get into the eyes of animals and cause severe injury.

Calves should also be protected from the rain until the caustic has done its work. A scab usually forms after six or eight hours.

A number of commercial dehorning compounds are on the market. These usually cost a little more to use than caustic potash, but most of them can be employed with greater safety and convenience. They should be used according to manufacturers' instructions.

Dehorning older animals

A number of tools and devices are used to dehorn older calves and mature cattle—hacksaws, powerful cutters with long handles, gouges and specially made chisels. In one effective method, a cone-shaped iron ring is brought to a cherry-red heat and slipped over the horn. The ring, which has a wooden handle on it, is then turned around so as to completely encircle the horn several times. This destroys the blood vessels in the horn and for lack of nourishment, the horn drops off about a month later. A hot soldering iron can be used instead of a ring.

The skin at the base of the horns should be removed with the horns, otherwise the horns will grow again.

Dehorning should be done in the cool weather when flies are not troublesome. Pine tar is usually applied after horns are removed.

Dehorning by elastration

The latest method of dehorning is by means of elastration. You slip a strong rubber ring over the base of the horn, cutting off the blood supply. In three to six weeks the horn drops off. A similar method is used in castration.

Electric dehorners

Another device for preventing the growth of horns is an electric dehorner.

The equipment consists of a 300-watt soldering iron with interchangeable tips, a soldering tip and a special dehorning tip. The dehorning tip has a hollow cone point. Applied over the budding horn button, it sears and cauterizes the tissues, killing the growth cells at the base of the horn. Within a few weeks the scab falls off.

How to tell the age of a cow

MATURE CATTLE have 32 teeth of which eight are incisors. All incisors are on the lower jaw. In place of incisors on the upper jaw, there is a thick layer of hard palate, called the dental pad.

At birth, a calf has two or more of the temporary or first set of incisor teeth. Within a month, all eight have appeared. These temporary teeth are gradually replaced by permanent ones.

At the age of five years, cattle have all permanent incisors. From then on, teeth start to wear down until at the age of 12 years only stumps remain.

The ages at which the various temporary incisors are replaced by permanent ones are shown at the right.

How to tell the age of a cow

Mature cattle have 32 teeth of which eight are incisors. All incisors are on the lower jaw. In place of incisors on the upper jaw, there is a thick layer of hard palate, called the dental pad.

At birth, a calf has two or more of the temporary or first set of incisor teeth. Within a month, all eight have appeared. These temporary teeth are gradually replaced by permanent ones.

At the age of five years, cattle have all permanent incisors. From then on, teeth start to wear down until at the age 12 years only stumps remain.

The ages at which the various temporary incisors are replaced by permanent ones are shown at the right.

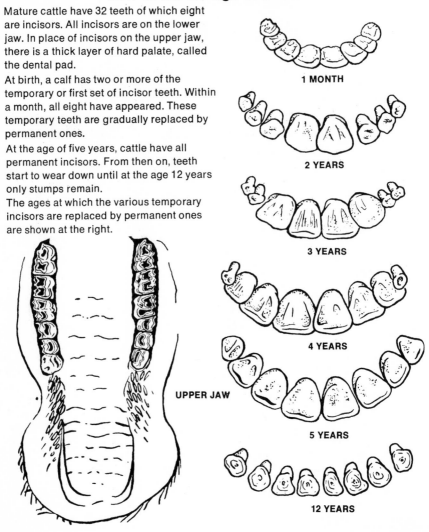

UPPER JAW

1 MONTH

2 YEARS

3 YEARS

4 YEARS

5 YEARS

12 YEARS

Bovine mastitis

BOVINE MASTITIS—inflammation of the udder—is the most costly disease of the dairy industry. It reduces milk production by permanent damage to the udder. It often contaminates milk with bacteria so that it is condemned by public health authorities. It lowers the butterfat content of milk as much as 20 percent and reduces the amount of milk sugar and casein. It makes cows unprofitable for dairy purposes and forces their sale for beef.

Older cows are more susceptible to mastitis than young ones. The disease does not attack heifers before they have freshened unless they have been sucked or have had their udders or teats injured. Before freshening, the teats of heifers are, by nature, well-sealed.

The most common organism present in mastitis is the *Streptococcus agalactiae*. This is like the "strep" that often causes people to have sore throats. The principal other organism present in the disease is a form of *Staphylococcus*, the same kind that often causes pimples. More than 20 other organisms have been identified as causes of the disease.

Symptoms

There are two forms of mastitis, acute and chronic. The acute form is commonly called *garget*. For technical purposes these two forms of the disease are further identified as being "peracute," "subacute," "subclinical," and so on.

In acute mastitis, the infected portion of the udder is reddened, swollen, hot and painful. The milk flow is reduced and varies from a watery, blood-tinged fluid to one that is thick, yellow and ropy.

At times these symptoms may be accompanied by depression of the animal's spirit, rough coat, dull eyes, loss of appetite, suspended rumination and possible constipation. Death may follow if the disease is caused by Staphylococci.

Acute mastitis is usually a flare-up of the chronic form already present in the udder. It may be brought on by exposure to cold or wet weather, sudden changes in temperature, injuries to the udder, feeding heavily for milk production, incomplete, irregular, or infrequent milking, or other health disturbances.

When an animal recovers from an acute attack, the disease usually returns to the chronic form.

An animal becomes infected with mastitis when the bacteria enter the opening of the teat canal, travel up and lodge in the milk cistern. Here they start a mild infection. Then they gradually spread to other parts of the gland until the whole quarter is infected. Acute attacks usually occur during this process, most often at the beginning or end of a lactation period.

The infection changes the tissue that secretes the milk. The quarter loses its soft pliable quality when scar tissue forms. In the advanced stages, the quarter becomes hard throughout and milk secretion may stop entirely.

With some animals the time required for this change may extend through a number of lactation periods. Others become useless in a comparatively short time.

Diagnosis

Early detection of mastitis is important. It is often impossible to apply drugs properly after the whole gland is infected and inflammation has closed the ducts. Diagnosis of the acute form is easy. The symptoms are unmistakable.

The California mastitis test

The California Mastitis Test (CMT) is a step-by-step plan with an unquestionable record of success in the control of mastitis. Although called a "test," actually CMT is a mastitis control program. Roughly, the CMT program may be divided into three parts:

1. Testing the milk to find out whether mastitis is present and, if so, determining its cause.
2. Testing the milking machine and its accessories and making repairs and alterations when necessary.
3. Establishing proper milking practices and routine testing procedures.

Method for testing milk

Heart of the CMT program lies in the milk test. This test is based on the fact that leukocytes (white blood corpuscles) always accumulate at the site of an inflammation and when the inside of an udder is inflamed, large numbers of them are released into the milk. The test reveals the relative number of leukocytes present—in other words, the severity of the inflammation—with surprising accuracy. Though highly sensitive, the test is easy to make.

The equipment used in making the test is simple, inexpensive and readily obtainable from agricultural supply houses. It consists of a white plastic paddle having four shallow cups and a purple reagent.

To make the test you draw less than a teaspoonful of milk from each quarter into a shallow cup, giving you a separate sample from each quarter. The samples are identified by "A", "B", "C", or "D" on the paddle, using a standard routine for identifying the quarters. You then tilt the paddle until it is almost vertical, and the proper amount of milk for the test remains in each of the cups. Then you squirt an amount of reagent from a plastic bottle equal to the amount of milk in each cup.

Within a few seconds you can tell whether the test is negative—no mastitis present—or, if positive, the severity of the inflammation. Upon stirring the mixture, positive reactions vary from a slight precipitate to the formation of a gel. A change in the color of the mixture to a deeper purple indicates that the milk is distinctly alkaline and a change to yellow signifies that it is strongly acid. The deep purple color may be caused either by inflammation or a drying off period of the gland. An acid reaction usually points to the presence of a distinct type of organism.

The problem of milking machines

A large percentage of the mastitis cases stem from improperly functioning milking machines.

Pulsations of milking machines of various makes vary between 45 and 70 per minute. Their vacuum levels vary between 10 and 16 inches of mercury.

When the vacuum is too high, it may draw the teat into the teat cup, the lumen may close and cut off the flow of milk. The vacuum inside of the teat causes it to shrink and more tissue is drawn into the teat cup This is called crawling of the teat cup.

The large-bore rubber liner is one of the principal causes of teat irritation. The purpose of the liner is to massage the teat so as to keep up the circulation of the blood. The pressure of the liner against the teat is in direct proportion to the diameter of the liner and the extent of the vacuum in the internal chamber of the teat cup.

With some liners, the diameter is so large that the rubber strikes the teat with such force that it pinches the teat instead of massaging it. The delicate tissues which line the teat are then rubbed together with each collapse of the liner. Injuries caused in this manner make the inner tissues an easy prey for invading bacteria.

Apparatus for testing milking machines

The greatest aid to detecting defects in the operation of milking machines is the strain gage amplifier. When plugged into a milking machine vacuum system, this amplifier records a wavy or jagged line on a moving strip of paper, showing even the smallest fluctuations in the vacuum. By interpreting the hills, valleys and jogs in this line, an experienced operator can tell with uncanny accuracy how a milking machine is operating by checking the following:

1. The rate and speed of collapse and recovery of the rubber liner against the teat.

2. Too-high or too-low vacuum.

3. If the air inlet to the shell is too small . . . if the pulsator is overloaded with too many machines . . . if the units are too far away . . . or if the pulsator is going too fast. If these happen, the liner will not close with sufficient force to relieve congestion brought about by the constant vacuum. (The purpose of the collapsing liner is to relieve congestion and prevent hard, red teats.)

4. The ratio of open time to closed time (liner recovery and collapse). This ratio influences, more than any other mechanical factor, the speed of milking. Some makes of machines, or defective machinery, have wider ratios on one side of the udder than the other.

5. The condition of the pulsators. When pulsators become worn they leak air, which interferes with teat cup liner collapse and recovery.

6.   Whether the releaser system in the pipeline is defective. A malfunctioning releaser may lead to surging milk in the line, improper milking, and vacuum fluctuations.

7.   The amount of pressure on the teat cup liner. When the number of units on a master pulsator system is varied, this pressure changes.

8.   Whether the vacuum is fluctuating. This may be due to faulty risers, restrictions, inadequate air in the claw, bending of milk tubes, or a host of other abnormalties.

Other tests for mastitis are the Hotis test, and the Whiteside test. These tests are a little more difficult than the strip cup but are much more sensitive. Special kits for testing for mastitis can be bought from agricultural supply houses.

Although these tests detect a larger number of diseased animals than the strip cup, they also should be used often to find every affected cow. The changes in the milk which these tests show are the result of bacteria in the quarter, but they do not tell the kind of bacteria present. This can be determined by making laboratory tests.

Mastitis bacteria remain in the udders of diseased animals at all times. Failure to find them does not of itself mean they are no longer there. Cows that have had mastitis should be checked as such as long as they remain in the herd.

Control and prevention

There is no easy way to keep mastitis out of a herd or to keep it from spreading after it has gained a foothold. Constant care is necessary. To keep the disease at a minimum, the following practices have been found most effective:

If the disease is present in your herd, sell or slaughter all badly infected animals. Divide those that remain into three groups: Place the healthy ones in the first, those suspected of having the disease in the second, and the slightly infected in the third. Those in the last group should be kept only temporarily. As soon as they are unprofitable, they should be sold.

Stable the members of each group together for convenience. Milk cows in the first group first. Then follow with those in the second and third. This is done because mastitis microbes are often spread from one cow to another on the hands of milkers or on the teat cups of milking machines.

Add first-calf heifers to the healthy group unless they show signs of mastitis at the time of calving. When animals freshen, they can be put back in their same group provided they have not contracted the disease. If they have, they should be put in the third group.

Do not bring new animals into the herd unless you know they are healthy. If there is any doubt, quarantine them until you are sure.

Disinfect udders before milking. This can be done by wiping them with a small piece of towel dipped in chlorine solution (Clorox and similar solutions containing chlorine are easy to use). Use a separate towel for each animal. These towels can be washed and used again.

Wash hands in the antiseptic solution and dry thoroughly before milking. Hand-milk all infected cows and never spill or squirt mastitic milk on the floor.

Handle cows so that they will properly let down their milk since attacks of mastitis can be brought on when milk is retained or not properly removed from infected udders. Avoid irritating incidents at milking time. Probably one of the most helpful things in the control of mastitis is to have people handle them who like cows and are liked by cows. The continual playing of a radio during milking helps to reduce the disturbance caused by other noises or changes.

Avoid injuries to teats or udders. A common injury results when a cow mashes her own teats or those of the cow next to her. This can happen where cows are stanchioned in stalls that are too narrow or short, where support posts are located between stalls, or where cement ridges are placed at the end of the stanchion row to keep bedding from spreading into the alleyway.

Promptly treat all injuries to teats and udders.

Provide adequate bedding for protection against cold and mechanical injury. Do not allow manure to collect behind the cows. Use lime or super phosphate on the floors several times weekly.

Milk each cow quickly and completely.

If a stall has been occupied by an infected cow, clean and disinfect it thoroughly before putting a healthy animal in it.

Keep your barn dry and well-ventilated. Let in as much sunshine as possible.

Dip the teat cups of milking machines in water and then in the chlorine solution before milking each cow. In a long-tube machine, leave the valve in the head open so that air can escape and the disinfectant will reach all interior parts of the teat cups.

Never operate more than two milking machine units per man at one time, and don't attempt any other chores while operating a milking machine.

When milk ceases to flow, remove the teat cups, since by that time the vacuum extends to the inside of the teat. Continued milking will injure the sensitive tissue lining the teat and the lower portions of the udder. Then the conditions are right for the invasion of organisms causing mastitis.

Pay particular attention to animals that milk out rapidly or have one quarter that milks out more rapidly or more slowly than others. It is very easy to forget and leave the milking machine on the easy-milking quarters or easy-milking cows when the milk has ceased to flow.

Be careful when cows are in the last stages of lactation and milk production is low. If you fail to remove the milking machine in time, mastitis may follow.

Always have the milking machine in the best operating condition. Hard or cracked inflations cause mastitis. Your milking machine service man can be of great help to you in keeping your milking machine in top operating condition. Many dairymen find it very satisfactory to have two complete sets of rubber inflations for each unit, alternating them week to week.

The milking machine should operate at at least 40 pulsations per minute. Pulsators that are not clean or are in poor condition provide varying rates in pulsation.

Between herd milkings, thoroughly clean all parts of the milking machine, using approved detergents and antiseptics. Hot water at about 180 deg. flushed through the machine is an excellent procedure after all of the milk has been washed out with cold water.

Treatment

Acute attacks of mastitis generally respond to the proper treatment, although the underlying cause will probably remain. Infected quarters should be milked every hour or two until the milk returns to normal. This should be accompanied by massage to work as much of the diseased material as possible into the milk cistern. It can then be removed by gentle stripping. This material should be disinfected and put out of reach of all animals. To decrease milk production, a diet of roughage is recommended.

Treatment of streptococcal mastitis includes the use of penicillin, usually in combination with other antibiotics such as Streptomycin, Aureomycin or Terramycin. Sulfa and other drugs are also used.

Since mastitis may be caused by a number of different organisms, no drug has been found that will cure all cases. To save dairymen the bother of finding out what kind of microbes are present, drug manufacturers making bougies containing several antibiotics, sometimes in combination with other drugs. Mastitis caused by Staphylococcus aureus is perhaps the most difficult to treat.

Milk fever

MILK FEVER is a noncontagious disease of dairy cows which occurs principally shortly after calving, though it may occur shortly before or during calving. It is technically known as hypocalcemia and is brought about by insufficient calcium in the blood.

It usually does not occur until the second calving, and happens most often at the births of the third to the seventh calf. The most susceptible animals are the heavy milk producers in good condition. Milk fever often occurs with painful, difficult or prolonged labor.

The underlying cause of milk fever is not fully understood. Authorities say that the lack of calcium in the blood is brought on by a disturbance of the parathyroid gland which is closely associated with calcium metabolism.

Symptoms

Contrary to its name, fever is not one of the symptoms of the disease.

Early symptoms usually begin between 12 hours and four days after calving. They are of two kinds. The animal may show signs of excitement, get a wild look in its eyes, switch her tail, tremble, weaken and stagger. Or she may become depressed, refuse food and not want to move about.

In either case, the first symptoms are followed shortly by collapse and loss of consciousness. The animal lies with its head turned to one side, the eyes are dull and expressionless, the muzzle dry and the temperature usually below normal.

The most frequent complication of the disease is pneumonia. This is often brought on when the animal inhales portions of its cud while lying down. To avoid this, the animal's body should be braced so that it rests on its brisket. The cud will then drop out of the animal's mouth instead of going down its throat.

An animal that does not get proper treatment for the disease will die within several hours to a few days after the loss of consciousness.

Treatment

Never try to drench a cow that has milk fever. Since she can't swallow, the liquid will go into her lungs and probably cause pneumonia.

Two methods are used to treat milk fever, both of which are remarkably successful when properly applied.

These treatments have the same object in view: to maintain the normal amount of calcium in the blood. This is done either by adding calcium to the blood to make up for the amount lost, or by not permitting so much calcium to be taken from the body in the milk.

By far the best method is to add calcium to the blood. This is done by injecting a 20-percent solution of calcium borogluconate. The usual dose is 250 to 500 cc. injected into a vein or 250 cc. intravenously and 250 cc. under the skin. It is better to distribute the subcutaneous portion by injecting it in several places. Since milk fever is often accompanied by acetonemia, an equal amount of 40-percent-dextrose solution is often given with the solution of calcium borogluconate.

Important: The solutions injected into the veins should be at body temperature and injections should be made slowly. Rapid injection of a solution may cause heart failure.

Care should be taken to introduce the injections into the blood vessels—not into the surrounding tissues—otherwise severe irritation will occur.

The injection of a calcium-gluconate solution returns the animal to consciousness in less than an hour and will have it on its feet in from two to four hours. When treated early, the cow may get up within a few minutes after the injection has been completed. In case of relapse, treatment should be repeated.

The other method of treating milk fever should be used only in case of extreme necessity—where the animal would otherwise die. The treatment is beset with great danger of infecting a cow with mastitis. Always remember that when you invade the udder you are engaged in surgical procedure and are not merely "doing chores."

The method consists in injecting filtered air into the udder. The air is pumped through absorbent cotton to a rubber tube and thence to a milking tube which is inserted in the teat. The cotton filters out the dust and germs.

The tube should be boiled for 10 minutes. The greatest care must be taken not to introduce microbes into the teat canal. Before beginning the inflation, the teats and udder should be washed with soap and water and dried with a sterile towel. The teats and their openings should be disinfected.

In case of emergency, a bicycle pump that has been thoroughly cleaned can be used for injecting the air.

As each udder quarter is fully inflated, its teat is tied with tape or bandaged to keep the air from leaking out. These tapes should be just tight enough to hold the air, and should not be kept on for more than three hours at any time. If the blood supply is cut off longer than this, gangrene may set in and then the ends of the teats will fall off.

The increased air pressure in the udder stops the secretion of milk and consequently the loss of calcium that this milk would contain. There is also reason to believe that the calcium present in the milk-producing glands is forced back into the blood by this pressure.

Prevention

Many things have been tried to prevent milk fever, with varying success. Partial or delayed milking may help some cows but is of little value in high-producing animals. Moreover, the practice helps bring on mastitis.

Giving limewater or a diet rich in calcium to a pregnant cow would seem to be the solution to the milk fever problem. Actually, research shows that it is of no benefit whatsoever.

Injection of calcium solutions right after a cow drops a calf is an effective preventive of the ailment, but is often impractical. You can't tell which cows are susceptible and to treat them all is very costly.

Milk fever can be prevented by adding vitamin D to the diet of a pregnant cow for the five to seven days before she freshens. Administer massive doses as per instructions of manufacturers.

Using four Jersey herds with previous records of milk fever, experiments were conducted which proved the effectiveness of a low-calcium ration in the two weeks before calving to ward off the disease. Of the 37 cows fed the deficient ration, none suffered from milk fever whereas 20 of the 60 cows on regular feed acquired the disease.

In brief, here's how research men hit upon this approach to prevent milk fever:

During the dry period, a cow's body demand for calcium is greatly reduced. As a result, the research men reasoned, the parathyroid gland is not needed for heavy calcium metabolism. It becomes inactive—out of practice, so to speak. Then when the cow freshens, the gland is not in shape to cope with the enormous demands made on it.

Feeding a cow a low-calcium diet while she is dry causes the parathyroid gland to remain active during the dry period to make the most of a bad calcium situation. When the cow freshens, the gland is in good working order and adequate calcium is made available in the blood for the increased demand.

Cattle brucellosis or bang's disease

IF BRUCELLOSIS should become established in your herd of cattle, on an average, here's what will happen:

Your calf crop will be cut 40 percent or more.

Milk production will drop at least 20 percent.

One out of every five cows that lose their calves will never calve profitably again.

ROUTE OF BRUCELLOSIS GERMS IN THEIR ATTACK ON CATTLE

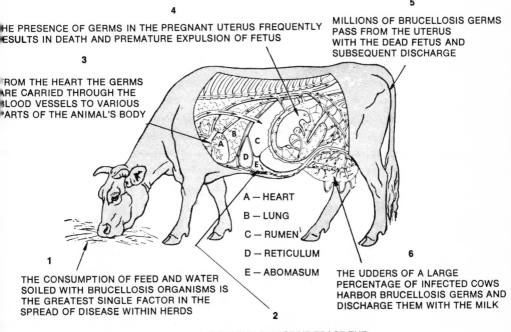

4
THE PRESENCE OF GERMS IN THE PREGNANT UTERUS FREQUENTLY RESULTS IN DEATH AND PREMATURE EXPULSION OF FETUS

5
MILLIONS OF BRUCELLOSIS GERMS PASS FROM THE UTERUS WITH THE DEAD FETUS AND SUBSEQUENT DISCHARGE

3
FROM THE HEART THE GERMS ARE CARRIED THROUGH THE BLOOD VESSELS TO VARIOUS PARTS OF THE ANIMAL'S BODY

A — HEART
B — LUNG
C — RUMEN
D — RETICULUM
E — ABOMASUM

1
THE CONSUMPTION OF FEED AND WATER SOILED WITH BRUCELLOSIS ORGANISMS IS THE GREATEST SINGLE FACTOR IN THE SPREAD OF DISEASE WITHIN HERDS

6
THE UDDERS OF A LARGE PERCENTAGE OF INFECTED COWS HARBOR BRUCELLOSIS GERMS AND DISCHARGE THEM WITH THE MILK

2
FROM THE DIGESTIVE TRACT THE GERMS ENTER THE BLOOD STREAM AND ARE CARRIED TO THE HEART

You and your family may get the disease in which case it is generally known as undulant fever. It is serious and sometimes fatal. You can get it by drinking raw milk from an infected cow or by direct contact with an infected animal whereby the microbes get into your food or drink.

You will not be able to sell your milk unless your herd is free from brucellosis.

Calves and unbred heifers seldom get brucellosis. When the microbe that causes it—*Brucella abortus*—enters the bodies of these animals, it is usually wiped out by the natural defenses in the blood.

Animals are generally infected through the digestive tract. The bacteria penetrate the intestines and enter the blood. Although calves are naturally immune to the disease, because the reproductive organs have not developed sufficiently to provide a normal place for the Brucella to multiply, still they often help spread it by drinking milk of infected cows. The *Brucella* organisms pass through the digestive tracts of the calves and are spread around in their dung. This usually stops within 30 days after the calves are weaned.

Pregnant cows and heifers are responsible for keeping the disease alive. For some strange reason, the bacteria attack the placenta, which is the membrane that covers the fetus, or unborn animal. *Brucella* organisms also invade the lymph glands and now and then the joints.

Many bulls acquire brucellosis, but only a few of them become spreaders of the disease. If the infection lodges in the testicles or other sexual parts, however, the *Brucella* organisms may be discharged with the semen and the bull becomes a dangerous carrier.

The purchase of infected animals is usually responsible for introducing the disease into a healthy herd. Upon abortion, the afterbirth and other discharges are laden with *Brucella* organisms. These may be spread around on feed, in water and on the skin of animals. The organisms will not pass through healthy skin, but cows use their tongues to wash themselves and so swallow the bacteria.

Brucella organisms are killed by all common disinfectants, by pasteurization and by four and one-half hours of direct sunlight. But in cold weather they have been known to live 75 days in an aborted fetus.

Following an abortion, the infection may disappear from the uterus but remain active in the udder for a long time. It is when the ovaries are involved that the animal becomes sterile or a difficult breeder. After aborting, some animals recover completely and thereafter remain immune or greatly resistant to further infection.

A healthy herd that becomes infected will have a run of abortions —called a storm—for perhaps two years and then the disease seems to disappear. Actually it becomes chronic. New animals introduced into the herd acquire it quickly unless precautions are taken.

The disease is unpredictable. Some animals will abort repeatedly, while others may have a normal pregnancy, only to be followed by another abortion.

The incubation period of brucellosis is quite variable. The minimum is about two weeks, but cases have been known where the disease did not appear until six months after infection. The usual incubation period is between 30 and 60 days.

Symptoms of the disease

Abortion is the most prominent sympton of cattle brucellosis, yet some animals do not abort. And abortion alone is not a sure sign that an animal is infected. About 15 percent of the abortions among cattle are due to causes other than brucellosis.

The symptoms of approaching abortion are similar to those of normal calving. But often a sticky, rust-colored, odorless discharge may be noticed a few days before abortion takes place.

There is no known cure for brucellosis, medicinal or otherwise.

Diagnosis of brucellosis

When an animal is infected with brucellosis, one of the antibodies formed in its blood to help fight the disease is called agglutinin. The amount present depends upon the extent and activity of the infection.

When such serum is brought in contact with an antigen composed of *Brucella* organisms, the organisms gather in clumps. They are said to be agglutinated, and this is the basis of the agglutination test for brucellosis. It requires laboratory equipment.

Like most tests of this kind, the agglutination test is not perfect. But its use in freeing thousands of herds of cattle from brucellosis is proof of its value.

The *ring test* is a quick method used to find out whether there are any animals with brucellosis in a herd. It is done most easily at the milk-receiving platform by taking a sample from each can or container, and then testing the composite sample. The test is comparatively simple and highly sensitive.

The antigen used consists of a mass of dead *Brucella* organisms which have been dyed a bright blue. Two drops of the antigen are added to about three-quarters of an inch of milk in a test tube. The mixture is then shaken and allowed to stand, either one hour and a half at room temperature or 30 minutes in a water bath at body temperature.

If there is a single animal in the herd with a positive test (a reactor), the stained antigen will rise to the top and will be concentrated in the cream layer, making a blue ring. If the test is negative, the blue color will remain evenly distributed in the skim. The cream will remain white.

With slight modification, cream may be tested instead of milk. The test will not work with milk that has been frozen.

With the ring test, a technician can make 50 to 100 herd tests a day as against four to eight with the blood test. When an infected herd is found, the blood is used to find individual reactors. There are several reasons why the ring test can't be used to find the individual reactors. Colostrum, the first milk secreted at the end of pregnancy, tends to give false positives. The milk of certain cows does not have good cream-rising qualities. Such milk will give a false negative when tested alone, but will react properly in a composite test. Only herds of dairy cows can be tested with the ring test; beef cows are missed.

Vaccination

Vaccination of heifers from six to eight months old is standard practice in well-managed herds where there is danger of infection. The vaccine used is a non-virulent type called Strain 19.

One complicating feature of vaccination against brucellosis is that about two weeks after injection of the vaccine, the blood reacts just as though the animal had gotten the disease from natural causes. This reaction persists for a variable period of time, but in animals vaccinated at the proper ages usually has disappeared by the time the animal is two years old, at which time the heifer would be bred. Immunity produced by vaccination of calves does not decrease as the animals become older, but is relatively stable throughout their lives.

Research and field evidence has shown that animals vaccinated at 6 to 8 months develop an immunity equal to that produced in cattle vaccinated at older ages. Vaccination of older animals produces a persistent reaction which cannot be distinguished from reactions caused by actual infections.

Vaccination of adult animals is only rarely, if ever, advisable. It has been demonstrated that any increased immunity produced by re-vaccination of adults is only temporary and of little value.

Bovine virus diarrhea

DUE TO VARIATION in symptoms occurring in different parts of the country, virus diarrhea was at one time believed to be caused by four different viruses, and was known as mucosal disease complex. Now it is known that only one type of virus is involved.

Bovine virus diarrhea (BVD) is primarily a disease of yearlings and up to 3-year-olds. It rarely occurs among adult cattle, presumably because most of them have already had it and are therefore immune. It is not known how the disease is spread, but when it starts, it spreads rapidly through a herd. Death losses are low on an average but in severe cases are high, especially among older calves and cows.

Symptoms

First symptoms are a rise in temperature to 104 to 106 degrees for two or three days, and then a drop to nearly normal. There is depression, lack of appetite, nasal discharge, and watery diarrhea. Later the diarrhea may become severe and frequently mixed with mucus and blood. Affected animals are markedly emaciated and dehydrated, with a rough, dry hair coat. Often there is drooling, a watery discharge from the eyes and clouding of the eye surfaces.

Ulcers often appear on nostrils, muzzle, lips, gums and in the mouth. Sometimes a foul-smelling discharge hangs from the nostrils and muzzle. In some affected herds there have been foot sores and severe lameness. These sores appear above the coronary band and there is a skin eruption between the dewclaws and heels.

Pregnant animals may abort when affected by the disease.

Dehydration is severe, with weight losses of as much as 1/2 to 1/5 total body weight. The coat of affected animals is dry and rough. Eyes may be inflammed.

The course of the disease may be light, lasting only about two to seven days, followed by recovery. Or it may become chronic, growing progressively more serious in its effects. Chronic cases are frequently fatal.

At the outset of the disease, digestive processes come to a halt, sometimes accompanied by mild bloat. Heart and breathing rates generally increase. It is usually difficult to grasp and pull the tongue from the mouth due to the greasy dead cells on its surface. The disease lasts up to three weeks in severe cases. Animals with the acute form of the disease may die within 48 hours.

If diarrhea is profuse, the animal should be salvaged at once. If an animal becomes dehydrated and emaciated, it has no sales value.

In addition to its observable symptoms, BVD is definitely associated with certain reproductive problems.

Control

A modified live-virus vaccine has been developed which provides immunity against the disease. When used, calves should be vaccinated at the age of six months. Such a vaccination program, however, may have a drawback. To quote from The Merck Veterinary Manual:

"The economic justification for vaccination is not well defined. The incidence of the fatal disease is so low in most herds, and the naturally protective antibody is so prevalent in most cattle populations, that the widespread vaccination does not seem warranted. Routine use has also been discouraged by reports that the vaccine can precipitate the clinical disease in certain circumstances.

On the other hand, many successful dairymen have their calves routinely vaccinated against BVD.

Bovine leptospirosis

LEPTOSPIROSIS is an infectious disease that attacks cattle, hogs, sheep, horses and even man. The kind that affects cattle, hogs and man is caused an organism called *Leptospira pomona*.

The disease is spread principally through the urine, where the organism is present in carrier animals. Contaminated bedding and tiny droplets of urine in the air, produced when animals urinate on a floor, no doubt contribute to the spread of the disease.

Symptoms

Leptospirosis may be severe, mild or even inapparent. In all three forms, pregnant animals may abort. In severe attacks, onset is sudden. There are fever, loss of appetite and a marked drop in milk flow.

Milk that is produced is thick and yellowish. This may at first be mistaken for a sign of mastitis. However, in leptospirosis the udder is not inflamed as in mastitis. The udder is limp and relatively empty.

In very severe cases the cow is jaundiced, the milk is pink and the urine the color of port wine. These symptoms usually do not appear until two or three days after the first signs of sickness. Abortion may occur at the height of the sickness but usually happens between 10 and 16 days thereafter.

Among affected animals about 5 percent of the older ones and 25 percent of the young ones die. Death occurs within the first two or three days after symptoms appear. In such cases the course may be so rapid that jaundice and discolored milk and urine do not appear, though other symptoms mentioned above are present. In addition there may be labored breathing, severe depression and shock. Fever reaches 104 to 107 degrees F.

In some outbreaks one-third to one-half the herd may be involved. The disease is more evident in mature cattle than in young ones. In many cases only one or two animals in a herd show symptoms. The disease occurs most often in warm weather. In the North it has seldom been observed earlier in the spring than April or later in the fall than November. It often shows greatest severity when cattle are on pasture and drinking from a slow-flowing stream.

A reliable, inexpensive blood test for the disease is used.

Treatment

Treatment of severe cases of leptospirosis is often unsuccessful because the course of the disease is extremely short. Blood transfusion is beneficial where anemia is pronounced.

Treatment with the antibiotics aureomycin, dihydrostreptomycin and terramycin may be of value but will probably not alter the course of the disease, especially in calves.

Prevention and control

Annual vaccination against the disease is necessary. The following control measures are recommended:

1. Isolate animals that show signs of leptospirosis.

2. Burn or bury bedding used for infected animals.

3. Avoid soiling hands and clothing when handling contaminated refuse or infected animals.

4. Bury aborted fetuses deep enough that they will not be dug up.

5. Do not feed milk from infected cattle to calves, swine or poultry, and don't use it in the house.

6. Keep infected animals out of streams and ponds and don't let them graze on marsh or bog pastures.

7. Do not pasture or house cattle, swine, sheep and horses together.

8. Do not buy replacements for at least 5 months after the last recognized case has been observed in the herd. Carrier animals, which appear normal may spread the disease to the susceptible new animals.

9. Consult your local veterinarian as soon as you suspect leptospirosis in your livestock. A diagnosis can be made quickly and treatment can start at once.

Vesicular stomatitis

VESICULAR STOMATITIS is a disease that affects cattle, horses and hogs. It closely resembles foot-and-mouth disease and vesicular exanthema.

The disease is caused by two different types of virus, called the New Jersey and Indiana types. The New Jersey type occurs more often in the United States and causes a more severe illness than the Indiana type. The exact mode of transmission has not been definitely established but seems to be through abrasions—slight cuts or scratches—of the mouth parts. Evidently biting insects often transmit the disease.

Vesicular stomatitis occurs principally during the late summer and early fall. Sometimes it spreads rapidly, affecting thousands of animals within a few weeks. It occurs most often among pastured animals.

The disease starts with an excessive amount of saliva and evident soreness and pain when the animal opens its mouth. Vesicles (blisters) that vary in size from that of a pea to as large as a hand appear on the tongue and other mouth parts, sometimes extending to the muzzle and nostrils. Often the teats and feet are affected in the same manner. Lameness occurs in both cattle and hogs. The vesicles break early in the course of the disease, leaving open sores.

Affected animals refuse to eat, or even drink in some instances. Calves under one year of age seldom contract the malady. There may be a rise in temperature with the appearance of the vesicles. In dairy herds the loss in milk production may be serious. Ordinarily there are no complications and animals recover completely. Return to normal flesh takes about a month from date of first symptoms. Immunity lasts less than one year.

There is no effective treatment known for the disease. Affected animals should be quarantined in an attempt to halt the spread of the disease. Positive diagnosis can be made with blood tests. Man is susceptible to the disease.

Bovine genital vibriosis

BOVINE VIBRIOSIS, also known as vibrionic abortion, is a venereal disease that causes infertility by destroying embryos. This usually occurs early in pregnancy in which case it is not noticeable. In a small percentage of cases abortion takes place after several months of pregnancy.

Symptoms

There is no fever or any other visible sign of illness. When the infection strikes a herd, it spreads rather quickly. Unless controlled, the disease will attack all females of breeding age.

Following the period of rapid spread, abortions are less frequent but the disease tends to persist among the one-to-three-year-olds. Affected heifers often require three or more services to settle. There are probably also undetected abortions.

Some animals are definitely non-breeders following an attack of the disease. Among older ones, the disease lasts only about three months.

Presence of the disease can be detected by means of a blood agglutination test although the test is not completely reliable. A vaginal mucus agglutination test is much better but, of course, can be used only with cows.

Bulls are often found infected with the disease and are believed to be the principal carriers. However, it has been demonstrated that the disease can be transmitted from one female to another. Other than this, not much is known on how animals become infected. Bulls show no signs of having the disease other than a positive reaction to the blood agglutination test.

Treatment

A heifer that fails to conceive on two or three services should be examined through the rectum for abnormalities. If none are present, a vaginal mucus agglutination test should be made.

Treatment with streptomycin is safe and effective at any stage of the heat cycle. Aureomycin and terramycin have also been used with good results. Treatment of heifers or cows, that have early abortions, with streptomycin in the uterus may permit quicker return to normal reproduction efficiency.

If the disease is found in a herd, all animals in it should be handled as if they were infected.

Where it is believed that the disease might be present, blood-test cows and bulls for additions to herds at time of purchase, and again one month later. Keep new animals separate during this period.

Keep cows apart from the herd at calving time so that the premises will not become contaminated with the microbes. Clean stall and disinfect thoroughly before using for another animal.

In infected or even in non-infected herds, breed artificially using semen containing streptomycin. Treated semen should stand three to four hours before use.

A rest period of two or three months will often bring about recovery of breeding efficiency.

Bovine trichomoniasis

BOVINE TRICHOMONIASIS is a venereal disease of cattle. It is transmitted during service and is usually introduced into a herd by a new bull or an infected cow. There is no evidence that animals can get the disease other than through sexual activities.

The disease is caused by a microscopic animal called *Trichomonas fetus*. It lives in the uterus of a cow and within the sheath of a bull's penis.

As a result of the disease, a cow may fail to conceive, conception may be followed by abortion, the fetus may die and remain in the uterus, or normal pregnancy and birth may occur despite the infection. When the fetus remains in the uterus it becomes macerated and the uterus becomes filled with a grayish-white, almost odorless fluid.

Animals that become infected but fail to get in calf may develop a vaginal discharge. This discharge may be continuous or intermittent, occurring chiefly during periods of heat, which may become irregular. There is no fever.

Abortion may occur at any time but usually takes place between the seventh and 16th weeks of pregnancy. There are no signs of heat during this period. Abortion may occur unnoticed, especially at night. A few days after abortion the animal usually comes in heat and this is often the first indication of the infection.

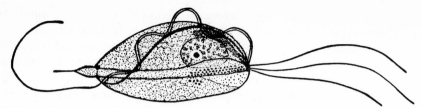

This awesome microbe causes trichomoniasis, the venereal disease of cattle. It is a tiny animal that can be seen only with the aid of a microscope

When the fetus is not expelled, the animal generally behaves like one normally in calf. Examination at the end of the gestation period shows the uterus to be filled with a whitish fluid.

Inflammation of the prepuce (foreskin) and pus are usually found in recently infected bulls. The penis is inflamed and may have many small nodules or elevations on it. In bulls the infection is usually chronic. It causes no noticeable discomfort.

The disease often follows the introduction of a new bull or cow into a herd. Laboratory diagnosis of trichomoniasis consists in microscopic examination of the discharge from the vagina or sheath. Unless large numbers of the microbes are present it is often difficult to find them.

Cows that abort early in the gestation period usually recover of their own accord. Such animals should be given a sexual rest period of about three months.

In cases in which the fetus dies and the uterus becomes filled with fluid, the cervix sometimes remains closed at the end of the gestation period. Veterinarians then open the uterus, remove its contents and douche the animal. Cows that fail to conceive after repeated services should be given additional sexual rest.

Treatment

No ordinary antiseptics for either cow or bull have proved reliable enough to prevent or eliminate infection. The treatment of bulls having the disease, with methods now in use, is not always effective. It may seem to be successful in the light of laboratory examinations but prove otherwise when the bull is bred to heifers. In case of a valuable bull, the treatment should nevertheless be tried.

Treatment consists in the application of bovaflavin ointment or other ointment containing 1 percent acriflavine in petrolatum (Vaseline). The ointment should be applied to the penis and to the inner surface of the prepuce under local anesthesia. Treatment should be continued at weekly intervals with frequent examinations to ascertain its effectiveness.

Prevention

To prevent occurrence of the disease, the following precautions are recommended by the United States Department of Agriculture:

No mature animal should be bought as a permanent addition to the herd without a thorough investigation of its breeding record and of the herd from which it comes.

No outside animals should be brought onto the premises for breeding purposes without the knowledge of their breeding history and that of the herds from which they come.

Cows should not be bred outside of the herd and away from the premises without taking similar precautions.

If breeding troubles and difficulties occur in the herd, a veterinarian should be consulted. If after examination and consultation it is determined that the trouble is due to trichomoniasis, breeding operations should be stopped for a time and available records should be studied in order to determine which animals are infected and which may reasonably be suspected of being infected.

The use of bulls known to be or suspected of being infected should be restricted to cows that have undergone an attack of the disease or have previously been exposed to infection.

A new bull should be provided for heifers coming to breeding age and for the cows that have not been exposed.

The use of artificial breeding is recommended, in case of infected herds, to prevent further spread of the infection.

The disease is rare in North America. Treatment of a bull is costly. In view of this, authorities generally recommend that an infected bull be slaughtered.

Leaky teats

CHRONIC LEAKING of a teat is in most cases due to weakness of the muscles that ordinarily hold the milk in the udder. It may also be the result of an operation performed to relieve a stricture or other obstruction.

Sometimes simple remedies are sufficient to overcome the defect. Among them are injecting Lugol's solution at several places around the teat opening, or rubbing the end of the teat with a small amount of glycerate of tannic acid after each milking. Often, however, only an operation will bring permanent relief. This consists in removing a V-shaped piece of the muscle that controls the size of the opening and sewing the parts together—a job for the experienced surgeon.

A teat fistula is a hole in the side of a teat, usually caused by barbed wire or other injury. The only remedy is to sew the hole shut. Except in emergency this should be done only during the dry period.

Bloody milk

THE COLOSTRUM and milk of a cow may be bloody for a short time after freshening. Bloody milk may also be caused by mastitis, injury to a teat or udder, or by leptospirosis.

The red corpuscles in bloody milk may be normal, damaged, or in the form of clots. If milk containing normal blood corpuscles is allowed to stand, the corpuscles will settle to the bottom of the container along with any blood clots, leaving the milk white. If the blood cells have been damaged so that the red substance, or hemoglobin, leaks out, this settling does not occur and the milk will be pink.

The bloody milk at calving time which occurs most often among first-calf heifers is usually caused by rupture of greatly distended small blood vessels. The corpuscles are not damaged and the condition will generally clear up of its own accord within a few days.

Bloody milk caused by mechanical injuries will also usually disappear in a short time. It may be necessary to use a milk tube in some teat injuries if blood continues to appear at milking time. Bloody milk which appears at calving time or is due to mechanical injury can often be relieved by applying ice packs to the udder and by not giving the cow an excessively rich diet. Gangrenous mastitis causes a dark red discharge that contains damaged red corpuscles.

Bloody milk caused by mastitis or leptospirosis calls for special treatment. Redness of milk that does not appear until several hours after milking is probably due to contamination of milk by one of the color-producing species of bacteria. Proper sanitation will stop it.

Calf scours, or infectious diarrhea

CALF SCOURS, also called white scours, or infectious diarrhea, attacks calves within the first ten days of their lives. Symptoms of the disease are often followed by death in 24 to 36 hours.

Many organisms, either alone or in combination, are believed to cause the disease. Once it begins in a barn, calf scours will attack nearly every newborn calf in the building unless rigid sanitation is practiced. Range cattle are seldom affected by it.

Calf scours should not be confused with ordinary diarrhea, caused by improper feeding.

Symptoms

The disease starts with a yellowish-white, greenish or light brown, very foul-smelling diarrhea. At the same time the calf becomes dull and weak. Its eyes become sunken, breathing becomes hurried and its temperature goes below normal. Before death, the animal lies on its side with its head on the ground. Occasionally, a chronic form of the disease develops. The calf becomes thin and potbellied and dies within a few weeks. When the symptoms of scours appear, call your veterinarian. Stop feeding infected animals and start giving them an electrolyte solution of three or four one-quart doses a day.

Prevention

The first food of a calf should be colostral milk. It is richer than the milk that comes later and also contains antibodies and substances that increase a calf's resistance against disease.

The greatest sanitation should be observed when a calf is born and for the first few days of its life. A large box stall, so constructed that it can be easily cleaned, should be provided for the cow when the calf is to be born. As soon as possible after birth, the calf's navel chord should be disinfected with tincture of iodine and ligated to prevent infection from entering through it.

Make sure that the calf gets three to four feedings of colostrum within the first 24 hours after birth, some within one half hour of birth. The antibodies in colostrum are not absorbed into the blood stream of the calf to any appreciable extent after 24-30 hours from birth. Colostrum is also high in vitamin A and contains about six times as much protein, three times as much mineral matter, and twice the dry matter concentration of normal milk. Small feeds of two to three pints per feeding are sufficient for the first 2 days.

Cows that have been milked for several days before calving will not produce colostrum at calving. Their calves must be provided colostrum from another source.

Limit milk to about 0.8 percent of body weight per calf daily. Eight pounds is the maximum amount of milk necessary to feed to any calf in an early weaning system for heifer replacements. The quantity of milk can be reduced to 4 pounds per day after 21 days of age and discontinued by 30 days of age.

Milk replacer may be substituted for whole milk as soon as the dam's milk is marketable. The milk replacer must be composed of high quality dry milk solids. Replacers containing ten percent or more animal fat are desirable. Replacers must also contain all necessary vitamins and minerals. Feed the milk replacer according to the manufacturer's directions. Dried skimmed milk and dried whole whey provide easily digestible high quality proteins and should constitute the protein in milk replacers. Sucrose (cane or beet sugar), vegetable protein, starch and cereal flour are unsatisfactory ingredients in milk replacers for newborn calves.

As set forth in bulletins on calve raising, calves fed milk or milk replacer once per day after the colostrum feeding period (2-3 days) grow as rapidly and are as healthy as those fed twice daily, the daily allowance being the same. Feeding once a day reduces the labor cost about 40 percent.

Milk replacers mixed at regular concentrations as recommended by the manufacturer have also been used successfully in once-a-day feeding. Keep fresh calf starter, hay and water before calves at all times. Be sure to check calves at least twice daily to see that starter, hay and water are fresh and clean and to help spot calves showing signs of illness.

Calf diphtheria

CALF DIPHTHERIA is a highly fatal infectious disease that principally affects suckling calves. In severe outbreaks, mature animals may be affected. The malady is also known by other names, including necrotic stomatitis, gangrenous stomatitis, ulcerative stomatitis, necrotic laryngitis and sore mouth.

The bacterium *Sphaerophorus necrophorus* is believed to be the principal cause of the disease but other organisms or factors may be involved.

Symptoms

First symptoms of the disease include refusal of feed and drooling of saliva. Later a grayish or yellowish deposit forms on the base or sides of the tongue, on the inside of the cheeks or on the lips. This diphtheritic membrane may spread to the hard palate, the gums near the back teeth, the vocal cords, the nasal passages, the windpipe and the lungs.

The toxins of the disease destroy the tissue, causing ulcers that are slightly raised, reddened and granular in appearance. The discharge from these ulcers combines with dead cells from the mouth and throat parts and forms a covering that gradually becomes dry, crumbly and cheesy in appearance. This sticks firmly to the surface and can be scraped off only with difficulty. In cases that drag along for some time, infected areas may be found in the stomach, intestines and liver.

Animals sick with calf diphtheria become depressed and even young suckling calves will often refuse feed, though swallowing movements may be observed. Animals lose weight and have a moist painful cough. Breathing is labored. Temperature usually reaches 105 degrees F.

In severe attacks of the disease, animals may die within a week after symptoms first appear. The toxins made by the microbes are absorbed into the blood stream. Death is thus caused by blood poisoning. In less severe attacks, animals may live for several weeks and then die. Mild cases may recover, especially if treated promptly.

Treatment

Where the disease has advanced to the extent of damaging the soft palate and windpipe, chances of recovery are not good.

Some of the sulfa drugs have been found effective against the disease if given in time. They are sulfamerazine, sulfamethazine and sulfa-pyridine. Penicillin either alone or in combination with sulfa drugs has also been found beneficial. As in all cases, drugs should be given in accordance with recommendations of their manufacturers.

Prevention

Prevention consists in separating sick from healthy animals at the first signs of the disease. This should be followed by cleaning and disinfecting contaminated stables and sheds. It is advisable to observe the apparently healthy group every day so as to detect any new cases promptly. Calves should not be fed coarse roughage or other things that might prick the mouth.

Calf pneumonia

PNEUMONIA is inflammation of the lungs. As in all such ailments, blood rushes to the inflamed parts. Some of the fluid portion of the blood breaks through the delicate walls of the lungs and fills the tiny air sacs. Parts of the lungs become solid and airless. In the end, the lungs become so filled with phlegm that the body blood can no longer give up carbon dioxide or take on oxygen. Temperatures range from 104 to 106 deg. F.

Calf pneumonia is caused by a virus and often stems from cold winds and rain, and from cold, damp quarters. Animals will get the disease when exposed to direct drafts when indoors. Overcrowding calves in winter until the air is foul and then releasing them outside is also said to bring on the trouble. On rare occasions the disease will break out under conditions that seem ideal.

The disease generally strikes calves between one and four months old. Resistance increases thereafter and after the age of six months a calf is seldom troubled with it. Mature cows, however, may act as carriers.

There are, of course, other kinds of pneumonia that attack young and old animals alike. It is often a secondary infection following some other illness. Inexperienced people sometimes drench an animal in such a manner that the medicine enters the lungs instead of the stomach and this brings it on.

Symptoms

The symptoms of calf pneumonia are dullness, lack of appetite, high fever, rapid breathing, roughened coat, and coughing. If coughing does not occur of its own accord, it can be brought on by pinching the upper part of the windpipe.

The animal distends its nostrils and may stand with forefeet apart, or rest on its brisket when lying down. It does these things to ease difficult breathing.

By listening closely, breathing sounds can be heard in the chest— a slight wheeze, gurgle or splash. There may be a discharge from the nostrils that varies from a small amount of clear fluid to a large quantity of sticky, pale-yellow material.

Death may follow in a few days after symptoms of calf pneumonia appear or the disease may last a few weeks. In the latter case, the animal usually dies. Calves that recover are often stunted in growth.

Treatment

Sick animals should at once be placed in dry quarters that are preferably warm. There should be fresh air but no drafts. Palatable foods in small amounts should be given often. Blankets should be provided where necessary.

If animals have been overcrowded, they should be broken up into smaller groups and given plenty of room. Separation by ages is desirable. After animals have been sick, they should not be allowed to mingle with the others until the youngsters are beyond the susceptible age.

Since various bacteria often become involved during an attack of the disease, no single drug is effective in all cases. Penicillin in full dosage is effective in many cases, Streptomycin in others. A wide spectrum can be obtained with a combination of these two or by combination of other antibiotics recommended by your veterinarian. Treatment with antibiotics should be continued for four days, or until the animal has been without fever for 24 hours. For good results, treatment should begin early, before the lungs are heavily involved.

Ketosis, or acetonemia

KETOSIS, also called acetonemia or hypoglycemia, is a malady that affects dairy cows almost exclusively. It appears within several days to a few weeks after calving and is not infectious. It occurs most often among high-producing cows in late winter and early spring. It often develops when a fat cow loses weight rapidly just after calving.

Most authorities think that the basic cause of ketosis is a glandular deficiency. The harmones that govern carbohydrate and fat metabolism are not produced in the body in large enough quantities. This lowers the sugar content of the blood. It also increases the number of so-called ketone bodies which would ordinarily not be produced in metabolism. These bodies appear in an affected cow's urine and milk.

Symptoms

Ketosis appears in at least three different forms. The most common symptoms are those of indigestion, as though the animal had swallowed a piece of metal or other indigestible object. The cow is constipated, listless and gradually loses her appetite.

In another form, the symptoms resemble those of milk fever. The animal has the symptoms of indigestion plus trembling and weakness. It finally collapses. In the third form, the animal is highly nervous. It may bellow, race around, and attack people.

In all three forms, there is a pronounced or complete reduction in milk flow, and the milk is off flavor. The animal loses condition rapidly. A fat cow may become thin within a few weeks after symptoms appear. Another characteristic of the disease is a sweetish, fetid odor of the breath—the smell of acetone.

Diagnosis

Ketone bodies can be detected in the urine by means of Rother's test or the "Acitest." But these tests have a serious fault: if no ketone bodies are present, certainly the animal does not have ketosis; but if they are present, the animal may or may not have the ailment. Pneumonia, metritis, mastitis and other diseases also give rise to the bodies.

A test without this fault consists in the use of a urine test in which a drop of urine is placed on an "Acitest" tablet. A color scale indicates the amount of ketones.

Treatment

Effective treatments for ketosis lie in the use of cortisone, hyprocortisone, prednisone, prednisolone or corticotropin (ACTH).

Within 8 to 10 hours after the injection of any one of these drugs (in accordance with instructions given by their manufacturers), blood sugar usually returns to normal. A marked improvement in appetite and general symptoms usually occurs within 24 hours. Milk production increases rapidly by the second or third day following treatment.

The older treatment for acetonemia consists in injecting glucose into the jugular vein, although it may also be given subcutaneously. The dose is one pint to one quart (500 to 1,000 cc.) of a 40-percent glucose solution, given daily. Treated animals usually recover completely in one to five days. The treatment is successful in about 60 percent of the cases.

A simple, inexpensive and fairly effective treatment for ketosis consists in feeding affected cows sodium propionate.

The substance is sold at drug stores. It has a bad taste but most cows will eat the drug if it is mixed in well with grain. If they do not eat it readily, try smaller amounts (an ounce) for the first few days. Then increase amount to $1/4$ pound daily (two ounces per feeding).

In mild cases a $1/4$-pound-daily dose seems sufficient. In more severe ketosis, $1/2$ pound daily in two doses is more effective. When the larger amount is given and when the cow is not eating grain, it is necessry to give it by capsule or drench. The material is soluble in warm water. It is not known how large a dosage can be given without harm.

Ten days of treatment are sufficient for most cows. Some cows, particularly the extremely fat ones, require a longer period.

Calcium gluconate is usually injected when it is difficult to determine quickly whether the condition is milk fever, or ketosis, or is ketosis complicated by milk fever.

Prevention

Animals susceptible to ketosis should be kept on a high-energy diet during the last few weeks of pregnancy. But they should not be excessively fat when they are getting ready to freshen.

In the two weeks following calving, high-energy rations should be further increased but roughage such as long hay or straw should be available. The addition of sodium propionate or propylene glycol to the ration is highly recommended. Abrupt changes in rations should be avoided during the ketosis-prone period.

Indigestion, or gastric impaction

IN COMMON INDIGESTION, the first two compartments of a cow's stomach are packed with food that won't digest. In rare cases, the third and even the fourth compartments are also overfilled.

Causes

The ailment can nearly always be traced to improper feeding. The affected animal has eaten an unlimited amount of indigestible, overripe or moldy feed, or has gorged on feed to which it is not accustomed. This often happens when an animal breaks loose from a pasture or stable and eats without restriction such things as apples, corn fodder, heated silage, green grain, corn meal or ground feed.

When a change of feed is responsible, it is usually because it was too abrupt—such as grain allowance has been increased, clover or alfalfa have replaced marsh hay, increased rations are given at calving time, or a change is made from a dry stable ration to lush pasture feed. An increase in choice feeds to speed up milk production often brings on the ailment.

Symptoms

A cow with indigestion goes off feed, stops chewing her cud, her milk production falls off and she shows evidence of constipation with few bowel movements. There are often moaning, kicking at the belly, arched back and grinding of teeth. Animals sometimes become paralyzed and go down in a stupor as happens with milk fever. Abortions may occur.

Treatment

If bloat accompanies the indigestion, the bloat should be treated first. Animals often recover suddenly without treatment. If not, the administration of five to ten gallons of warm water through a stomach tube, followed by vigorous kneading of the ruman will usually activate digestion.

Recommended laxative is magnesium hydroxide (Epsom salts), for mature cattle 1 to 1½ lbs. dissolved in a few quarts of warm water and given by means of stomach tube; or mineral oil, two to three quarts, also given by means of stomach tube. The stimulant and laxative are usually given at the same time.

Intravenous injection of calcium gluconate is also beneficial. This should be a 20 percent solution and 250 to 500cc. should be injected slowly.

After treatment, cattle should not be put back on feed until the rumen again becomes active.

In very severe cases it may be necessary to operate and remove the undigested feed from the paunch.

Bloat

BLOAT, also called tympanites, often causes heavy losses of cattle. It occurs when the rumen, and reticulum (first and second stomach), become swollen with the gases of fermenting feed. Sometimes it comes on suddenly without warning; in other cases it appears regularly after each feeding.

Usually bloat is brought on when cattle or sheep are first turned onto young, lush grass or clover; particularly when it is wet with dew. The animals eat greedily and overload their paunches. Turnips, potatoes, apples, pulp from sugar beet factories and other easily fermented feeds also cause the ailment.

The reason gas accumulates in the rumen is because it cannot be released in the usual way, that is, by belching. Instead of rising to the top of the rumen, the gas remains mixed with the feeds to form a foam or froth, also called frothy bloat.

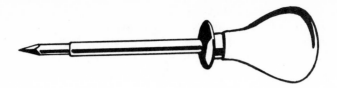

The trocar is used to relieve cattle bloat. This one is shown encased in its cannula. This is the part that remains in the cow's loin to allow gas to escape after the trocar is withdrawn

There are a number of theories as to the basic cause of bloat. Among them are: (1) Tickle theory—Roughage is necessary in the diet because it tickles the lining of the paunch and makes a cow belch. (2) Toxic theory—Young plants form gases in the paunch that paralyze the nerves which control belching. (3) Feed density theory—Lush legumes make heavy boluses that sink to the floor of the cow's paunch instead of floating. This raises the fluid level above the outlet where gas is ordinarily released. (4) Failure in the animal's digestive mechanism.

Symptoms

The most characteristic symptom of bloat is the swelling of the left flank. In severe cases, the upper part of the flank rises above the level of the backbone. When this surface is struck with the tips of the fingers, a drumlike sound can be heard.

An animal with bloat move uneasily. It breathes with difficulty. Sometimes it has a rupture of the stomach. Death may come within a few hours after the first symptoms appear unless relief is obtained.

Treatment

Treatment consists in releasing the gas at once. First, pass a stomach tube through a speculum into the stomach, reaching the gas pockets. If much froth is present, this will be disappointing. Next, pass about a pint of a defoaming agent, such as vegetable oil, corn oil, peanut oil, soybean oil, or household detergents through the tube into the stomach. If it won't go down, inject it into the paunch with a syringe having a large extra-long needle. Work fast.

Where absolutely necessary to save an animal's life, you can release the gas by puncturing the paunch with a knife, or a trocar—a sharp-pointed instrument encased in a sheath called a *cannula*. This procedure is called "tapping." The insertion is made at a point equally distant from the last rib, the point of the hip and the edge of the loin. It a trocar is used, the skin at this point is first cut with a knife. To penetrate the rumen, the knife or trocar is directed downward and slightly forward.

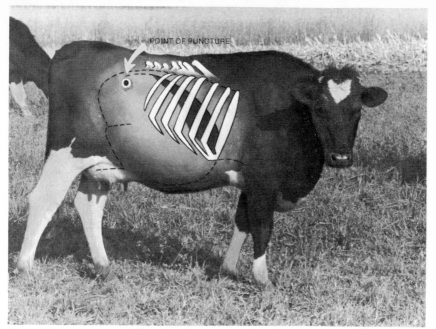

POINT OF PUNCTURE

Arrow shows approximate position where cow with bloat should be tapped. A knife can be used for this purpose but it's better to use a trocar

The part of the trocar with the sharp point is withdrawn from the sheath after insertion. The sheath, or cannula, then serves as a tube through which the gas escapes.

It may be necessary to leave it in for several hours, in which case it should be tied in place with a stout cord. When it is certain that all gas has been released, the instrument can be removed.

Do not let the animal drink any water until at least three hours after the bloat is relieved.

To prevent more formation of gas, an ounce of creolin in two quarts of water may be given as a drench, or poured into the paunch through a cannula.

The gas that escapes when an animal is tapped nearly always brings with it some of the stomach contents. This usually causes infection and the wound often takes weeks to heal.

Prevention

To prevent bloat, feed animals dry hay before turning them loose on legume pasture. In this way they will not gorge themselves on the green forage.

Keep some good palatable hay in the same field, to make sure the animals can get enough coarse or rough material for good paunch function.

Pasture legumes only after they are in full bloom.

Fields with at least 50 percent grasses are usually safe. However, climate and other factors may make it hard to keep a dependable pasture with the two kinds of plants in the right proportions.

Keep cows off legume pastures during and just after moist weather, especially in early spring and the wet season of the fall. When plants are short and the weather favors rapid leaf growth, the danger of bloat is greatest.

Chronic bloat appears regularly after each meal and principally affects cattle that are kept in a stable all winter. The bloat is not enough to cause alarm, but nevertheless lowers milk production and disturbs the well-being of the animal. Treatment consists in giving laxatives, such as Epsom salts, Glauber's salt or mineral oil. Daily exercise will help overcome the condition.

Choke

CHOKE OCCURS when feed or some foreign body clogs the gullet of an animal. In cattle, apples, ears of corn, turnips, beets, cabbage stumps and potatoes are the principal causes. Pieces of metal, glass or balls are also sometimes responsible for choke.

In cases where an animal has an esophagus that is narrower than normal, even soft feeds like bran or pulp when dry will sometimes clog a gullet. This is specially true when such an animal eats rapidly through hunger or is naturally a greedy eater.

Symptoms

Symptoms vary somewhat depending on the size of the obstruction and its location. If the object is in the chest portion of the esophagus and does not completely block the passage, early symptoms are usually not alarming. An affected animal may even attempt to eat and drink. In its doing so, however, the feed and water will be ejected back into the mouth accompanied with coughing and an attempt to vomit.

If the object is lodged in the neck portion of the esophagus the animal seldom tries to eat or drink. The obstructing object may often be seen and felt along the neck. Common symptoms, when the obstruction is in either location, are coughing, slobbering, forced swallowing movements and attempts to vomit even when no food or water is swallowed.

If the gullet is completely or almost completely blocked, the animal will refuse food and water, will soon become bloated and show all the symptoms of bloat so as to avoid puncturing the esophagus by passing beside the obstruction instead of pushing it down.

Treatment

If the animal is seriously bloated, it may have to be tapped before an attempt is made to relieve the choke. The method used for tapping cattle is described in the chapter on bloat.

If the obstruction is in the upper-neck part of the gullet, it can be felt from the outside. In such cases it should be forced into the throat by placing a hand on either side of the gullet and working the obstruction gently upward. It can then be removed by reaching it through the animal's mouth. Two men can do this job much better than one.

When the obstruction is in the chest portion of the gullet, two methods of relief are in common use: pushing the obstruction into the paunch, or snaring it out through the mouth. The latter method is often used, regardless of the location of the obstruction.

It is necessary to hold the animal's mouth open while removing the obstruction. The best way to do this is to use a mouth *speculum*, commonly called a jaw spreader. If you do not have one of these, the mouth can be held open with a large clevis. This should be put into the mouth flat and crosswise, then turned so as to keep the jaws apart.

To push the obstruction into the paunch, a *probang* is used. Such an instrument can be made by inserting a smooth wooden plug into the end of a piece of rubber tubing, five feet long and from one half

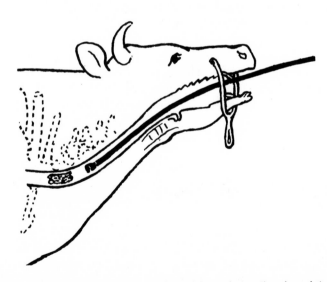

Drawing shows how a *probang* is used to push an obstruction down into an animal's paunch. The mouth is kept open with a *speculum* during the process. Actually, the *probang* is nothing more than a piece of rubber tubing that terminates in a smooth wooden plug

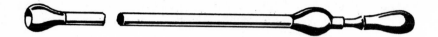

The probang is used to dislodge an obstruction in an animal's gullet by forcing it into the stomach.

to one inch in diameter. Probangs used by veterinarians have cup-shaped ends.

When a probang is inserted into the throat, the animal will always try to lower its head and plunge forward. If it succeeds in doing this, the free end of the probang may strike something, driving the other end through the wall of the gullet. To guard against this, the animal's head should be firmly secured over some fixed object, such as a stout post or fence. Hold the head high enough to provide a straight channel through the mouth and pharynx into the esophagus.

The probang should be lubricated with linseed oil or some other harmless oil before inserting it gently through the mouth into the gullet. When the obstruction is encountered use firm but gentle pressure, being careful not to injure the animal. It may be necessary to make a number of attempts at intervals of several hours or even on successive days before the obstacle is dislodged.

To snare an obstacle out of a gullet, a piece of fairly stiff wire is bent in half so as to form a loop. The loop end is inserted into the gullet so as to snare the obstacle and pull it out through the mouth. The wire should be lubricated, and great care should be used to avoid injuring the animal.

Foot rot of cattle and sheep

FOOT ROT of cattle and sheep is caused by an infection that destroys the tissues. Authorities do not agree on the microbe involved. What is known is that the organisms thrive in wet dark places, especially mud, which probably means that they are anaerobic—they thrive in the absence of air.

The microbes enter the tissues of the feet through small cuts or bruises and multiply under the skin and in the outer tissues. Other organisms then move into the wounds and increase the infection.

A good way to bandage a cow's foot

After treating wound, rip a bandage down the center from the end about a foot. Tie a loose knot where the ends join, to keep bandage from ripping further. Tie the two ends of the bandage around the pastern as shown at the right

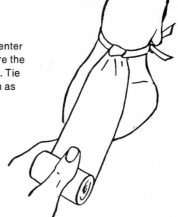

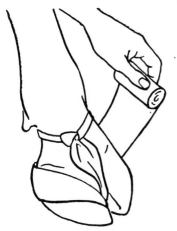

Lift animal's foot and bring bandage down between toes as shown at the left

Wrap the toes alternately, overlapping the layers, until the foot is covered as shown at the right

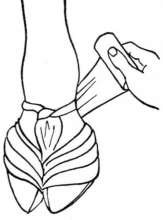

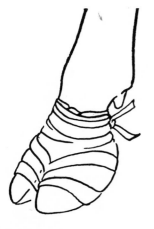

When the job is finished, sew the layers of bandage firmly together. If the first tie around the pastern feels tight, cut the two tied ends off so as not to interfere with the circulation

Symptoms

Symptoms are lameness, heat, and often intense pain which can be noted by touching the infected area. The pain keeps animals from moving around for food and as a result they lose weight. The milk production of cows falls off. When sheep have the infection in both forefeet, pain is often so great that they kneel when eating. A watery fluid oozes from the affected area. The tissues rot away as the disease progresses and this is accompanied by a grayish, cheesy discharge. There is always a foul odor present.

Treatment

The standard treatment consists in carefully trimming away the rotting portion with a sharp knife or pruning shears. The infected parts are then treated with antiseptics, such as a 10 to 30-percent copper-sulphate solution or a 2 to 10-percent solution of formaldehyde. These washes are corrosive, and the wound should be examined carefully before each succeeding treatment to see that they do not eat into the flesh. Otherwise healing will be difficult. A number of very good salves and ointments specially prepared for treatment of foot rot are available. Sulfathiazole ointment is widely used.

The sulfa drugs also are given either by mouth, or the sodium salts of the drugs are injected into the jugular vein. Sulfaquinoxaline or sulfa-pyridine have been highly successful when given as drenches. Sulfapyridine combined with penicillin as an injection is also excellent.

When using the sulfa drugs, relief often comes to the animal with astonishing rapidity—sometimes in 24 hours. In mild cases, cutting is unnecessary.

In treating badly infected feet, it is sometimes wise to remove one of the claws at the top of the hoof. The pus is then drained off. This allows the air to enter so the microbes can no longer live. The hoof is then treated with an antiseptic solution or salve, bandaged and soon heals. The animals seem to get along just as well with one claw. A simple bandage can be made by cutting a corner of a burlap bag in such a way that a pocket 6 inches square remains and has ribbons left to wrap around the fetlock under the dewclaws.

Prevention

Dry pastures and clean, dry barns constitute the best way to ward off the disease. Wet or muddy places should be drained or filled. If the foot rot gets a start in a herd, treatment should be followed by disinfection of the premises, otherwise animals may become reinfected. Another precaution consists in clearing premises of broken glass, tin cans, etc.

"Hardware disease"

CATTLE like to swallow pieces of metal and other foreign objects. As a result, many adult animals have nails, keys, pieces of wire, staples or even pocket knives in their paunches. Technically, the disease is known as reticuloperitonitis.

These objects ordinarily do little or no harm while they lie in the rumen, but the normal movement of the contents carries the heavy particle forward and into the reticulum (the second compartment, also known as the honeycomb). As it contracts in its normal way, sharp objects penetrate the wall and may puncture the diaphragm or the liver. Once imbedded in the diaphragm they slowly move forward until they also puncture the heart sac—the pericardium—and even the heart itself.

The metal objects interfere with the heart action, causing a severe trouble known as *traumatic pericarditis*. This means an injury to the heart covering or sac. Usually an inflammation of the inside wall of the abdomen, peritonitis, also occurs.

Symptoms

Symptoms of hardware disease are often not easy to recognize. An affected animal may show loss of appetite, decreased milk production, arched back and tucked up abdomen, as is the case with certain digestive troubles. In advanced cases a pulse may be seen in the jugular vein, where there should be none.

Evidence of hardware disease often shows up after calving. Straining in delivery may force a piece of wire or a nail through the stomach wall into the heart or liver.

In advanced cases, sounds caused by friction in the heart can be heard at a distance of several yards. Animals may die without apparent cause until a post-mortem examination is made.

Metal detectors have come into limited use for detecting metal objects in cows. These instruments are not always dependable because most older cattle pieces of metal in their stomachs and these lie there without doing any harm.

Treatment

Two methods of treatment are used. One consists in operating to remove the metal object. In the other method, the animal is placed on an inclined platform, built to fit a stall, with the forepart of the animal's body higher than the rear. This causes the metal to lodge in a place where there is little likelihood that it will do any harm. The animal is kept on the inclined platform for at least three weeks, during which time stomach tissue grows around the metal and holds it in place.

To build an inclined platform, place a 2 x 6-in. plank on edge across the stall at the stanchion. Nail strong boards to it, long enough to reach to within a foot of the gutter. For added strength and support, nail a 2 x 4 on edge to the bottom of the boards at a point where the boards are exactly 4 inches above the floor. Use other supports if necessary. Nail half-inch cleats crosswise at about 6-in. intervals on the platform to keep the animal from slipping.

Never give laxatives to an animal suspected of having hardware disease. Laxatives will weaken the animal and will do no good.

Prevention consists largely in not letting small metallic objects lie around where cattle can get at them. Further prevention embodies the use of permanent bar magnets, weighing a few ounces. Lodged in the reticulum, or second stomach, such magnets hold sharp magnetic objects in such a position that they cannot cause injury.

Lumpy jaw

LUMPY JAW is usually spoken of as one disease. Actually it is two, caused by two different microbes. The outward appearance of the animal is almost the same in both cases. Usually one or both jaws have tumor-like swellings in the region of the throat.

Both diseases are chronic. They start slowly and continue for life unless the animal is treated. They seldom cause death.

Lumpy jaw principally affects cattle, but other farm animals are somewhat susceptible. Human beings are slightly susceptible. The malady occurs most often in the West and Southwest. Although it is caused by germs, it is not communicable, that is, one animal will not readily get it from another except through transfer of pus from a diseased animal.

The diseases are known technically as *actinomycosis* and *actinobacillosis*.

Symptoms

Actinomycosis is caused by the so-called ray fungus. This organism is found in barley awns, oat stubble and various grasses. It enters the body through abrasions in the skin or inside of the mouth.

As a rule, actinomycosis is confined to the bones of the jaw and head, but soft tissues may also be attacked. The bones become large and spongy. They are full of a sticky pus that contains yellow particles called "sulphur granules."

The growth may expand until it breaks through the skin and the pus then gives forth a foul odor. The growth may also extend inward and involve the palate and gums. Then the teeth may become loose and later fall out.

Actinobacillosis, on the other hand, is confined to the soft tissues of the neck, jaws and head. Movable swellings appear that vary in size from a walnut to an egg, or larger. These growths also finally break through the skin and discharge a creamy pus. This also contains yellow granules but they are smaller and more numerous than those in the pus of actinomycosis.

The tongue is often infected in actinobacillosis. It may become hard and protrude from the mouth. The animal has difficulty in moving it and constantly drools saliva. This condition is called "wooden tongue." In severe cases the animal is unable to chew. It finally becomes weak and dies of exhaustion.

Treatment

Treatment of actinomycosis is not very satisfactory. It is not easy to reach the germs in the hollows of the bones. Injection of streptomycin or sylfa drugs around the infected areas helps if the disease has not advanced too far. The dosage is 5 grams daily for three days or two to six grams every other day for five treatments.

Actinobacillosis yields readily to treatment, with a high percentage of cure. The drug used is either sodium or potassium iodide. It is dissolved in water and given as a drench. The dose is $1^1/2$ to $2^1/2$ drams a day. When the tongue and upper throat are affected, particular care must be taken to pour the drug in such a way that none of it goes into the lungs. Otherwise pneumonia may follow.

After a week or 10 days, an animal that has been given the remedy may show signs of getting too much iodine. This is revealed by flow of tears, catarrh, loss of appetite and scurfy skin. Treatment should then be discontinued for a few days or a week, after which time it can be resumed.

The animal is generally cured in from two to six weeks. But some cases do not respond to the remedy. If no improvement is noticed in three or four weeks, further treatment is useless and should be abandoned.

Iodine may easily be administered by injecting sodium iodine into the blood vessels. This is a quicker and more convenient method, but requires greater care. The size of the dose must be governed by the weight and condition of the animal treated.

Iodine appears in the milk during treatment and this makes it unsalable. The drug should not be given pregnant cows because it may cause abortion. A small percentage of animals suffer shock when given the iodine remedy, so cannot be treated with the drug. These and other animals that can't be cured should be fattened and sold for beef. Treatment of the disease with oxytetracycline, streptomycin, or erythromycin is also effective.

Prevention

There is no known way to prevent the ailment completely, except perhaps to avoid feeding coarse, stemmy hay or feed which contains foxtail, needlegrass or similar plants. Elimination of overgrazing will help to some extent. Seeding pastures with more desirable plants may also help.

Although lumpy jaw is not communicable, careful cattle owners keep infected animals away from others, particularly when pus comes out of open wounds.

Animals with lumpy jaw are subject to rigid inspection when slaughtered for beef. Infected parts are, of course, cut away. If infection is general, as sometimes happens, the whole carcass is condemned.

Shipping fever, or pneumatic pasteurellosis

SHIPPING FEVER is technically known as pneumatic pasteurellosis. It is principally a disease of cattle but it also attacks sheep and other livestock.

The disease occurs most often while animals are being shipped by rail or truck or immediately thereafter. And if these sick animals are allowed to mingle with healthy ones, the latter may also contract the disease.

Greatest losses occur among young or poorly nourished stock, indicating that the physical condition of the animals has a great deal to do with their susceptibility. Overcrowding, irregular feeding and watering, and the stress brought on by traveling are largely responsible for bringing on the disease. These things lower an animal's resistance. When the disease occurs on farms or cattle ranges, it can nearly always be traced to abrupt changes in feeding or weather.

Shipping fever may occur at any time of the year but is most common in cold and changeable weather. Fall, winter and early spring are the worst times of the year for it.

The primary cause of the disease is obscure. *Pasteurella multocida* and related organisms are present in large numbers in infected animals. But these are always present in the throats and other air passages of healthy cattle. For this reason, many authorities believe shipping fever is caused by a virus, as yet unidentified. *Pasteurella*, they say, causes a secondary infection.

Symptoms

The outward symptoms of shipping fever resemble those of the "flu" in human beings. It lasts from two to eight days or longer. Animals have a high fever (104 to 107 deg. F.), loss of appetite, a discharge from the nose, an occasional hacking cough, swollen and watery eyes, a crestfallen and gaunt appearance, a stiffened gait as though their joints ached, and sometimes diarrhea.

Other symptoms may also occur, such as soft swellings beneath the skin of the head, throat or dewlap. The tongue is sometimes swollen and the animal drools and slobbers because of tongue and throat irritation. There may be difficulty in breathing, bloody discharge from the nostrils, and strings of mucus that hang from the mouth.

There is also an intestinal form of the disease with diarrhea, staggering gait and extreme weakness. This is less frequent than the pulmonary form. Both kinds may occur at the same time.

Within three to eight days after the first symptoms appear, animals may develop pneumonia and die. In mild attacks of the disease, animals recover within a week or two.

Unless an animal dies suddenly of an acute attack of the disease, post-mortem examinations reveal hemorrhages in one or more organs of the body, depending upon the seat of the disease. Swellings of doughy consistency, tinged with blood, may be found under the skin. Lymph glands may contain blood. Hemorrhages may be found in the fatty tissue around the kidneys, and in the intestines and heart walls.

Shipping fever is sometimes difficult to diagnose because many of the symptoms resemble those of anthrax, malignant edema and blackleg.

Prevention and Treatment

Two types of biological products are used against shipping fever. Bacterins and aggressins are used for its prevention; and antiserums for its cure and for temporary protection.

For best results, feeder and stocker cattle should be treated with a bacterin or aggressin at least 10 days before shipment. It produces immunity for a period of several months to a year. Treatment while in transit or immediately preceding it is of no value.

Immune serum, on the other hand, produces immediate resistance against the disease. This immunity may last only a few weeks and should not be depended upon for more than four days. Serum is used to treat animals while in transit, or upon arrival at their destination if any animals in the shipment are sick with the disease. Serum also has curative value.

The sulfa drugs are widely used in the treatment of sick animals. These are given through the mouth in doses ranging from $3/4$ to $1^1/2$ grains per pound of body weight. Sulfamerazine, sulfathiazole and sulfadiazine are the ones used most often. When attacks are severe, sulfamerazine is sometimes given in combination with penicillin. The penicillin is injected intramuscularly every three hours in doses of 100,000 units.

In the *Special Report on Diseases of Cattle*, prepared by the U.S. Bureau of Animal Industry, the following recommendations are made to shippers and others who handle cattle:

Avoid hard driving and allow ample time for rest before loading. On arrival at the pens, the animals should not be allowed to fill up on water but should first have rest and be fed grass or nonlegume hay.

Avoid overcrowding cattle in the cars. In cold weather, bed the car well. In very severe weather, in northern latitudes, it may be well to line the hide walls of the car with heavy paper.

Give feed and water at proper intervals en route. When unloaded for feed, water and rest, the cattle should have plenty of time to become well-rested.

Under the 28-hour law, five hours' rest is the minimum specified time, and the railroads ordinarily allow that period, exclusive of the time of unloading and reloading. It is better, however, to give stocker and feeder cattle special care, allowing at least eight hours for feed, water and rest. Plenty of rest and regular feeding and watering are essential if animals are to arrive at their final destination in the best possible condition.

The common practice of withholding water from animals until they are very thirsty so that later they will take a heavy fill is harmful. The practice tends to upset the digestive system so seriously that the animals are slow in resuming normal feeding and gain in weigh. It is therefore recommended that this damaging practice be discontinued.

In stocker and feeder cattle that pass through the public market, the same attention should be given to the shipments back to the country that has been outlined for the shipments to market. After the arrival of cattle at their final destination in the country, they should receive attention and care.

On arrival, feeder cattle should be given a fill of dry roughage, such as timothy hay, or corn stover. After having access to this roughage a few hours, they should have water but not all that they will drink. By the end of the first day, give free access to dry roughage and water.

Most feeder cattle are raised on grasses different from those found in the fattening areas. Therefore, if they are to be pasture fed, let them become accustomed to the new grasses gradually, giving them at first only a few hours' grazing each day.

If feeder cattle are intended for dry-lot feeding with no pasture available, give them access to cornstalk fields or feed them on corn fodder and hay for 10 days to two weeks before starting them on the fattening rations.

If the cattle arrive in cold weather, especially if it is wet and stormy, provide adequate, dry shelter.

Anaplasmosis

ANAPLASMOSIS is a blood disease of cattle that prevails in the South and West. But cases have been reported in 32 states, including Illinois, Indiana and Pennsylvania. The malady occurs mostly in the summer and fall, although in the South, animals are occasionally affected in the winter.

How the malady is spread

The disease is believed to be spread by blood-sucking insects such as ticks and flies that carry it from animal to animal. It is often transmitted during castration, dehorning, vaccination and blood sampling when the instruments used are not properly sterilized between operations.

Anaplasmosis is seldom severe in animals under one year of age. Between 30 and 50 percent of the older infected animals usually die. Now and then, for some unexplained reason, the percentage of deaths is quite low.

Animals that recover from anaplasmosis remain carriers of the disease. The microbes that cause the malady remain in their blood in small numbers but the animals seem healthy. The infection can be transmitted from the dam to the unborn calf, which then becomes a carrier although it may never show any outward signs of the disease.

The incubation period of anaplasmosis is between 15 and 40 days.

Symptoms

The microscopic parasite that causes anaplasmosis attacks and destroys the red blood cells and brings on a severe anemia. The blood becomes pale and watery. The malady occurs in several forms.

The mild form is confined to calves under five months old. Often its presence can be determined only by examination of the blood under a microscope, since there are few if any outward symptoms.

In the acute form, the animal at first has a high fever which is followed by subnormal temperature shortly before death. Breathing is fast and labored. Other symptoms are exhaustion, a wobbly gait, suspended rumination and loss of appetite. Usually there is jaundice, which can be observed by yellow discoloration in the eyes, inside the mouth, on the brisket, udder and vagina.

Sometimes animals with anaplasmosis show a depraved appetite by eating dirt and chewing bones. Urination is frequent. Usually there is constipation. Dung is blood-tinged, or dark in color, and partly covered with mucus. Death may follow within 24 hours after the appearance of first symptoms, but the average fatal case lingers two or three days. Animals that do not die recover in several weeks.

The peracute (highly acute) form attacks mostly milk cows that are high producers. It is less common than either the mild or acute forms. Its course is so rapid that the animal is usually dead before symptoms are noticed.

In the so-called chronic form, the animal may linger for weeks or months before dying or recovering. This type is believed to be more common among range stock than among dairy or feed-lot animals.

Anaplasmosis is sometimes mistaken for tick fever in areas where the latter disease occurs. One difference between them is that in tick fever the urine is bloody while in anaplasmosis it is clear.

Diagnosis

An accurate test for anaplasmosis is used whereby both carrier animals and those with active infections can be detected.

Methods for prevention

It is believed that anaplasmosis could be wiped out if we can stop the transfer of blood from sick carrier animals to healthy ones. It should be remembered, however, that ticks might act as reservoir hosts of the disease organisms.

Where the disease is not widespread, it is sound practice to fatten and sell for slaughter all animals that recover from the disease, thus checking its further spread.

The utmost care should be used to disinfect instruments that come in contact with the blood of animals. Such instruments should first be washed in clean water, then boiled for several minutes in water containing 2 percent of washing soda. When there are no facilities for boiling the instruments, they may be immersed for at least 15 minutes in a 2-percent lye solution. This should be kept tightly covered, and a fresh solution made every day, because it loses its strength when exposed to the air.

When removed from the lye solution, hypodermic needles may be dipped in a 2-percent compound solution of cresol, 2 percent formalin, or 60 to 70 percent alcohol.

The disease can be prevented by adding small amounts of chlortetracycline to the feed through the seasons when infections are at their height.

Treatment

Transfusion of 8 to 12 quarts of normal bovine blood is the best single treatment and is often enough to start a very sick animal back on the road to recovery, according to *The Merck Veterinary Manual.*

Afflicted animals should be kept in the shade, protected against biting insects and given green feed. Rough handling should be avoided. It has been observed that diseased animals that drink large quantities of water usually recover, while those that drink only a small amount or none at all, usually die. If an animal refuses to drink, water should be administered into the animal's stomach through a stomach tube.

Johne's disease, or paratuberculosis

JOHNE'S DISEASE, also called paratuberculosis, is a chronic dysentery. It affects principally cattle but also attacks horses, sheep, deer and goats. There is no cure.

The disease is spread in the dung of infected animals. The organisms contaminate the feed and water of healthy animals. When the organisms arrive in the intestines, they attack its walls and set up such an infection that food can no longer be absorbed into the blood.

The bacteria resemble those which cause tuberculosis, and have been known to live 163 days in a water ditch and six months in cow dung.

Johne's disease infects principally young animals, but death may not follow until years after the animal becomes infected. Calves that acquire it when a few weeks old may not show symptoms until they are three or four years old.

Symptoms

The first symptom of Johne's disease is a general loss of condition, even though the appetite remains good. Diarrhea occurs without straining. There are a rough coat and dry skin. Later appetite fails and the affected animal refuses all feed.

There is no fever. Death may occur within a few weeks from the time diarrhea begins, or the animal may cease to scour and seem to recover. But then, in another week or perhaps even a year later, diarrhea starts again and the animal dies. Besides killing animals and making them unthrifty, Johne's disease causes a decline of 20 to 30 percent in breeding efficiency.

Symptoms often appear after calving, abortion, pneumonia or garget. Purebred animals, placed on official test for milk production, are often victims. These things all lower the vitality of animals and make them more susceptible to disease.

Diagnosis with the johnin test

Diagnosis of Johne's disease is difficult since many animals that are active spreaders show no symptoms. Veterinarians employ the johnin test when the presence of the disease is suspected. This is similar to the intradermic test used in diagnosing tuberculosis.

The johnin test is not perfect but it is nonetheless extremely valuable in ridding a herd of the disease.

Indemnities are paid to cattle slaughtered on account of the disease. For information about this, ask your state livestock officials.

No satisfactory treatment is known

At present there is no satisfactory treatment for Johne's disease. Practically all animals that develop symptoms die within a period of one month to two years.

Diseased animals should be sold for beef while they are still in good condition. Since man is not susceptible to the disease and no edible parts are involved, the carcass passes inspection as wholesome food.

Control and eradication

It is not easy to control the spread of Johne's disease. But unless the disease is stopped, a herd will become unprofitable, and may even be completely wiped out. In one Illinois herd there were so many reactors that the owner found it cheapest to sell them all.

To protect against Johne's disease, herd owners are advised to:

Have the herd tested with the johnin test once a year.

Sell all reactors at once for slaughter.

Exercise utmost sanitary measures. Premises that were occupied by diseased animals should be thoroughly cleaned and disinfected, including drinking troughs and anything else that might have become contaminated. Manure of infected animals and even some of the top soil on which it lay should be removed and buried. Care should be taken that this does not contaminate nearby streams or other water supplies.

If it is necessary to introduce new animals into a herd, buy only from reputable breeders and have the animals tested with johnin for possible infection.

Blackleg

BLACKLEG is a disease that usually attacks young cattle only—those between six months and two years old. Animals younger than four months and older than three years are practically immune.

Death usually occurs between 12 and 36 hours after the symptoms first appear. Rarely does an animal recover from the disease.

Sheep and goats are susceptible to blackleg, swine slightly, but the other domestic animals and man are immune.

Blackleg is caused by the *Clostridium chauvoei*, a microbe which forms spores that are highly resistant to destruction by heat, cold, drying, or chemical disinfectants. They may lie for several years in a pasture or barn, a constant threat to cattle. This is why the disease occurs year after year on certain farms or in certain areas.

The bacteria usually enter the body of an animal through small abrasions or punctures of the skin, like those made by barb wire fences, thorns or burrs. The germs are anaerobic so will not develop or multiply in air. They don't enter the body nearly as easily through open wounds or cuts because there is too much air present.

Purebred or high-grade stock is much more likely to acquire the disease than low-grade. In this country, blackleg began to increase when cattle were improved. Some say it is because better cattle have thinner hides.

Cattle seem to be more susceptible when they are rapidly improving in flesh, as in the spring when they start eating fresh grass. On the other hand, in some localities the change from grass to hay in the fall also seems to have a bad effect. But the disease is not confined to particular seasons.

Symptoms

The symptoms of blackleg are easy to recognize—high fever, loss of appetite, lameness, rapid breathing and listlessness.

Following these symptoms but sometimes preceding them, gas-filled swelling—like tumors—appear on the neck, shoulders, chest and flanks. The inside of the mouth becomes a dark red and in 12 hours changes to a dirty leaden or purplish color.

At first the tumors are small and painful, but they increase in size rapidly. Two or more that are close together will unite to form one big one. When the tumors are stroked or pressed lightly, they make a peculiar crackling sound under the skin. This is caused by gas that is formed when the organisms multiply. Just before death, the animal is unable to rise, the muscles twitch and there may be violent convulsions.

The carcass of a blackleg victim soon becomes distended with gas to such an extent that the two legs on the upper side of the carcass stick straight out in the air instead of resting on the ground.

The symptoms of blackleg resemble those of anthrax, but the swellings of the latter are hard and do not contain gas. Also, blackleg kills more quickly than anthrax.

Malignant edema is also like blackleg and the swellings are filled with gas. But blackleg starts with pinpoint openings in the skin, while malignant edema usually can be traced to the infection of a large wound, such as follows an operation or serious injury.

The positive way to tell one disease from another is by microscopic examination of the organisms.

Protection against the disease

Where blackleg is apt to occur, animals should be protected against the disease through vaccination. Calves vaccinated when over six months old do not generally require further treatment. Animals vaccinated when younger than this should be vaccinated again for complete protection.

It is difficult to rid pastures of blackleg. This makes it of utmost importance to wipe out sources of infection as soon as they are known. Carcasses of animals that die of the disease should be burned at once, if possible. If this is not practicable, then they should be buried deep in the ground and covered with lime before the earth is filled in. If an animal dies in a stable, the animal and all litter should be removed, and the stable thoroughly and repeatedly disinfected.

Outbreaks of blackleg have been reported as developing in pastures where no animal had the disease in the proceding 11 years, and there was no apparent source of outside infection. This shows the persistence of the spores and the need for immediate action when the disease appears. Spores may be carried to marshy pastures by rivers that overflow.

It is comparatively easy to kill the germs in their active or so-called vegetative state, but after they form spores it sometimes seems almost impossible.

Treatment of sick animals

Vaccination is often used in treating animals in the early stages of the disease. When the malady appears in a herd, fever among apparently normal individuals is taken to indicate that these animals are coming down with the disease. Penicillin or broad-spectrum antibiotics in addition to vaccine are often used in treatment of more advanced cases but these measures are often unsuccessful.

Red water disease

KNOWN technically as bacillary hemoglobinuria, red water disease occurs principally in the poorly drained valleys of California, Idaho, Nevada and Oregon. It has also been reported in many other states even as far north as Wisconsin.

Floodwaters sometimes seem to carry the disease from infected localities to ranches previously free of the disease, and cause sudden outbreaks. Rarely does the malady appear in upland areas. The so-called "red water season" is between June and November.

Symptoms

The symptoms are uniform and easily recognized. The onset is sudden, with high fever and loss of appetite. A sick animal often stands away from the rest with arched back, and moves with reluctance. Milk flow and rumination stop. Bowel evacuations are at first scanty. Later, bloody diarrhea may appear. The muzzle is dry and hot; pulse is fast and weak. But the most pronounced symptoms is foamy urine of port wine color. This symptom has given the disease its common name.

The disease can be distinguished from others with similar symptoms, such as anaplasmosis, by the rapidity of its progress. Anthrax is the only other disease with which it might be confused.

Among affected untreated animals the death rate may be as high as 95 percent. The duration of noticeable illness varies from 10 hours to three or four days.

Immunization and treatment

A bacterin used against red water disease affords practically 100 percent protection. For best results, it is injected about four to six weeks before the disease appeared in the area during previous years. Protection lasts about a year.

Sick animals are treated with an antitoxic serum. If treatment is given early, recovery is often dramatic. The color of the urine becomes normal in 12 hours. In localities where the disease prevails, the serum is often injected at the first sign of fever or dullness, instead of waiting until the disease is more advanced. Penicillin and other antibiotics are beneficial in the early stages of the disease.

Feed should be withheld from sick animals until they are well on the road to recovery but ample water should be supplied.

Anthrax

ANTHRAX is a highly fatal disease that attacks nearly all warm-blooded animals, including man. Herbivorous animals—those that eat plants and plant seeds—are more susceptible than those that eat meat. Fowls, however, are not susceptible under ordinary conditions. The cause of the disease is a germ known as *Bacillus anthracis*.

Animals become infected through feed, water, openings in the skin, bites of infected insects, and even by breathing the spores into their lungs. Scavenger animals, such as buzzards, carry the malady from one area to another. Men become infected by handling hides, wool, furs or the carcasses of animals that have died of the disease.

Anthrax occurs most often when animals are on pasture. But stabled animals also get it, particularly if they are fed contaminated hay.

The disease may start anywhere, but is usually confined to certain areas where it appears year after year. In low-lying marshy land, or in soil rich in decayed plant and animal matter, the spores of the microbes live for a long time.

Dried spores have been known to survive and cause disease after being stored for 40 years. The bacilli themselves, though, have little resistance to heat or drying when not in the spore form.

The southeastern part of South Dakota, northeastern Nebraska, a belt along the Texas Gulf Coast, California and the delta region of the Mississippi, including parts of Arkansas, Mississippi and Louisiana, are areas where serious outbreaks of the disease formerly occurred.

Symptoms

Anthrax occurs in four forms: peracute, acute, subacute and chronic.

In the peracute form there are usually no outward symptoms. An animal, apparently in perfect health, staggers, collapses, has a few convulsive movements and dies. Close examination often shows blood-stained discharges from the nose, mouth and rectum. This form is common among sheep, cattle and horses. It appears at the beginning of an outbreak.

In the acute form, death occurs in a day or two; in the subacute form, death may occur in three to five days or the animal may recover completely. In these forms the animal is at first excited and then becomes depressed. It lags behind the herd, its head hangs low, it refuses to eat and prefers to stand still or lie down. Breathing is labored and rapid. Pregnant cows may abort. A high fever sets in. Bloody discharges usually come from the natural body openings. Small hemorrhages appear inside the mouth. Swellings that can be depressed may develop over the body, but more commonly are found around the genital organs or the lower wall of the abdomen. The tongue may be discolored and swollen. As in the peracute form, the animal finally staggers to its death.

Chronic anthrax occurs mostly in swine. Presence of the disease is revealed in post-mortem examinations by infection of certain glands and by other symptoms. Swine are more resistant to anthrax than other farm animals. When they contract the disease by feeding on infected carcasses, some of the swine may die without having any outward symptoms. Others may have swellings about the throat that cause death by suffocation. Many hogs with such swellings recover.

When swine develop anthrax from sources other than from contaminated carcasses, they have the same symptoms but they seldom die suddenly.

Anthrax occurs in sheep and goats most often in the peracute form. Symptoms are similar to those in cattle: unsteady gait, trembling, restlessness, difficult breathing, bloody discharges from the natural body openings and convulsions before death. Anthrax in sheep may be mistaken for blackleg or malignant edema.

In man, anthrax usually occurs as an infection of the skin, resembling a carbuncle, or as an infection of the lungs known as woolsorter's disease. Medical attention is most important when anthrax is suspected.

Diagnosis

Where the outward symptoms of the disease are not sufficiently pronounced to justify a positive diagnosis, then a post-morem examination should be made. This is a dangerous operation and should be done only by someone who knows how to protect himself against infection. When the tissues and the bacteria are exposed to air, they quickly form spores, and these are very difficult to kill or control.

Carcasses of animals dead of the disease decompose rapidly and soon become greatly bloated. Dark blood escapes from the natural openings of the body. The spleen and other organs show signs of the disease. The microbes that cause the disease are present in the blood. They can be identified easily under a microscope.

What to do when anthrax strikes

Anthrax is one of the most dreaded of diseases. The heavy toll that it takes, the long time that it contaminates the soil, and the many ways in which it can be spread, make necessary the most rigid control measures.

A livestock owner should notify a veterinarian or a livestock sanitary official at once if the disease appears or is suspected in a herd.

When a diagnosis of anthrax has been made, the U. S. Department of Agriculture suggests the following measures for its control:

1. Prompt and proper disposal, either by complete burning or deep burial, of animals dead of the disease, together with all the manure, bedding, blood-stained soil and similar material that has been contaminated by these animals.

2. Careful examination of the herd for animals showing early symptoms of the disease, prompt isolation of sick animals, and immediate treatment with large does of anti-anthrax serum.

3. Vaccination of the apparently well animals in the herd as soon as

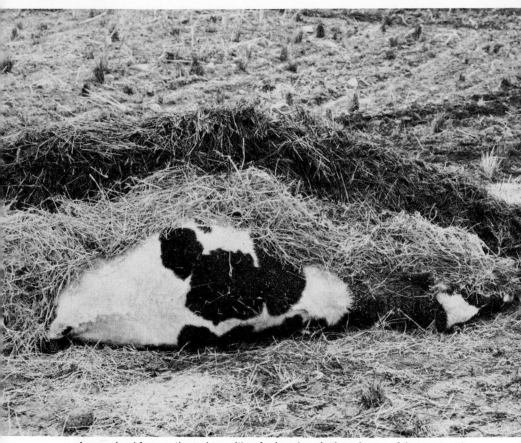

A cow, dead from anthrax, in position for burning. Anthrax is one of the most serious of animal diseases. Dead animals should promptly be disposed of by burning or by deep burial

possible for prevention, in accordance with methods recommended by the state livestock sanitary officials and other experienced veterinarians.

4. Immediate change of pastures if practicable. This precaution alone in many instances has helped to reduce losses. If the outbreak occurs during the fly season, it is best to move the herd at night so that most of the infection-carrying flies will be left behind.

5. Strict quarantine of premises, rigidly enforced, to prohibit positively the movement of livestock or other commodities of a contraband nature within, out of, or into the infected area.

Prevention and Treatment

A large number of biological products are available for combating anthrax, all with special uses and limitations. They have three general purposes: to immunize animals against the disease, to protect them in the face of outbreaks and to treat those that are sick. In most states a special permit is necessary to obtain the vaccines.

Foot-and-mouth disease

FOOT-AND-MOUTH disease is a highly contagious plague that affects all cloven-hoofed animals, but principally cattle, swine, sheep and goats. It may also spread to deer, elk, and moose from range or pasture animals.

The disease is caused by at least three different types of virus. Immunity against one of them will not give protection against the others. Outbreaks occur with such suddenness that often all susceptible members of a herd show symptoms at practically the same time. The period of incubation is between 18 hours and three weeks.

Here is the head of a cow affected with foot-and-mouth disease. One of the big problems is that all animals in a herd may show symptoms at virtually the same time. One of the symptoms is that the saliva increases

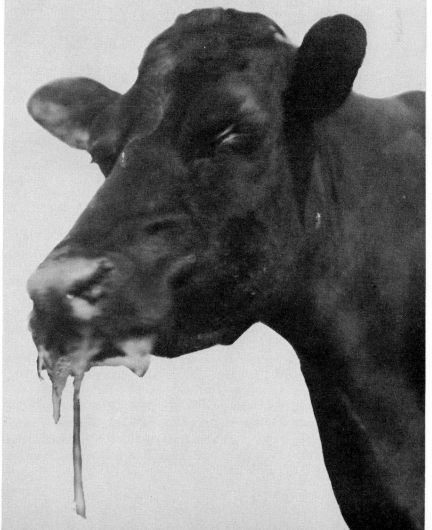

USDA photos

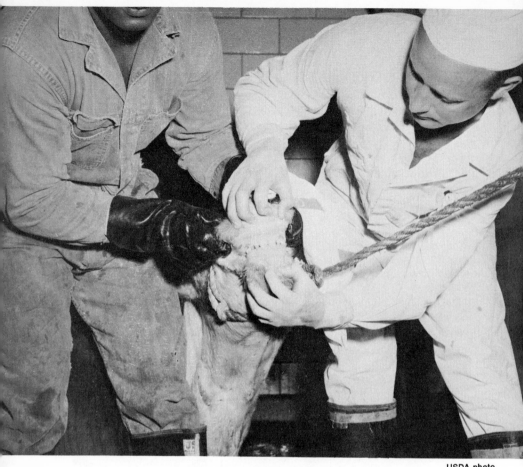

Eroded areas on the upper lip of a steer infected with foot-and-mouth virus are typical lesions of the disease. This animal is being examined in Plum Island Animal Disease Laboratory

Symptoms

The virus attacks the mouth, tongue, stomach, intestines and the skin around the toes, upper part of the hoof and the coronary band. A blister, or vesicle, forms where the infection first starts. In one or two days, the infection spreads through the blood, causing a fever. Thereupon blisters appear at the foot and mouth, on parts not previously infected, and around the coronet. They also occur on the teats of cows.

At this time the fever usually disappears but the animal is visibly sick. Milk flow is reduced. Lameness appears and increases in the following days.

The blisters soon break and give forth a fluid which may be either clear or cloudy. The broken blisters are painful and may become infected with other organisms. The flow of saliva increases. Drooling occurs freely and stringy saliva hangs from the mouth. The saliva, the "water" from the blisters, the milk and the urine are all laden with the virus.

The intensity of the disease varies widely. In the mild form, losses may be only 3 percent of the animals affected, while in severe forms losses may reach 30 to 50 percent. Greatest losses occur among young animals that are fed infected milk.

On the average, mortality is low. But the total financial loss from the disease is enormous if it is allowed to run its course. The value of dairy cattle often is permanently impaired. Udders are ruined by abscesses, and lameness sometimes continues throughout life. Abortion is frequent.

Animals that survive an attack of the disease usually recover in 10 to 20 days. In the more virulent forms, recovery sometimes takes three months to a year.

Control and eradication

Because the disease can assume plague proportions, it is controlled by the U.S.D.A. and the states. Treatment of foot-and-mouth disease is absolutely forbidden by federal law.

When foot-and-mouth disease is suspected, the area is at once quarantined. If the malady is present, all affected animals and those directly exposed are slaughtered and buried or burned.

Rabies, or Hydrophobia

DOGS are the principal spreaders of rabies, or hydrophobia. Outbreaks also occur among coyotes, foxes and other beats that attack livestock and fowls. All warm-blooded animals are susceptible, including squirrels, raccoons, opossums, and other park animals.

The infection is caused by a filtrable virus that attacks the nervous system. It is transmitted in the saliva of a diseased animal that bites its victims. Upon entering the blood stream, the virus infects the nerves, follows their course to the spinal cord, and finally involves the brain.

Greatest losses occur among cattle. From 15 to 45 percent of the bites of rabid animals result in death to the victim. So far as is known, there is no natural immunity against rabies. Where the bitten animals do not get the disease, it is presumed that the virus did not enter the wound, or was washed out by profuse bleeding.

Symptoms

There are two typical symptoms of rabies: apparent insanity, called *furious rabies;* and signs of paralysis, called *dumb rabies.* Symptoms appear between two and 12 weeks after an animal is bitten.

Dogs—In a dog, the first symptom is usually restlessness, as though the animal had a foreboding that something is wrong. The character of the animal may change—a friendly dog becomes vicious and a vicious one, friendly. The animal's voice changes and takes on a dismal, hoarse quality. Froth may appear at the mouth.

If the furious form follows the first symptoms, the dog becomes aggressive, roams aimlessly about and snaps at anything that moves. If put in a cage, it may bite iron bars until its teeth break.

When the dumb form follows the first symptoms, the dog is not excited, in fact, it is quite the opposite. It does not roam. The muscles of its lower jaw become paralyzed and its mouth hangs open several inches. The mouth can be pushed shut but will not stay that way unless held in place.

Dog owners often mistake this condition for a bone in the throat, try to remove it and thus expose themselves to the disease. It should be noted that a dog with an obstruction in its throat will attempt to remove it with its paw or otherwise, whereas a dog with a paralyzed throat will not make such an effort. This leads to the name hydrophobia, which means hatred of water.

Whether the disease assumes the furious or the dumb form, the throat muscles become paralyzed. The animal tries to drink but cannot. In the end paralysis sets in and the dog dies.

Because city and park animals become infected, and may change temperament, children especially must be taught to avoid squirrels and other animals which are unusually tame. They may bite when they are handled.

Cattle—Both the furious and the dumb form of rabies strike cattle, the former being more common. An exact line of distinction cannot be drawn between the two because the furious form often turns into the dumb type before the animal dies.

The first signs of the disease are loss of appetite, restlessness, stoppage of milk flow and change in disposition. In the dumb form this is followed by paralysis and death.

In furious rabies, the first symptoms are followed by excitement, with vicious attacks on other animals, violent butting and pawing of the ground and loud bellows in a weird tone of voice.

Rabid cattle may bite, but the tendency is not so pronounced as in the case of dogs. Loss of flesh is rapid. The animal becomes more quiet about the fourth day when paralysis starts. Death occurs not later than the sixth day.

Other animals—Rabid animals of all kinds attack other animals or people. Horses show signs of violent itching. One strange turn of the disease is that beasts try to eat dirt, stones, pieces of wood or other indigestible substances.

The loss of domestic animals bitten by rabid foxes has been large since 1939 in Southern and Southeastern states. "When an outbreak occurs in a community, fantastic things may happen," says Stanley P. Young of the United States Fish and Wildlife Service. "Foxes chase dogs and attack persons. The rabid animals may be found anywhere, in a farmyard or the middle of a town. One was killed on the second floor of a county courthouse."

Positive proof of rabies can be established by microscopic examination of a section of a dead animal's brain or spinal cord. Such examinations are made by public health authorities whenever possible. The matter is attended to by veterinarians and livestock sanitary officials. They should be called at once when rabies is suspected.

Prevention

Rabies has been completely wiped out in northern European countries, including Great Britain, Denmark, Sweden and Norway. The disease could be practically eradicated by enforcing a few simple precautions. They are:

1. Impounding or disposing of all stray dogs.

2. Muzzling all dogs in areas where the infection exists or is suspected.

3. Greater restraint of farm dogs, especially at night.

4. Enforcing strict quarantine measures over a wide area whenever the disease appears.

Public Health officials require vaccination of dogs in areas quarantined for rabies, and many cities require annual rabies vaccination of all dogs.

Treatment

Once the outward symptoms of rabies appear, there is no effective treatment. When a person is bitten by an animal suspected of having the disease, the Pasteur treatment should be given at once. Only 15 percent of the people exposed to rabies acquire it. But no one who has been bitten can afford to take a chance. An untreated person risks his life.

Farm animals respond to the Pasteur treatment, but it usually costs more than the animal is worth except where valuable purebred stock or family pets are involved. In experiments where animals have been purposely given the disease, some of the animals recovered of their own accord.

Tuberculosis

MANY ANIMALS are susceptible to tuberculosis. There are three kinds of tubercle bacilli. They are known as the human, bovine and avian. The principal reason tuberculosis is so hard to cure is that the microbes have a wax-like covering that protects them against destruction by certain of the white blood cells. The malady commonly ends with a slow wasting away of the tissues especially in old animals.

How the disease is spread

The disease is spread in feed, water and air. A cow with tuberculosis of the lungs may spread it as she drinks from a common trough. The discharge from her lungs comes into her mouth and she slobbers it into the water, which is drunk by other cattle. The microbes pass through their intestines unaltered and may remain alive in dung for a year. Thus pools, small streams and fodder are often contaminated.

Tuberculosis may attack almost any part of the body. In poultry, the liver and spleen are most often affected and the disease is spread largely through droppings. In other farm animals, tuberculosis of the lungs is most common, followed by infection of the udder. In the latter case, large numbers of the bacteria appear in the milk. A calf can get the malady by a single feeding on a tuberculous udder.

The incubation period of the disease is indefinite. The bacilli multiply so slowly that several months may elapse from the time of infection until a test indicates that the animal is diseased. Outward symptoms may not appear for years, so slow is the course of tuberculosis.

Symptoms

Usually the first noticeable symptom of the malady is loss of weight. When the lungs are affected, cattle develop a cough, but one strange thing is that the most heavily infected animals often seem to be in prime condition.

Often the first symptom of tuberculosis in poultry is lameness in the left leg, although both legs may be affected. Tuberculous birds have a ravenous appetite, yet derive no benefit from their feed. Their flesh wastes away. This can be noticed by feeling the breastbones. In the last stages of the disease a mature hen may weigh only a pound. Other symptoms are pale comb and wattles, swollen joints and diarrhea. Their eyes usually remain bright.

Since most swine are marketed before they are two years old, symptoms in them are seldom noticed. When older animals have tuberculosis, they gradually lose weight and condition and their joints become enlarged.

Susceptibility of various animals

Man and animals both show a marked difference in their resistance to the three kinds of tubercle bacilli.

Cattle are the principal victims of the bovine type. Only rarely do they become infected with human or avian tuberculosis. Horses and mules are resistant to all three types. Chickens are susceptible only to the avian type. Sheep and goats are practically immune to the disease.

Swine are susceptible to all three types. The bovine type causes the severest disease, but nine-tenths of swine infections are caused by the avian type.

Dogs may get human tuberculosis, but rarely acquire the bovine type and are immune to the avian form.

Man is, of course, susceptible to the human type. Ordinarily he is quite resistant to the bovine type, but with frequent exposure, such as daily drinking of unpasteurized milk from infected cows, he is likely to acquire the disease. Children are more susceptible than adults to tuberculosis. Infants have the least resistance of all.

One common type of bovine tuberculosis in humans is tuberculosis of the bone, especially of the vertebrae; and disappearance of the hunchback is a tribute to the eradication of tuberculosis in cattle.

Diagnosis

In many diseases, the body becomes allergic, or reacts to the poisons produced by that malady. In tuberculosis that is particularly true, and it is the basis of an extremely sensitive test used to determine its presence.

To obtain the poisons produced by tuberculosis, the microbes are first grown on a suitable culture medium. This is then filtered and processed to yield a clear fluid called *tuberculin*. It contains no living microbes and has no effect on animals free of tuberculosis.

When tuberculin is injected under the skin of an animal having tuberculosis, the injection is followed in a few hours by a fever which gradually subsides. If the injection is made into the skin, a red swelling appears at the spot between 24 and 72 hours later. If tuberculin is dropped in the eye, a milky discharge follows within a few hours.

Prevention

In 1917, one cow in every 20 was infected with tuberculosis. By 1950 this had been reduced to less than one cow in 200. The decrease was brought about through the efforts of the United States Bureau of Animal Industry, the state livestock sanitary officials and the livestock owners. The task entailed making over 300 million tuberculin tests and slaughtering more than four million animals.

Today the disease is rare but outbreaks are still possible. When an infected animal is found in a herd, the whole herd is quarantined and tested. Reactors are slaughtered. The herd is then retested every 60 days until no reactors are found. A final test is made six months thereafter.

Indemnity payments are made to the owner for the positive reactors that were slaughtered.

Swine—Except where pigs feed on infected udders, they do not contract tuberculosis from one another. They almost always acquire it by consuming feed contaminated by cattle, fowls and human beings. When these sources of infection are eliminated, tuberculosis among swine dies out. Tuberculin tests are applied mainly to purebred herds where hogs are kept beyond the usual slaughtering age.

Swine should not be permitted to mingle with poultry where the malady is present or suspected, nor eat the dung of infected cattle. They should not be fed milk from tuberculous cattle. Milk from unaccredited sources should be pasteurized.

Coccidiosis

COCCIDIOSIS is one of the most widespread diseases among farm animals. Only the horse is immune.

The ailment, also known as bloody scours or red diarrhea, causes major losses to poultry and serious losses of calves and lambs. The amount of damage done through stunted growth and the lowered production is enormous.

The microbes causing the disease are called *coccidia*. They are parasites and get into the body in food and water. There are many different kinds. All of them are specific in their action, that is, the ones that attack cattle will not affect fowls, and so on.

When *coccidia* get into the intestines in large enough numbers they multiply rapidly and invade the intestinal walls. If the infection doesn't kill an animal, the disease reaches a peak, or climax, and then dies out. The *coccidia* form what are called *oocysts*. These are discharged by the millions in the dung. After an animal becomes infected, it takes between one and three weeks before the oocysts appear in the dung. The larger the number of *coccidia* taken into the body at the time of infection, the more severe will be the disease, and of course the more oocysts will appear in the dung.

Outbreaks of coccidiosis appear often when cattle are crowded together. Groups of calves in feed lots are more susceptible than the same number in pastures. There are two reasons for this: overcrowding lowers the resistance of the animals, and it exposes them to large numbers of coccidia.

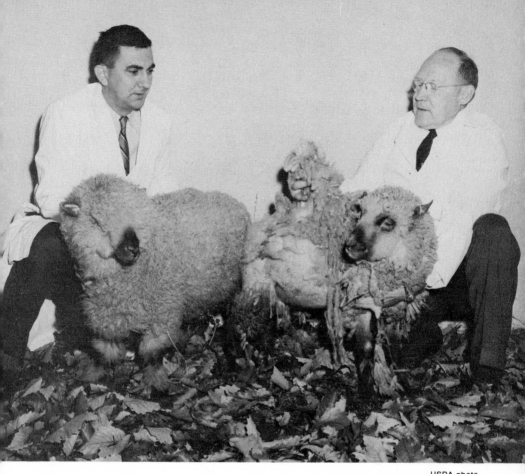

USDA parasitologists demonstrate "wool breaking" in sheep, a condition resulting from coccidiosis infection. The wool becomes thin as a result of the infection and is easily rubbed off the skin. All poultry and livestock are subject to coccidiosis infection

Symptoms

Coccidiosis thickens the wall of the intestines and thus reduces their ability to digest and absorb food. It causes inflammation and pin-point hemorrhages of the membrane.

Symptoms of the infection are bloody diarrhea, anemia, loss of weight and general weakness. Severe straining accompanies excretion, and dung is stringy and full of mucus. In calves, pneumonia often develops as a secondary infection. Delirium and nervous symptoms, such as twitching of the muscles, appear near the end of fatal attacks. Animals that do not die in the first two weeks of the illness may be expeced to recover.

Calves sometimes get a severe but non-fatal form of the malady in the second month of life. They have a non-bloody diarrhea that is often mistaken for the continuation of white scours.

Control

Coccidiosis is said to be born of filth, but it sometimes occurs under the most sanitary conditions, and where there is no crowding of animals.

It has been found almost impossible to raise cattle completely free of the disease. But since its severity depends largely upon the number of organisms that enter the intestines at the time of infection, cleanliness plays an important part in keeping down losses.

Under favorable conditions, it takes several days from the time the oocysts are discharged with the dung until the infective stage of the parasite develops. While still in the spore stage, the oocysts resist freezing and disinfectants, but are killed by sunlight, drying and putrefaction. Under moist conditions, particularly in manure, they will remain alive for a year or two.

It is of prime importance to prevent contamination of water and feed. Manure and contaminated bedding should be removed daily.

A number of procedures have been developed to reduce coccidiosis and other calf diseases. In the portable-pen system the calf is removed from the dam within 24 hours after birth and placed in a portable pen by itself. Moving the pens once a week prevents build-up of sporulated oocysts and thus allows light infections to induce immunity. A method of successfully starving the coccidia has been reported as follows:

As soon as diarrhea starts, withhold all energy feeds for 24 hours. Allow no milk, replacer, calf pellets, hay, or bedding. At the same time, let the calf suck a solution of one heaping teaspoon of table salt and one rounded teaspoon of sodium bicarbonate (baking soda) per gallon of water. Give up to three quarts at a time, four times daily. Parenteral vitamins, antibiotics, or intravenous fluid therapy can be given at the same time.

After 24 hours and at least an hour after the last feeding of the salt-bicarbonate solution, start to feed replacer or milk at a volume of not more than 2.5 percent of body weight per feeding four times daily, in the morning, at noon, in the evening, and at night. Follow this regimen for three or four days. At the resumption of milk feeding, begin therapy with an oral antidiarrheal medicine of proven efficacy. Your veterinarian can recommend one.

The young calf can live 24 hours without energy feeds but most bacteria in the gut wil be starved out during this time and washed out of the digestive tract.

Calves with diarrhea lose vital amounts of salt, carbonate, and water. Dehydration and acidosis result. The salt-bicarbonate solution counteracts the two conditions. The electrolyte solution is absorbed gradually and retained well by the system when given orally. Other, more sophiticated electrolyte solutions have advantages but lack on-the-farm availability.

Winter dysentery, or black scours

WINTER DYSENTERY, also known as infectious diarrhea, black scours and vibronic enteritis of calves, occurs among stabled cattle, chiefly from December to March.

The disease is usually mild and only rarely causes a death loss. Yet it causes heavy losses in milk production and rapid loss in condition. It affects principally cows, though calves are also attacked by it.

It generally apears by first attacking a few herds in the same neighborhood, then it often spreads until herds within several miles have been infected. Visiting stockmen presumably carry the microbes from one place to another on their shoes and clothing. Or movement of birds and dogs may spread the infection widely and quickly.

Symptoms

Winter dysentery usually appears suddenly, first affecting only a few cattle, then spreading rapidly until 50 to 100 percent of the adults and a smaller percentage of calves and young stock are affected.

The first symptom is a watery foul-smelling diarrhea which is usually brown but may be black. In severe cases the diarrhea may be tinged with blood. Temperature often remains normal but may go as high as 103 degrees Fahrenheit. Pulse and respiration are usually normal. Appetite and milk production fall off and in a few days affected animals acquire a gaunt apearance. The disease runs its course in from three days to a week. Scouring usually stops by the end of the third day.

Treatment

Several kinds of drenches are in use but none of them are very effective in reducing the course of the disease. Among them are catechu, zinc phenosulphenate and ferrous sulphate. These are used alone or in combination.

In severe cases, blood transfusions with salt, electrolytes and glucose have been effective. No vaccine or other immunizing agent has been developed.

Cattle mange

CATTLE MANGE, also called scab, scabies or barn itch, causes losses in the livestock industry by reducing the weight of animals, making calves unthrifty and lowering milk production of cows. It also brings about the death of animals by lowering their vitality so they can't resist other diseases. Cattle mange is caused by mites, of which there are four different kinds.

Mange may be confused with ringworm, X-disease, allergies or infections due to filth.

Sarcoptic scab or mange is the most severe form of scabies. The mites, called *Sarcoptes*, penetrate the outer layer of skin and create burrows, or galleries, where they mate and lay eggs. After this, the female dies in the burrow. Mites are mature two weeks after the eggs are laid.

The disease is more common in winter than in summer but may occur at any time, particularly in crowded stables where animals often come in contact with one another. Mites and eggs die in a few weeks when removed from animals.

Sarcoptic mange can be transmitted to other animals and to man. But each kind of animal has its own type of mite, and the type that thrives on cattle, for example, will soon die on swine.

Sarcoptic mites prefer places where the hair is thin and the skin tender. First symptoms are usually severe itching around the eyes, face and neck, but it may start elsewhere on the body. Animals affected continually rub themselves on stanchions or other rigid structures. Dandruff is abundant. Hair falls out. Scabs appear. After a few weeks, the skin becomes wrinkled and hangs in thick folds. It may become hard and leathery. If not treated, the mange will spread over the whole body.

Psoroptic mange, or common cattle scab, is caused by *Psoroptes*, small white or yellowish mites. When full grown, the males are about one-fiftieth of an inch long and the females a little longer.

These mites attack parts of the body where the hair is thick. They live on the surface of the skin. Each female lays 15 to 24 eggs which hatch in three or four days. The young reach maturity and start laying eggs when 10 to 12 days old. The life span is 30 to 40 days.

The first symptoms are itching around the withers, on top of the neck just in front of the withers, and at the base of the tail. If skin is scraped off at the infected areas with the blunt edge of a knife and the scrapings are put on a piece of black paper or cloth, the mites can be seen moving. Warm sunshine or other warmth will increase their movements so they can be more easily seen.

The mites puncture the skin and suck lymph. This sets up an inflammation and causes eruptions and crusts to form. The animal loses its hair on infected areas. If not treated, these areas become larger until the whole body is involved. In such cases the animal may die.

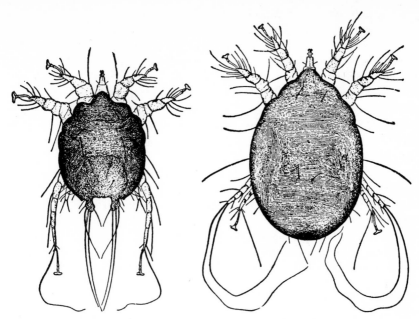

Male (left) and female psoroptic-mange mites, enlarged about 75 times

During its course, the ailment may seem to disappear in the summer, only to come back worse than ever the following winter.

Chorioptic, or *symbiotic*, scab attacks cattle occasionally but is of minor important. The *Chorioptes* can be seen under a high-powered magnifying glass and resemble those of common scab. They spread slowly, live on top of the skin, and usually attack the legs or tail. For purpose of treatment, the disease need not be distinguished from common scab.

Demodectic mange occurs in cattle, swine and horses but does very little damage. The mites enter the hair follicles and cause nodules or small lumps, principally on the shoulders, neck, or breast and dewlap. These lumps vary in size from a pinhead to a hazelnut. They finally break and discharge a thick pus.

The disease may progress rapidly until nodules appear all over the body or it may spread slowly with no apparent increase for several years. Chief damage is to the hides of older animals.

There is no known practical remedy for demodectic mange, although frequent clippings keep it from spreading.

Treatment

There are several effective treatments for sarcoptic, psoroptic and chorioptic mange. The use of lindane is preferred in treament of cattle mange but in states where its use is prohibited, lime-sulfur dips are most widely used. In treating dairy cattle, make sure that the drug you use is approved by the Food and Drug Administration.

Solutions are sprayed on, and when there are many animals, they are dipped. This is done by causing animals to swim through vats filled with the solution.

Spraying or dipping animals with these mange killers is done at six to 10-day intervals for sarcoptic scab and 10 to 12-day intervals for psoroptic scab. The first application kills the mites but not the eggs. The second kills the mites that have hatched in the meantime but before they are old enough to lay eggs.

Benzene hexachloride can be used on range cattle but is not good on dairy cows. It has a disagreeable odor which lasts for several days and contaminates milk. Lindane has practically no odor. It is a more highly refined form of benzene hexachloride. These products should be used as recommended by their manufacturers.

The leathery condition of the skin caused by mange may last for weeks after the parasites have been killed.

Screwworms and blowflies

PRIMARY SCREWWORMS eat the flesh of living animals and in this manner formerly caused tremendous livestock losses in southern and southwestern states. Cattle, sheep, hogs, horses, mules and dogs are attacked in about the order named.

The primary screwworm is the larval, or maggot, stage of a certain kind of blowfly. As adults these flies are bluish-green, with three dark stripes along the back between the wings and a yellowish-red face.

The flies choose the open wounds of warm-blooded animals as places to lay their eggs. In cattle these wounds are often caused by branding, castrating, dehorning, blood-sucking insects, cacti and barbed wire. Infestation of the navel cord of newborn animals is common.

The eggs are laid at the edges of wounds and are cemented in oval, shingle-like clusters. Each mass consists of 50 to 300 eggs. The flies lay eggs at four-day intervals and one female may lay 3,000 eggs.

The maggots emerge from the eggs in about 11 hours and at once burrow into the living flesh. Here they feed and grow for a period of four to seven days. In this short time the destruction of flesh is so great that a large percentage of infested animals die.

The maggots change skins twice while gorging themselves on the meat. When fully grown, they are pinkish in color and leave the wound and drop to the ground. They then dig into the earth, become inactive and turn into hard-skinned, dark-brown pupae. At the end of this stage, which lasts from seven to 60 days, the blowflies emerge and work their way to the surface.

The youngsters are grayish but assume their gaudy coloration in about five days. In warm weather the life cycle is completed in about 20 days. In cold weather the cycle may require nearly three months.

Primary blowflies, no matter which stage of the cycle they may be in, are killed by frost and when temperatures average below 50 degrees for as long as three months. This is why they seldom appear very far north. Now and then when weather conditions are unusually favorable, outbreaks of the pest have occurred as far north as Iowa, Illinois and Indiana. It is believed these outbreaks followed the shipment of infested animals from the South.

Blowflies that breed on dead animals

There are a number of other kinds of blowflies with practically the same life cycle as the one that requires living flesh, but these others lay their eggs on dead flesh. The maggots later attack living animals. Most of the important kinds have a metallic luster which varies from almost black, such as the wool-maggot fly, to the light green of the green-bottle species. The more harmful kinds are widespread over the continent. They do the most damage in the areas inhabited by the screwworm fly and in the Pacific Northwest.

How to control losses

Three measures can be used to prevent losses from screwworms: so far as possible, keep animals from getting wounds; treat wounds that do occur; kill screwworms that infest wounds.

Operations that cause wounds, such as castration, should be done during the winter whenever, possible. Blood-sucking flies and other insects should be controlled. Projecting boards and nails in stables, fences and corrals should be eliminated. Dogs should not be used for catching animals.

Treatment

Wounds that occur should be treated and covered until healed. The best treatment known was developed by the U.S. Department of Agriculture. It is called EQ-335.

To make EQ-335 add by weight 3 parts of lindane, 35 parts of pine oil, 42 of white mineral oil, 10 of an emulsifier, and 10 of silica gel. It is applied to wounds with a small paintbrush. The treatment kills maggots deep in the wounds, young maggots as they hatch from eggs, and flies attracted to the wound to feed or lay more eggs.

The active ingredient of EQ-335 is lindane. Any screwworm remedy that contains three to five percent lindane is effective against the pests. The area around the wound should be gently massaged so that the remedy will contact all larvae present. Use caution in treating young calves since they are susceptible to lindane. Always follow directions.

Killing less destructive blowflies

Since the less destructive blowflies breed principally in dead animals, control of them consists in burying carcasses and killing flies by insecticides, traps and poisoned baits.

Poisoned baits may be prepared by placing pieces of meat or the carcasses of small animals in shallow water containing one-half ounce of nicotine sulphate to the gallon in suitable containers exposed to the flies. The dead flies accumulate on the surface of the bait and it is necessary to remove them occasionally to obtain the best results. Care should be taken to prevent chickens, hogs and other animals from having acesss to the bait.

Sterile males help eradicate screwworms

A female screwworm fly mates only once and when this occurs with a sterile male, naturally the eggs won't hatch.

This fact underlies the highly successful screwworm eradication program, started in the 1950's, which has now practically wiped out the screwworm menace. The project, carried out jointly by the U.S.D.A. and the states, consists in sterilizing millions of screwworm flies by exposing them to gamma rays of Cobalt 60 and then distributing them over infested areas by plane. The sterile males greatly outnumber their native brethren and effectively compete in wooing the native females.

Unfortunately the areas along the Mexican border are periodically reinfested with the flies. Sterile flies are distributed along both sides of the border but strong south winds can blow unsterilized flies as far as 200 miles.

Veterinarians are lending their utmost cooperation in reporting immediately cases of suspected screwworm infestation.

Cattle grubs, or warbles

THE DAMAGE done by cattle grubs, commonly called warbles, is estimated at about 50 million dollars a year. The grubs come from eggs laid by heel flies. Infested animals do not gain weight as they should, milk production falls off, hides are damaged, and animals often injure themselves trying to escape from the flies.

The flies are large and sturdy-looking and resemble small bumble bees. Although they do not bite, they have a way of terrorizing cattle as they dart and buzz around. This often causes animals to stampede, and in so doing, cut themselves on barbed wire or otherwise injure themselves.

Heel flies usually lay their eggs just above the feet or on the bellies of cattle. The eggs are neatly attached to hairs, sometimes one to a hair, sometimes a string of eggs on one hair, depending upon which of the

COMMON CATTLE GRUB

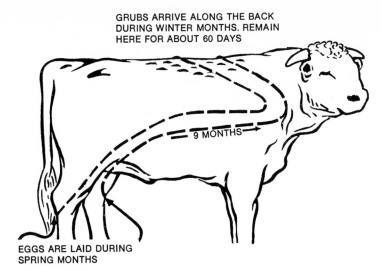

GRUBS ARRIVE ALONG THE BACK
DURING WINTER MONTHS. REMAIN
HERE FOR ABOUT 60 DAYS

9 MONTHS

EGGS ARE LAID DURING
SPRING MONTHS

Cattle grubs cause a great deal of economic damage. They are caused by large flies (see drawing below) which resemble bumble bees. The eggs are laid just above the feet or on the belly, and nine months later the grubs arrive on the animal's back, where they live for about 60 days and do considerable damage to the animal

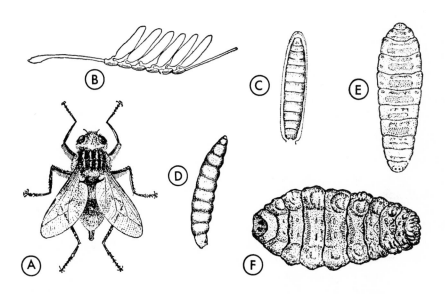

The heel or warble fly. A, adult female. B, eggs attached to hair. C, larva as seen in eggs. D, larva from gullet of cow. E, later stage of larva from beneath the hide of back. F, larva or warble at the stage when it leaves the back of cattle and falls to the ground

two kinds of heel fly is involved. The life cycle of these flies is about the same and so is the method for killing them.

The eggs hatch in a week or less and the tiny grubs that emerge burrow through the skin of an infested animal and enter the muscles. They then work their way upward until they reach the flesh on the animal's back. The trip takes from six to nine months.

When the grubs reach the back, they puncture a hole in the hide in order to breathe. In 35 to 60 days, when they are nearly one inch long, they force their way through the hide and drop to the ground.

About five weeks later—in the early spring—they become flies which may mate within an hour and are then ready to spend the rest of their short lives terrorizing their bovine victims. They have no mouth parts with which to eat so on an average they live only about a week.

While living in the backs of animals, grubs form painful swellings. The number of warbles per animal may run as high as 200. Calves become most heavily infested and the number becomes increasingly less as cattle grow older.

If you have a small herd, extract the grubs with a small instrument or by hand-squeezing. Try not to crush the grub under the skin. To do so can cause soreness and a severe reaction.

The skinned carcasses of cattle infested with warbles show greenish-yellow areas in the loins and the meat may be down-graded on inspection. Hides are sometimes made valueless by the pests.

Treatment

The pests can be killed by dusting the backs of the animals with 5 percent rotenone. This should be rubbed well into the hair with the hands or a brush. To contact all grubs, treatment should be repeated every four weeks or oftener during the warble season. Treatment should be started 25 days after the first warbles appear.

If a spray is preferred, proceed as follows:

Add 7½ pounds of 5 percent rotenone dust and 2 pounds of a wetting agent (Dreft, Vel, Swerl, etc.) to 100 gallons of water. Nozzle pressure should be 60 pounds or more—the higher, the better. Apply 1 gallon of spray per animal and repeat at 30-day intervals. (Do not spray directly into the eyes of an animal). Several other equally effective insecticides are available.

A newer method for controlling cattle grubs consists in adding a drug to the feed, thus killing the young grubs before they start their trip to an animal's back. Use of this method is prohibited in dairy herds.

Drugs of this kind should be used only in strict compliance with instructions by manufacturers.

The horn fly

HORN FLIES are about half the size of houseflies. They get their name because they gather in great numbers around the base of the horns of cattle. But they also feed on the backs, shoulders, withers and bellies.

They do a lot of damage because they are blood-suckers and breed in such large numbers. Experiments have shown that young cattle not preyed upon by horn flies gain an average of a half-pound more per day than cattle that are infested with them.

Horn flies spend the winter in the resting or pupal stage in or under cattle dung. They emerge in the spring as flies and spend all of their time on cattle except when mating. A female fly lives about seven weeks and lays 400 eggs. In the North, the flies remain active until killed by frost.

Since horn flies live almost continuously on their hosts, they are easily controlled. Malathion, methoxychlor, toxaphene, and ronnel are excellent sprays for beef cattle.

To avoid residues in milk, the only sprays permitted on dairy cattle are dichlorvos, crotozyphos and coumaphos. These are mixed with oil. When dust sprays are used great care must be taken to avoid contaminating milk.

Horn flies can also be controlled through use of "back rubbers," available in stores. These consist of bags saturated with oil-base insecticides suspended between two posts in such a way that cattle rub their backs against them.

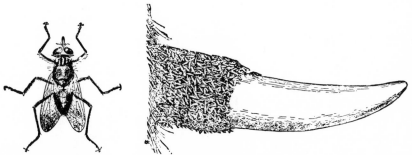

Horn flies suck the blood of farm animals and annoy them so they don't eat properly. This lowers meat production an estimated ten million dollars a year

Cattle lice

FOUR kinds of lice infest cattle. Three of them suck the blood of animals, the other bites off pieces of skin for food or eats particles of hair and scales. They all cause itching and result in lowered milk production.

Two species of the lice that suck blood commonly are called "blue lice," while the one that bites is known as the "red louse." The life history of these pests is practically the same. The eggs or "nits" are firmly attached to the hairs and hatch in from 5 to 18 days.

The number of lice infesting cattle increases slowly during the fall months and much more rapidly during the winter and spring. If animals are not treated, they sometimes become covered with lice and their eggs before hot weather comes. Then the number of lice begins to decline. But some lice remain through the summer and again start to increase with the coming of cooler weather.

The presence of lice sometimes goes unnoticed until they have become firmly established. This is particularly true of young stock. But even in small numbers, red lice loosen hair so it can be pulled out in bunches. These biting lice usually are found first on the withers or around the root of the tail. When present in large numbers, they form colonies that may be as much as five inches in diameter, and produce a raw-skin condition that resembles scab.

Since sucking lice live on blood, a large number of them often cause anemia among cattle. Lousy cows produce 10 to 15 percent less milk than they would otherwise.

Treatment

Cattle lice can be killed by dusting, spraying or dipping. Dusting is best in cold weather. Treatments should be given in the fall before the lice become numerous and repeated in 16 or 18 days if necessary.

Treatments for lice are the same as those for horn flies as discussed in preceding chapter.

Lungworm disease of cattle

THE LUNGWORMS that attack cattle are white, threadlike and between two and three inches long. While in the body of an animal, they live principally in the small and medium-sized bronchial tubes—air passages in the lungs. They attack calves more often than older animals.

Female lungworms produce eggs that usually hatch in these air passages. The resulting larvae are coughed into the mouth and then swallowed by the animals. Unhatched eggs are also coughed up and

Life cycle of the lungworm

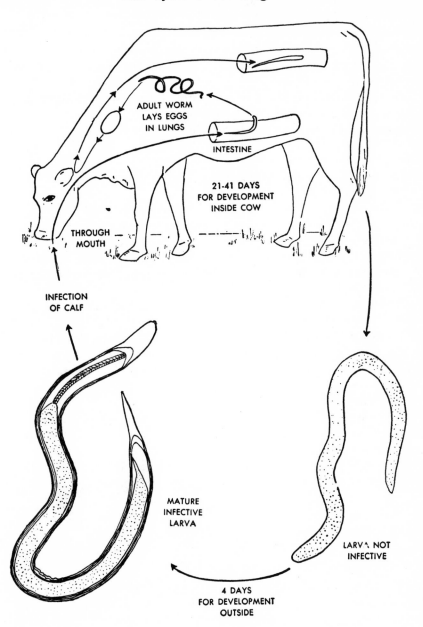

ADULT WORM
LAYS EGGS
IN LUNGS

INTESTINE

21-41 DAYS
FOR DEVELOPMENT
INSIDE COW

THROUGH
MOUTH

INFECTION
OF CALF

MATURE
INFECTIVE
LARVA

LARVA NOT
INFECTIVE

4 DAYS
FOR DEVELOPMENT
OUTSIDE

swallowed, sometimes to hatch in the stomach and sometimes not. The larvae and remaining unhatched eggs are eliminated in the dung.

When conditions are favorable, in four days to a week the parasites reach a third stage of development in which they are infective. In this stage they contaminate grass and infect cattle. They can also be spread through hay and drinking water.

Upon reaching the intestines, lungworms burrow through the walls and reach the lungs by way of the lymph glands and blood stream. They may live in the lungs as long as four months, producing eggs and inflammation, before they die.

Lungworm disease occurs when weather is mild. In the South it may occur the year around. In the North it may start when calves are first turned to pasture and reach its height in July and August.

Symptoms

In light cases of lungworm disease, the only symptoms may be an occasional dry cough and poor condition. In severe cases animals cough often, breathe with difficulty and become weaker and weaker as the disease progresses. Frothy phlegm drivels from the mouth. When the lungs are heavily involved, shallow breathing, lowered head and protruding tongue occur. Pneumonia and other secondary diseases often follow.

Diarrhea may develop when larvae penetrate the intestines in large numbers.

The larvae of lungworms can usually be found in the droppings of infected cattle. When they cannot, laboratory methods are often employed. One of these is called the "flotation method." It consists in putting dung in a solution of zinc sulphate. Under proper conditions, the lungworms float while the rest of the substance settles to the bottom.

Control and treatment

Since lungworms are generally expelled of their own accord, further treatment is often unnecessary. Vaccination against the disease is practiced in some European countries.

A number of drugs are available for treatment of the disease. Perhaps the most widely used are methyridine and tetramisole.

Stomach and intestinal worms of cattle

THREE KINDS OF ROUNDWORMS commonly infest the abomasum, or fourth stomach, of cattle. One of them is the *Haemonchus contortus*, often called the large stomach worm or twisted wire worm. Another is the *Ostertagia ostertagi* or lesser stomach worm, and the third is the *Trichostrongylus axei*.

Cattle stomach worms occur most often among young stock, although occasionally animals up to three years old are affected. Most cases appear in the fall and winter.

The large stomach worm

The large stomach worm of cattle is the same kind that affects sheep. It is one-half to three-fourths of an inch long and about as thick as an ordinary pin. Its life history is described under *Internal parasites of sheep*.

Symptoms of large-stomach-worm disease are loss of condition, weakness and anemia. The anemia, which is caused by the blood-sucking habit of the worms, is evident from paleness of skin and membranes of the mouth and eyes, and by a watery swelling of the underjaw. This so-called edema of the jaw is especially noticeable after an affected animal has had strenuous exercise.

The lesser stomach worm

Ostertagia ostertagi is a hairlike worm a little more than one-quarter inch long. It attacks cattle and sometimes sheep. Its life history is like that of the large stomach worm.

These small worms burrow into the lining of the stomach, causing small lumps, or nodules. These lumps appear as small white patches. Since the worms are bloodsuckers, small clots of blood may be present.

Deaths may occur in outbreaks among yearlings. Principal symptoms are loss of condition, anemia, rough coat, watery diarrhea and bottle jaw. Temperature is generally normal, appetite is normal, but thirst is greater than normal.

Trichostrongyles

The worm called *Trichostrongylus axei*, or minute stomach worm, is very slender and one-fifth of an inch or less in length. Little is known of its life cycle. It occurs in the stomach and sometimes in the small intestine of cattle. It also affects sheep and horses.

This worm often produces severe gastroenteritis, that is, inflammation of the stomach and intestines. Principal symptoms are diarrhea, loss of condition and a thickened stomach lining that is thrown into folds.

Diagnosis usually depends upon microscopic examination of scrapings from the stomach lining.

Treatment for stomach worms

A great many drugs are available for combatting stomach worms. Among those in wide use are thiabendazole and levamisole Phenothiazine is in wide use but is less effective than some of the newer preparations.

In giving drugs the instructions of manufacturers should be followed exactly. Toxic reactions to it are not common and seldom serious. Nevertheless animals under treatment should be watched for unfavorable reactions.

Sometimes temporary blindness occurs following use of the drug. In such cases affected animals should be kept in a darkened stable, or at least in dense shade, until they recover. Constipation frequently follows the use of phenothiazine in which case a laxative should be given. The temporary red color of the animal's urine does no harm.

The life cycle of intestinal worms is similar to that of stomach worms. The symptoms are also similar, except that some intestinal worms are not bloodsuckers and so do not cause anemia.

Treatment for intestinal worms

Phenothiazine is effective against the nodular worm, *Oesophagostomum radiatum*, found in the intestine and cecum. It is also somewhat effective against hookworms, but it has not proved effective in the treatment of *Cooperia*, whipworms, threadworms and tapeworms, al of which may be found in the intestines.

Many drugs to combat intestinal worms are in use but due to the number of organisms involved none are perfect. Among those used most widely are the organophosphates such as Coumaphos and Haloxon. Lead arsenate and niclosamide are effective against tapeworms in cattle and sheep.

Prevention of worm diseases

Worm diseases can be largely if not completely prevented by using certain precautions. These include good feeding, using only well-drained pastures, supplying drinking water from wells or flowing streams (preferably in troughs that are raised above the ground) and separation of young and old animals. Damp places should be fenced off. Hay and grain should be fed from racks and troughs, not from the ground. Pastures should be rotated as much as possible and should not be overstocked. Pastures that can't be drained should be used only for mature cattle.

Urinary calculi

URINARY CALCULI in animals are the same as kidney stones in people. They are formed mostly from calcium and magnesium salts. They affect all kinds of animals but are most common among cattle and sheep. Hogs are seldom affected.

Males are much more often affected than females and castrated animals are said to be particularly susceptible. Greatest losses occur on the range and in feed lots.

Urinary calculi are believed to be the result of faulty metabolism and nutrition but their exact cause is unknown. The technical name for the disease is urolithiasis.

Symptoms

A calculus may cause no apparent discomfort in an animal so long as they remain in the bladder or are small enough to pass readily through the urethra. But serious symptoms and death occur when one or more of them obstruct the passage of urine. In such cases the first symptoms are frequent attempts on the part of the animal to urinate, dribbling or stoppage of urine and restlessness.

In cattle, kicking at the belly, winding the tail and backing up are common symptoms. Later, an affected animal acquires a characteristic straddling gait.

Unless the obstruction is removed, the urine generally breaks through the bladder wall and accumulates in the abdomen, forming what is called "water belly." Less often the urine breaks through the wall of the urethra and forms a large swelling between the scrotum and the sheath.

Treatment

By the time symptoms of urinary calculi are observed, obstruction is so far advanced that only a surgical operation can restore an animal to normal life. Removal of the calculi requires skill and such an operation is often unsatisfactory. In steers and wethers an opening is often made in the urethra above the point of obstruction. This lets the urine drain out and allows time for the animal to recover and improve in condition before slaughter. Where blocking of the urethra is incomplete and urine still dribbles, many cases will respond to treatment consisting in half-ounces doses of ammonium chloride given three times a day.

Prevention

Various investigators have reported trouble that seemed to be associated with certain feeds. Sorghum feeds, both grain and fodder, have been blamed. Such reports have come from Nebraska and Texas and other States in the Great Plains. Wheat bran has been blamed. Alfalfa hay, corn, barley and beet tops generally have not caused difficulty.

Vitamin A deficiency has been suspected as responsible for calculi formation. Laboratory tests on rats have shown that certain diets lacking vitamin A may produce calculi. In cattle and sheep, however, there is little evidence of any association of vitamin A or carotene intake with occurrence of water belly.

Ammonium chloride was first tried as a means of reducing alkalinity in mink feeds and has become a practical means of keeping down calculi in those animals. Apparently it is just as effective in ruminants as in non-ruminants.

Insufficient water to drink tends to produce the trouble, as the urine is then much more concentrated, and solids are more apt to separate out. Therefore it is important that the animals have access at all times to a good supply of water. Salt should also always be available, as animals tend to drink more when they have plenty of salt.

Mad itch, or pseudorabies

MAD ITCH, also called pseudorabies and Aujeszky's disease, is a comparatively rare, infectious ailment caused by a filtrable virus. Cattle and swine are susceptible.

The first symptom is intense itching. Animals lick their thighs and buttocks until they are cleaned of hair. As the disease progresses, they rub themselves against posts, barbed wire or anything solid or rigid. There is usually drooling. Death occurs in 12 to 48 hours in nearly all cases. The disease in swine is mild but it is definitely known that they act as carriers.

The manner in which mad itch is spread is not known. It also affects rats but they do not act as carriers as was formerly believed. Outbreaks among cattle and sheep are halted when they are separated from hogs.

Q fever

THE DISEASE known as Q fever is principally an occupational disease of man. Cattle, sheep, goats, and turkeys act as carriers. Although anyone coming in contact with infected animals may acquire it, the disease occurs principally among persons concerned with the slaughter and handling of livestock. It can also be acquired through drinking raw milk of infected cows or goats.

Q fever is caused by an organism called *Coxiella burnetii*, a rickettsia which occupies the position between the viruses and bacteria. It causes no observable symptoms in animals but the presence of the disease can be determined by laboratory tests both in animals and in man.

Dairy cattle and sheep are highly susceptible. The disease is spread principally through dust containing pulverized dung from infected animals. The organism is abundantly present in the afterbirth of infected sheep.

Symptoms

The infection resembles that of mild influenza. Fever is present but there is no rash, as is the case with other rickettsial diseases such as typhus, Rocky Mountain spotted fever and trench fever. Outbreaks have occurred in southern California, Chicago and Texas.

Treatment of Q fever is a medical problem. The drug used is tetracycline.

Pinkeye, or infectious keratitis

PINKEYE, or infectious keratitis, is a contagious eye disease of cattle. It causes practically no deaths but results in general inefficiency of animals as producers of food. It may spread through an entire herd.

Animals of all ages are susceptible but those less than two years old are principally affected. Symptoms usually include sensitivity to light, weakened eyesight, watery eyes and swelling of the lids. Either or both eyes may be affected. The eyeballs may become covered with a white film. Animals may bellow with pain.

Cattle with the disease should be kept in dark stalls if possible. Since flies may spread the ailment, they should be kept away from the animals.

Treatment

Several antiseptics are used in treating the malady. A 1-percent solution of silver nitrate is often used as an eye lotion. It should be applied without rubbing every other day with a piece of cotton, until improvement is noted; then every third or fourth day until the animal is cured. The solution should be fresh, since it deteriorates.

Pinkeye is commonly treated with penicillin, chloramphenicol, tetracycline or mitrofurazone. Treatment should be started early to be effective.

Ringworm

RINGWORM is a disease of the skin. It is caused by a fungus and can be transmitted from one animal to another on halters or by other direct or indirect means of contact. Man may also become infected.

The disease can usually be cured by applying tincture of iodine about every three to seven days. Before applying the iodine, scrub the affected parts thoroughly with mild soap and warm water. This is done to remove scabs and loose skin so that the iodine can reach the fungus that may be underneath. For ringworm in horses, shave the area and apply tincture of iodine twice a day for two weeks.

Other medicines, applied in the same way to cure the disease, are an alcoholic solution of salicylic acid, or a 20 percent solution of sodium-caprylate.

Strict cleanliness and good grooming will usually prevent ringworm and other skin diseases. Applying whitewash to stables and caustic soda to grooming brushes and harness helps to destroy the source of infection.

Ringworm can be controlled with good sanitary procedures and medical treatment

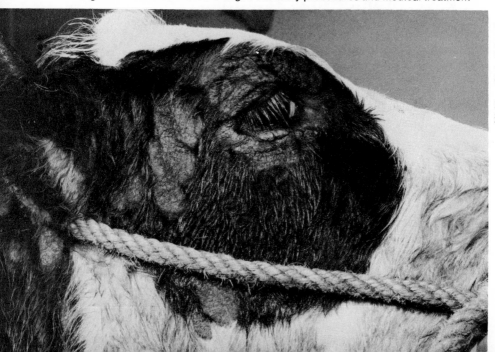

Michigan State University

Common warts

WARTS ON CATTLE may reduce the value of hides 25 percent or more. Warts vary greatly in size and there are two kinds, soft and hard. The large ones are usually soft, resemble cauliflowers, and often bleed and slough off. Also, they frequently have an offensive odor.

Experiments have shown that warts are infectious. The cause is a filtrable virus. In view of this, they should be done away with to stop them from spreading. Warts sometimes disappear of their own accord. Young animals especially are apt to lose them when they grow up.

Small warts can be removed by clipping them off with scissors or by tying a strong thread tightly around the base of the wart and leaving the thread there for a few days. The wart then sloughs off.

Tying-off is also considered best for removing large warts that contain blood vessels, since cutting in such cases often results in excessive bleeding. Scissors or thread should be sterilized before using. Tincture of iodine will serve for this purpose. The stumps of warts should be touched with either glacial acetic acid or with tincture of iodine.

When an animal has many warts that cover a large area of the body, special vaccines are often injected. These are prepared by manufacturers from the virus that causes warts.

The spread of warts can be controlled by removing all warty animals from a herd. Stables, pens, chutes and rubbing posts used by them should then be disinfected.

If treatment for warts is begun when they are small, it may not be necessary to cut them off. They may be destroyed by daily applications of glacial acetic acid or tincture of iodine. Before the acid is applied, the healthy skin surrounding the wart should be greased thoroughly with petrolatum or lard. Care should be taken, of course, not to apply the grease to the wart itself, otherwise the acid will not come in contact with it.

Small warts on the udders of cows will sometimes disappear if kept soft by applying castor oil or sweet oil after each milking.

Cowpox—true and false

TRUE COWPOX seldom occurs in the United States. When it does, it can almost always be traced to a person who has recently been vaccinated against smallpox and has infected the cow with smallpox virus, presumably during the act of milking.

However, there is another disease whose symptoms are similar to those of true cowpox but which is caused by an entirely different organism. This disease occurs fairly often and is commonly called false cowpox or pseudo-cowpox. Presumably it is caused by *Actinomyces*, an organism closely related to the one that causes foot rot, but there is some evidence that a virus may also be present.

Symptoms

False cowpox occurs most often in the spring. Once it gets started, it has a way of sweeping through a herd until nearly every cow has been infected.

The pox usually occur only on the teats and udder and at first appear as small red pimples or swellings. These develop into blisters which may be broken during milking and leave raw tender areas that may become infected with bacteria. If undisturbed, pus forms within the blisters. This shortly dries up and a scab forms which later falls off.

Here's the difference between true and false cowpox: In true cowpox, the area surrounding the pox is inflamed and the disease leaves pits or so-called pock marks. This is not the case with false cowpox.

Control

Animals can be vaccinated against cowpox but the disease is usually not sufficiently prevalent or serious to justify the expense. Infected animals should be isolated at once. There is no effective treatment available but spread is greatly reduced by milking the infected cows last.

Brisket disease

BRISKET DISEASE is brought on by high altitudes where the thinness of the air taxes the heart of an animal and causes it to get larger. The blood doesn't get the normal amount of oxygen, so the heart pumps more blood to make up the difference.

Symptoms are dullness, diarrhea, loss of appetite and weight, increase in heart beat and fast breathing. Palpitation of the heart, coughing and nosebleed appear upon exercise. Later, a swelling appears in the region of the throat and brisket. This may extend to the limb and lower part of the abdomen. Death may come in two weeks to three months. Calves may die without swellings.

Animals recover when brought to lower altitudes.

X-disease, or hyperkeratosis

X-DISEASE, or hyperkeratosis, is a malady of cattle that is often fatal—particularly to young calves. Once the disease is well on its course, there is little hope of curing it, though some animals recover.

Symptoms

First symptoms of the disease are reddeing of the mouth parts, excessive shedding of tears, slobbering, licking into the nostrils and loss of appetite. Wartlike growths appear on the tongue, dental pad and cheek. These symptoms are followed by depression and progressive thickening of the skin.

The skin changes occur over the withers, on the sides of the neck, on the cheeks, and back of shoulders. The hair is lost and the skin becomes dry, leathery and deeply creased. Diarrhea is sometimes present, most commonly late in the course of the disease when the animal is almost dead.

Pregnant cows with the disease often abort or drop calves prematurely. The disease may continue several weeks to three months or more before a severely affected animal finally dies.

Cause of the disease

The disease is caused by highly chlorinated naphthalene, a manufactured wax used in certain lubricants. This chemical is used to lend body to greases and oils used under heavy pressures and at high temperatures.

Until the cause of X-disease was determined greases and oils containing highly chlorinated naphthalene were widely used to grease pellet machines and other machinery used to process and harvest livestock feeds. Thus they found their way into the stomachs of cattle and may still do so unless precautions are taken.

Prevention

Cattle owners can prevent the occurrence of the disease by observing the following:

1. Keep cattle away from machinery so they canot lick or come in contact with oil or grease that might contain highly chlorinated naphthalene.

2. Fence off drain pits for oil or places where crankcase oil is dumped.

3. If used motor oil is employed in devices against which cattle rub to oil themselves, care should be taken not to use "break-in" oil from new motors or oil from vehicles in which a cylinder lubricant has been added to the gasoline.

Acorn calves

AN "ACORN" CALF is one that is born deformed because of certain improper feeds. The head of such a calf may be short, usually with an undershot jaw, or it may be long and narrow. Usually the long bones of both fore and hind legs are noticeably short.

Victims of the ailment are often unable to stand alone, suffer from incoordination, may have arched backs and frequently have a chronic tendency to bloat. The last malady is often fatal to calves that have been weaned. Symptoms that occur less often are twitching of the muscles, turning in circles and falling over backwards.

Acorn calves occur frequently in the Sierra Nevada foothills, in dry years. They differ from bulldog calves found in Dexter cattle in that bulldog calves are born dead whereas acorn calves are born alive and with good care reach adult life. The acorn condition is not hereditary whereas bulldog condition is.

The malady is not caused primarily by eating acorns as was formerly supposed. The exact cause is not known but experiments indicate that it is due to lack of vitamins A and D. These can be supplied by supplementary feeding of pregnant dams with legumes, high grade leafy hay of current year's crop, good quality silage or new high-grade alfalfa meal or by feeding vitamin supplements in grain or in range pellets.

Although acorns are not the principal cause of acorn calves, they may be partly responsible for it. One authority believes that the tannic acid in the acorns may destroy some essential in the diet or prevent its formation from other feeds.

Plants that poison livestock

MORE THAN 40 plants are known to be poisonous to livestock. Losses caused by eating them occur most often in the western range country. There are fewer poisonous plants in the East because plowing of the land has kept them in check.

For most kinds of plant poisoning there is no effective remedy. Prevention consists in destroying the poisonous plants or keeping animals from eating them. A number of poisons in these plants have been identified.

Hydrocyanic acid poisoning

Hydrocyanic acid, also known as prussic acid, develops under certain circumstances in a number of plants, including the wild chokeberry, wild black cherry, sorghum, Sudan grass, Johnson grass, wild flax, arrow-grass, wild lima beans and California desert almond.

Normally the sorghums, including Sudan and Johnson grass, are good feed. The acid develops when the growth of the plants has been retarded or stopped by drought, frost, bruising, trampling, wilting or mowing. It may develop in Sudan grass hay that gets wet in the stack or in the mow.

Symptoms of hydrocyanic acid poisoning include a brief period of stimulation followed by depression and paralysis. Stupor, difficult breathing and frequent convulsions result from action of the poison on the brain centers that control breathing.

Hydrocyanic acid often kills animals in a few minutes, although sometimes an animal may live several hours after symptoms first appear. Where there is still a chance for recovery, the U.S. Department of Agriculture suggests the injection of methylene blue, sodium nitrate, or sodium thiosulphate, preferably into the veins. Another treatment consists in the injection of a combination of sodium nitrate and sodium thiosulphate. For cattle, two to three grams of sodium nitrate in water followed by four to six grams of sodium thiosulphate in water has been found effective.

For sheep, up to one gram of sodium nitrate and two to three grams of sodium thiosulphate are recommended. This treatment may be supplemented by other measures such as injections of atropine, inhalation of ammonia or injections of glucose.

Other plant poisons

Alkaloids, such as morphine and strychnine, occur at times in larkspurs and certain lupines, such as bluebonnets.

Saponins are irritant poisons which cause vomiting. They are found in bitter rubberweed, pingue, corncockle seeds, bullnettle and bittersweet.

Resinoids are found in various plants and some of them are very poisonous. Among them are a few of the milkweeds, rhododendrons, azaleas and water hemlock, said to be the most poisonous plant in the United States.

Oxalic acid is contained in greasewood to the extent of being poisonous to livestock and harmful amounts have been reported when sugar beet tops are pastured after wilting.

Important facts about the principal poisonous plants

From *A Pasture Handbook*, U. S. Dept. Agr. Misc. Pub. 194.

Common and scientific names of plant	Location	Parts of plant that usually cause poisoning	Animals most commonly poisoned	Conditions under which poisoning usually occurs, and minimum quantity required	Characteristic effects
Arrowgrass (*Triglochin maritima* L.)	Salt or alkaline marshes and wet places throughout the United States	Leaves and stems	Cattle and sheep	Eating about 1 percent of animal's weight of green plants in a few minutes	Difficult breathing, spasms, coma, illness of short duration
Aster, Parry (*Aster parryi* A. Gray)	Dry flats of Wyoming	Leaves and Stems	Sheep	Eating 125 pounds of green plants in a day when animals are hungry	Weakness, prostration, rapid weak pulse, increased urination, and cyanosis
Azalea, western (*Rhododendron occidentale* (Torr. and Gray) Gray)	Moist places in Coast Range and Sierra Nevada Mountains of California	Leaves	Sheep	Eating a few ounces of leaves	Salivation, vomiting, and weakness
Baccharis (*Baccharis ramulrosa* (DC.) A. Gray)	Hillsides of western Texas and southern New Mexico and Arizona	Leaves	Cattle	Scarcity of feed in fall and early winter	Extreme prostration, severe inflammation of stomach
Black laurel (*Leucothoe davisiae* Torr.)	Springy ground in Sierra Nevada Mountains of California	Leaves	Sheep	Eating 0.2 pound in a day's feeding	Salivation, vomiting, weakness
Bracken (*Pteridium* sp.)	Thickets, hills, and rich woods throughout the United States	Fronds	Horses and cattle	Eating 5 pounds daily for about a month	Horses: lack of control of legs, weakness. Cattle: hemorrhages in various parts of body
Cherry, wild (*Prunus* sp.)	Hillsides, along streams, in woods throughout the United States	Leaves	Sheep and cattle	Eating 1 percent of animal's weight of green plants in a few minutes	Difficult breathing, spasms, coma, illness of short duration
Cocklebur (*Xanthium* sp.)	In fields and waste land of the eastern half and low wet places of the western half of the U.S.	First or primary leaves of seedlings	Pigs and cattle	Eating 0.75 percent of animal's weight of green plants in a few minutes	Prostration, inflamed stomach
Copperweed (*Oxytenia acerosa* Nutt.)	Colorado Basin in Colorado, Utah, and New Mexico to southern Calif.	Leaves	Cattle and sheep	Eating the plant in the fall when other feed is scarce	Loss of appetite, depression, weakness, and coma
Deathcamas (*Zygadenus* sp.)	Gravelly hills, depressions, and meadows in western half of the United States	Leaves and stems	Sheep and cattle	Eating 0.5 percent of animal's weight of green plants in a day	Vomiting, frothing and weakness
Drymary, thickleaf (*Drymaria holosteoides* Benth. *D. pachyphylla* Wooten and Standley)	Denuded areas in western Texas and southern New Mexico	Leaves and stems	Cattle	Eating 0.5 percent of animal's weight of green plants in a day	Depression, weakness, inflamed stomach and intestines

Important facts about the principal poisonous plants—*Continued*

Common and scientific names of plant	Location	Parts of plant that usually cause poisoning	Animals most commonly poisoned	Conditions under which poisoning usually occurs, and minimum quantity required	Characteristic effects
Dutchmans-breeches (*Dicentra cucullaria* (L.) Bernh.)	In woods, eastern half of United States north of Georgia	Leaves and stems	Cattle	Feeding on plant, particularly in spring and early summer	Trembling, frothing at the mouth, and convulsions
Greasewood (*Sarcobatus vermiculatus* (Hook.) Torr.)	Somewhat alkaline fields in western part of the United States	Leaves	Sheep	Eating 1.5 pounds in a few minutes	Depression, kidney lesions
Horsebrush (*Tetradymia glabrata* Gray; *T. canascens* DC.)	Principally in Utah, Nevada, and eastern Calif.	Leaves and small stems	Sheep	Usually eaten by hungry animals while being trailed	May cause bighead as the result of sensitization to light
Horsetail (*Equisetum* sp.)	Wet meadows throughout United States	Tops	Horses	Eating the plant in hay	Weakness, craving for the plant, diarrhea, loss of flesh, lack of control of legs
Larkspur (*Delphinium* spp.)	Mountains and plains throughout United States	Leaves of young plants	Cattle	Eating 0.5 percent of animal's weight, especially of young plants, within a few minutes	Weakness, trembling, constipation
Laurel, sheep (*Kalmia angustifolia* L.)	Moist soil, hillsides, and swamps, Maine and New York to Georgia	Leaves	Cattle, sheep and goats	Eating 0.2 percent of animal's weight of green plants in a day	Salivation, vomiting, and weakness
Locoweed (*Astragalus* sp[1]; *Oxytropis* sp.)	Plains and some mountain valleys, western half of United States	Leaves and stems	Cattle, horses, sheep, goats	Feeding for several days or weeks on the plants	Constipation, craving for the plant, rough coat, incoordination and peculiar actions
Lupine (*Lupinus* sp.)	Throughout United States	Leaves of young plants, and fruit	Sheep and cattle	Eating 0.5 percent of animal's weight of green plants or fruit in a day	Sheep: nervousness from some species, depression from others. Cattle: weakness and trembling
Milkweed (*Asclepias labriformis* M. E. Jones)	Southeastern Utah	Leaves	Sheep and cattle	Eaten by hungry animals often during the fall and winter	Weakness, shallow respiration, spasms, violent struggling
Milkweed, broadleaf (*A. eriocarpa* Benth.; *A. latifolia* (Torr.) Raf.)	*A. eriocarpa:* dry valleys in southern half of California. *A. latifolia:* dry plains of Southwest; along ditches, in abandoned fields and dry places, Colorado to Mexico and California	Leaves	Sheep	Eating 0.1 percent of animal's weight of green plants in a day	Depression, weakness, inflamed stomach and intestines

Important facts about the principal poisonous plants —Continued

Common and scientific names of plant	Location	Parts of plant that usually cause poisoning	Animals most commonly poisoned	Conditions under which poisoning usually occurs, and minimum quantity required	Characteristic effects
Milkweed, whorled (A. gallioides H.B.K.; A. mexicana Cav.)	Dry plains and foothills—A. gallioides: Kansas to Utah and south to Texas, Arizona, and Mexico; A. mexicana: Southern Mexico northward to Washington, Idaho, Utah, and Arizona	Leaves and stems	Cattle and sheep	Eating 0.2 percent of animal's weight of green plants in a day	Incoordination followed by severe spasms
Mountain-laurel (Kalmia latifolia L.)	Woods and hillsides	Leaves	Cattle, sheep and goats	Eating 0.4 percent of animal's weight of green plants in a day	Salivation, vomiting, and weakness
Nightshade, black (Solanum nigrum L.)	Waste ground from Maine to California	Green fruit and leaves	Cattle, sheep, goats, chickens, ducks and geese	Feeding on green plant	Thirst, diarrhea, loss of appetite, weakness, lack of coordination
Oaks, shin and Gambel (Quercus spp.)	Sand hills and lower mountains of Colorado, Utah, and Southwest	Leaves and leaf buds	Cattle	Feeding largely on oak for 2 weeks or more, especially in spring	Emaciation, scabby nose, constipation, followed by diarrhea and weakness
Oleander, common (Nerium oleander L.)	Fields, roadsides, edge of woods in southern part of United States	Leaves	All animals	Eating small quantities	Stupor, trembling, convulsions, paralysis, vomiting, and diarrhea
Paperflower, greenstem (Psilostrophe sparsiflora (A. Gray) A. Nels.)	Northern Arizona and southern Utah	Leaves and flowers	Sheep	Eaten during the early spring or late fall when other feed is scarce	Depression, weakness, emaciation
Peganum, Harmel (Peganum harmala L.)	Texas and New Mexico	Fruits, leaves and stems	Sheep and cattle	Scarcity of desirable feed	Nervousness, incoordination, and paralysis
Poisonbean (Daubentonia drummondii Rydb.)	Coastal plains of Florida and Texas	Seeds	Cattle, sheep and goats	Eating small quantities of seeds	Depression, diarrhea, and rapid pulse
Poisonhemlock (Conium maculatum L.)	Widely distributed	Fruits and leaves	Sheep and cattle	Seldom eaten when other feed is available	Nervous tremors, weakness, and respiratory paralysis
Poisonvetch (Astragalus spp.)	Mountains, foothills, and valleys of Intermountain States	Leaves and stems	Cattle and sheep	Eating considerable quantities during a day's feeding	Difficult breathing, nausea, and weakness
Ragwort, or groundsel (Senecio spp.)	Throughout United States	Leaves and stems	Cattle and horses	Feeding for several days on one of the poisonous species	Jaundice, scabby nose, discomfort, loss of appetite, uneasiness, and loss of flesh

Important facts about the principal poisonous plants—*Continued*

Common and scientific names of plant	Location	Parts of plant that usually cause poisoning	Animals most commonly poisoned	Conditions under which poisoning usually occurs, and minimum quantity required	Characteristic effects
Rayless goldenrod (*Applopappus heterophyllus* (A. Gray) Blake)	Fields along ditches in western Texas, New Mexico, and Arizona	Leaves and stems	Cattle, sheep and horses	Feeding on the plant frequently for several days	Marked weakness and trembling, especially after exercise
Rubberweed, bitter (*Actinea odorata* (DC.) Kuntze)	Western Texas to southeastern California	Leaves, stems and flowers	Sheep	Eating small quantities daily for several days	Vomiting, weakness
Rubberweed, Colorado (*A. richardsoni* (Hook.) Kuntze)	Gravelly hills and flats in mountains of Colorado, New Mexico, Utah, and Arizona	Leaves and stems	Sheep	Eating small quantities during several days	Vomiting, weakness
St. Johnswort (*Hypericum perforatum* L.)	Fields, waste places, and hills across northern half of United States	Leaves	Animals with areas of white skin and hair	Feeding on the plant and being in bright sunlight	Sore, scabby areas on white skin, itching, rapid respiration
Snakeroot, white (*Eupatorium rugosum* Houtt.)	Rich woods and ravines in eastern half of the United States	Leaves and stems	Cattle and sheep	Feeding on the plant for several days	Marked trembling and weakness, especially after exercise
Sneezeweed (*Helenium hoopesii* Gray)	Mountains, meadows, and valleys from Montana to Arizona	Leaves	Sheep and cattle	Feeding on the plant for 2 weeks or more	Profuse vomiting and weakness
Tarweed (*Amsinckia intermedia* F. and M.)	Northwest, principally in eastern Washington, eastern Oregon, and northern Idaho	Seeds	Horses, cattle and swine	Eaten when mixed with wheat chaff or screenings	Loss of appetite, jaundice, emaciation, and, in horses, a tendency to walk continuously
Waterhemlock (*Cicuta* sp.)	Wet places throughout the United States	Roots and root-stocks	Sheep and cattle	Eating very small quantities	Violent spasms

[1] Some poisonous species of *Astragalus* are not locoweeds.

Tremetol is an oily alcohol that is found in white snakeroot and rayless goldenrod (jimmyweed). It causes "trembles" in livestock and milk sickness in human beings.

The poisons in some plants have not been identified. Among them are those that occur in locoweed, copperweed, paper flower, littleleaf horsebrush, the spineless horsebrush and bracken. With exception of the locoweed and bracken, these plants are the principal causes of range bighead of sheep.

Locoweeds, of which there are seven definitely known varieties, make animals "go loco," or crazy. These differ from the other poisonous plants in that they are habit-forming. After animals have eaten them for a while they prefer them to other feed and so actually become "dope fiends." Addiction is accompanied by loss of condition. High-spirited horses become dull. They seem to lose control of their muscles. In stepping over slight obstructions, they lift their feet much higher than necessary. Later they become solitary in their habits. If someone approaches, they may pay no attention at first, then rear and perhaps fall over backwards. Tails and manes of locoed horses become very long. Locoed cattle act in a manner similar to horses.

Algae, or "water bloom," forms a powerful poison, as yet unidentified, when it decomposes—becomes bad-smelling. Animals eating it or drinking water containing it may die suddenly. Staggering, weak hind quarters, deep breathing, and convulsions are mong the early symptoms.

Methods of control

Most poisonous plants don't taste good to animals. They eat them by accident or because there is nothing better to be had.

To avoid having animals eat poisonous plants, the U.S. Department of Agriculture recommends the following:

Don't allow overgrazing, and particularly avoid putting animals on drought-stricken ranges and pastures.

Use care in turning hungry animals onto a range with poisonous plants after they have been shipped or driven a long distance without feed.

Try not to harvest poisonous plants with hay, or the seeds of these plants with grain.

So far as practicable, wipe out the poisonous plants on pastures and ranges. Where the cost of doing this is too great, at least eradicate them along trails and around watering places where they are likely to be eaten.

Where poisonous plants get an earlier start in the spring than good forage plants, animals should not be turned out too early.

Where poisonous plants are present that injure one kind of livestock more than another, use this area for grazing animals that are injured least.

The few poisonous plants that animals like to eat should be wiped out or the areas where they grow should be fenced off.

Sweet clover poisoning

WHEN SWEET CLOVER, in hay or silage, becomes moldy or otherwise spoiled, it contains a substance, called *coumarin*, that keeps blood from clotting. Animals eating such spoiled feed may die from hemorrhages. These may be internal and spread throughout the body, or a single severe hemorrhage may occur following a bruise, or because of a cut made during castration, dehorning or other operation. When a cow while affected with the ailment drops a calf, both the calf and the dam may die.

The disease affects chiefly cattle under three years old. Pigs are also susceptible; sheep only slightly so, and horses hardly at all. The malady is never caused by grazing on sweet clover in the pasture. It is impossible to tell by the amount of mold or other spoilage how severe the disease that it may cause will be. A solid moldy mass of clover may do little or no injury, whereas a slight spoilage may cause severe illness. The offending mold grows readily in the hollow stems of large plants.

Symptoms

Animals with sweet clover disease are dull and move with difficulty. Swellings may be found anywhere on the body but particularly around the hips, chest and neck where bruising is most likely to occur. These swellings contain blood. They do not pit when pressed, nor do they crackle like the swellings present in blackleg.

The mouth parts are pale. Appetite is good and temperature and breathing are normal. Pulse is normal until hemorrhages become serious; then the heart rate and the strength of the heart beat increase greatly.

Treatment

Immediate change of feed is, of course, necessary. But even when this is done, new cases of the disease may develop for a week or 10 days after the feed has been changed.

Quick recovery of a sick animal follows the intravenous infusion of one to two quarts of defibrinated blood per 1,000 lbs. body weight from an animal that has not been fed sweet clover. Recovery will occur even when the affected animal is down and apparently almost dead.

Blood can be defibrinated or oxalated by shaking or stirring it for a few minutes and then straining it through gauze or cheesecloth. Another method consists in mixing 50 cc. of 2.5 percent sodium citrate solution with each pint of whole blood. This can be strained and used instead of defibrinated blood.

Coagulation of the blood is restored in half an hour or less and animals are back to normal within a week or 10 days. A change of feed alone is not enough to save animals when they are already bleeding to death.

Veterinary treatment often includes the injection of synthetic vitamin K.

Substances that poison livestock

LEAD KILLS more farm animals than any other metallic substance, and the greatest losses from lead occur among cattle. The principal reason is that most good paints contain white lead and cattle like to lick freshly painted surfaces.

Some other causes of lead poisoning are lotions, ointments and salves containing lead. These are often applied to wounds or inflammations or to the skin to kill external parasites. The lead is licked off by the animals or may even cause poisoning by absorption through the skin. Lead poisoning is also caused by the eating of vegetation coated with lead arsenate in orchard sprays, by breathing tetraethyllead (ethyl) gasoline fumes, by eating lead shot and bullets while grazing on target ranges, and by inhaling smelter dust containing lead.

Calves sometimes die from lead poisoning after eating old dry paint from boards.

Symptoms

First symptoms of lead poisoning are slobbering, choking, colic, and loss of appetite and milk secretion. Constipation is common; diarrhea or bloating may occur. Often there are trembling, champing of jaws, walking in circles and apparent blindness. Death may occur during such an attack, or animals may fall into a stupor and die while in this condition. Animals with such symptoms seldom live more than a few days.

When small quantities of lead are absorbed over a long period of time, chronic lead poisoning sets in. This often results in stiff joints, convulsions, skin eruptions, loss of weight, abortions and failure to conceive.

Treatment

The most common treatment for lead poisoning is a purgative dose of Epsom salts. Certain "chelates" can also be injected intravenously to form insoluble compounds of lead which can be excreted from the body. These combine with the lead so that it is excreted from the body. Lead poisoning is nearly always the result of carelessness or lack of previous knowledge concerning this danger.

Miscellaneous poisons

Other common substances that sometimes poison livestock are the following:

Sprays containing cresylic acid in strong solutions are poisonous to livestock.

Seed grain treated with mercuric compounds may cause poisoning when eaten. Seed grains so treated should be destroyed rather than fed to livestock.

Sodium chlorate, used to kill Canadian thistles, will also kill cattle.

Nitrate fertilizers are poisonous to animals, yet cattle like to eat them. Watch out so cattle don't get at fertilizer bags, heavily fertilized spots in a field, or sweepings from places where fertilizer has been kept.

Copper sulphate, carbon tetrachloride and tetrachlorethylene should be used properly and not left where animals can get at them. Rat and woodchuck poisons should be placed where domestic animals can't reach them.

Carelessness in handling preparations containing arsenic, such as paris green, arsenical dips, organphosphate sprays and grasshopper bait, may poison animals, particularly horses and mules. Horses are not so susceptible to lead poisoning as cattle.

Nutritional diseases of cattle

IF CATTLE get the right feed, the addition of vitamins or minerals to their ration is not necessary, with the exception of common salt. But the right feed is not always available, and sometimes even feed that seems to be good is lacking in the proper minerals.

The so-called nutritional diseases are usually not fatal. Yet they cause greater financial loss than is generally believed. Animals lacking the proper minerals and vitamins do not have the rate of growth that they should, are more susceptible to diseases and have reproduction difficulties.

Dramatic results often follow the addition of minerals or vitamins to animal diets. Certain well-defined diseases disappear and unthrifty animals gain condition.

This has led many farmers to believe that these substances to some extent take the place of wholesome feed. But this is not true. Only when otherwise nutritious feeds are lacking in minerals and vitamins should these substances be supplied. To give animals more of them than their bodies need is always a waste of money and sometimes injures the health of livestock.

The minerals that enter into nutritional ailments are phosphorus, calcium, magnesium, iodine, iron, copper, cobalt, selenium and common salt. Other minerals such as zinc and fluorine are also necessary to animal health, but they are almost always present in sufficient quantities in ordinary feeds and seldom if ever need be supplied as ration supplements. A few other minerals are essential in certain rations compounded from highly refined or so-called purified nutritional factors.

Calcium and phosphorus deficiency

When cattle do not get enough calcium and phosphorus, their appe-

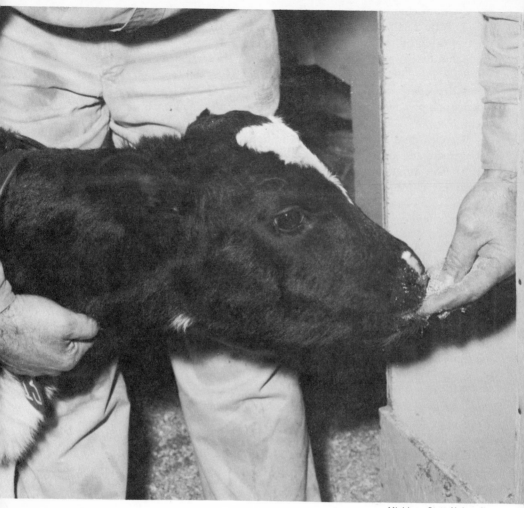

Getting a taste from the fingers. Encourage the calf to eat grain at an early age

tites become depraved. They chew and eat bones, wood, hair, rocks and many other things.

As the deficiency becomes greater, animals lose their appetites, become thin, and have weak bones and stiff joints. Cows have decreased milk flow, do not come in heat regularly or settle when they should. Cases have been reported, however, where calcium-deficient cows remained in good condition and did not show the stiffness that accompanies phosphorous deficiency.

Cattle require more calcium and phosphorus in periods of rapid growth and heavy lactation than at other times. During heavy lactation periods, dairy cows often give up more of these elements in their milk than they obtain in their feed. The difference is taken from their bones, which are weakened as a result.

Where mineral nutritional diseases occur

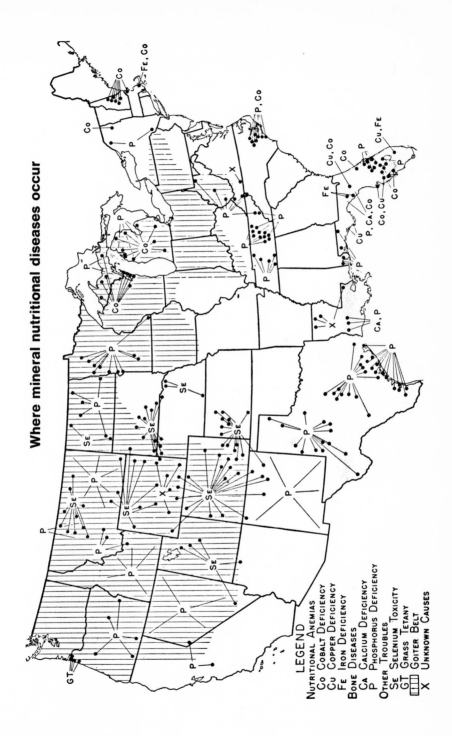

LEGEND

NUTRITIONAL ANEMIAS
Co COBALT DEFICIENCY
Cu COPPER DEFICIENCY
Fe IRON DEFICIENCY
BONE DISEASES
Ca CALCIUM DEFICIENCY
P   PHOSPHORUS DEFICIENCY
OTHER TROUBLES
Se SELENIUM TOXICITY
GT GRASS TETANY
    GOITER BELT
X   UNKNOWN CAUSES

Calcium should be added to a ration that consists only of poor grass or grain hays. Leguminous plants such as alfalfa, the clovers, the vetches, soybeans and peas are rich in calcium. Where the ration is lacking in such feeds, calcium may be supplied by adding finely ground limestone to a grain mixture at the rate of 40 pounds to a ton of grain.

Unlike calcium, the phosphorus in cattle rations comes largely from grain.

Phosphorus deficiency occurs where a ration consists of low-quality roughage with little or no grain or mill feed. The problem is often complicated by underfeeding. It occurs in many areas in the West and Southwest.

The phosphorus supplement that is considerered best in bone meal. This is often supplied by adding one pound of steamed bone meal to every hundred pounds of grain mix. Some bone meal is sold for fertilizers. Only bone meal prepared for livestock should be used. Cattle will usually refuse the kind that is intended for fertilizer.

For range cattle, a mineral "lick" or block is usually provided. This consists of equal parts of steamed bone meal and common salt. The mixture is placed in a stout shallow trough or box fastened to a tree or between two posts. It should be protected so that the rain will not wash away the salt and leave the less-palatable bone meal.

The phosphorus requirement of lactating dairy cows needs particular attention. This is especially true in areas where there is lack of the mineral in the soil.

Lack of magnesium

If a young calf is fed on milk without forage or grain for more than a few weeks, it becomes nervous and irritable and loses its appetite. If the animal is continued on this feed it develops convulsions. It will become temporarily blind and will turn in circles until it loses its balance. There is frothing at the mouth.

Such attacks may last several minutes and be repeated later. Young calves usually recover but older ones nearly always die with the first attack.

The malady is caused by lack of magnesium in the blood. Ordinary diets of forage and grain contain enough magnesium so that the disease is not likely to occur. Feeds rich in magnesium are legume and grass hay, cottonseed, linseed and soybean meal, wheat bran, wheat middlings, beet pulp and hominy feed.

Too little iodine

Cows that do not get enough iodine in their feed often give birth to weak calves with goiters, a condition known as "big-neck." Some of these calves are so weak that they die within a few days. Others may have normal vigor and have no noticeable symptoms other than enlargement of the thyroid gland in the neck and difficulty in breathing.

Pressure of the goiter on the windpipe causes the breathing difficulty.

Lack of iodine in feed is caused by the absence of enough of this element in the soil on the feed or water. Areas that are deficient in iodine are known to exist in Montana, Idaho, Oregon and Washington, and in parts of Utah, Wyoming, North Dakota, Minnesota, Wisconsin and Michigan. Sections of California, Nevada, Colorado, Nebraska, Iowa, and Texas have also been reported to be deficient in the element.

Cattle owners in these areas usually feed their animals iodized salt. Where large quantities are required, stockmen may save money by preparing their own mixtures in the proportion of one ounce of powdered potassium iodide to every 300 pounds of granulated stock salt. However, careful mixing is important.

Not enough iron, copper, cobalt

Iron is a necessary part of hemoglobin, the principal component of the red blood corpuscles. Copper and cobalt are necessary for the formation of the red cells but do not become part of them. They are known as catalysts. They perform a service in making hemoglobin that is not completely understood. A deficiency of iron, copper and cobalt can occur singly or in combination.

The red blood cells in the body are constantly being made and destroyed. Whenever cattle do not get enough iron, copper and cobalt, the dead cells are not replaced in sufficient numbers, or the newly made ones do not contain enough hemoglobin. This condition is known as nutritional anemia.

Animals with anemia gradually lose their appetites and become thin and weak. Diarrhea or constipation may occur. Young cattle fail to grow as they should. Sexual development is delayed. Among cows, lactation is unsatisfactory.

In Florida, a condition occurs which for many years has been known as "salt sick." In Michigan the same disease is called "Grand Traverse," or "lake shore disease." Both of these ailments are now recognized as nutritional anemia.

In Michigan, some cases of Grand Traverse respond well to cobalt alone; in others, it is better to use iron and copper also. In Florida, whenever animals fail to respond to the usual supplement of iron and copper, cobalt should be added to the mineral mixture.

For advanced cases the following treatment is recommended:

Dissolve 10 grams of cobalt chloride or cobalt sulphate in one gallon of water. Give mature animals six ounces as a drench once weekly for three or four weeks. Calves should be given three ounces, and other animals in proportion.

For prevention of the disease:

Add one pound of cobalt chloride or cobalt sulphate to each ton of the regular salt-lick mixture (100 pounds of salt, 25 pounds of red oxide of iron, and one pound of powdered copper sulphate). A recommended manner of making this addition is to dissolve 22 grams of the cobalt salt in a small amount of water and spray it over 100 pounds of the salt-lick mineral with a fly sprayer or atomizer. It should be mixed thoroughly so that animals taking it will secure a uniform amount. This should be offered in protected mineral boxes at all times. The necessary minerals have been compressed into a block, and may be purchased with or without salt.

Animals must have salt

Common salt is a necessary part of the diet of animals. The common feeds, such as grains and grasses, do not contain enough salt to sustain normal vigor, so the substance must be supplied as a ration supplement.

The salt requirements are said to be about one-fourth to one-half an ounce a day for calves and sheep and perhaps three ounces a day for high-producing cows.

Symptoms of salt deficiency are loss of appetite, rough coat, salt hunger, a rapid decline in condition and decreased milk yield among dairy cows.

It is common practice to add salt to grain mixtures and mineral licks, but in addition farm animals should have free access to salt at all times. On the range, boxes containing salt or salt mixed with minerals should be provided so that even the most timid animals will get all they need. Water must always be available when salt is provided after a period of deprivation.

Animals that have been deprived of salt for some time and then are given all they want may eat so much that they get sick or even die. Salt-hungry animals should be given small quantities at first until the intense craving for it disappears.

So far as is known, cattle and other ruminants usually get all the vitamins they need in their regular diet with the exception of vitamins A and D. Most cattle feeds, such as green grass, hay, silage of good quality and grains are rich in vitamins. If these feeds are supplied in the rations in sufficient quantities, vitamin supplements are unnecessary.

Vitamin-A deficiency

Vitamin A is derived from carotene, which is contained in green and yellow plants. Cattle of all ages may suffer from this deficiency, but young animals are particularly susceptible. New born calves do not have a reserve supply in their bodies, even if the pregnant mothers receive more than they need in their feed.

One of the first symptoms of vitamin-A deficiency is night blindness. Animals with this ailment cannot see well in dim light, and are dazzled and keep blinking their eyes in bright sunlight. If cattle with night blindness are driven about a corral at dusk, they bump into fences or stumble over objects placed in their way.

Swelling of legs and forequarters, rapid breathing, stiffness, lameness, loss of appetite, loss of weight and convulsions are other symptoms of vitamin-A deficiency. In severe cases, cows and bulls may lose their sexual desires and their ability to reproduce, but this damage is usually temporary. The vitamin A requirement for normal reproduction is much higher than the amount needed to ward off night blindness.

The principal cause of vitamin-A deficiency is lack of carotene in the diet. This condition arises in feed lots where animals are fed very little roughage or roughage of poor quality, in the winter when animals are fed poorly cured hay or straw, and among calves fed on skim milk without good sources of carotene. Vitamin A supplements are widely used, even when no symptoms of deficiency appear. Improved production and growth often justify the added cost.

Vitamin-A deficiency disappears promptly when animals are given the proper feed. Feeds rich in carotene are pasture grass and legumes, high-grade leafy hay of the current-year's crop, well-made silage, and new high-grade alfalfa meal.

Vitamin D prevents rickets

The presence of vitamin D in the body is necessary for proper assimilation of calcium and phosphorus.

Bone deformities are the symptoms that are most easily recognized in vitamin-D deficiency. But this ailment is not always caused by lack of this vitamin. It also occurs when animals do not get enough calcium and phosphorus.

Deficiency of vitamin D does not occur often and when it does, it is easy to cure. One or two pounds of sun-cured alfalfa a day usually will prevent rickets in calves up to 195 days old. Two pounds of good sun-cured timothy hay a day have been found to prevent vitamin-D deficiency in calves up to nine months old. However, there is a great variation in the Vitamin-D content of sun-cured forages, determinable only by chemical means. Because of this, the practice of adding irradiated yeast or cod-liver oil to the rations of young dairy calves and lambs is quite common. Vitamin-D deficiency occurs most often in the winter when animals do not get enough direct sunshine.

Wheat-pasture poisoning

Wheat-pasture poisoning occurs principally in the winter and particularly in the Texas and Oklahoma Panhandles, when cattle graze on growing wheat. Poisoning occurs most often when growth is lush and moisture is plentiful.

The first symptoms are unusual excitement, incoordination and loss of appetite. Viciousness, staggering and falling come later. Nervousness becomes apparent with muscular twitching, particularly in the legs. The animal may grind its teeth and saliva flows freely. The third eyelid will protrude or flicker. The next symptoms are labored breathing, unconsciousness, followed by convulsions and death.

The most commonly used treatment is the intravenous or intraperitoneal injections of a solution of calcium gluconate. The solution should contain not less than 17 percent of calcium gluconate. It may be fortified with magnesium or phosphorus or both. Calcium gluconate solutions with added magnesium and phosphorus seem to speed recovery and lessen the need for a second injection. Prepared solutions are available at drug stores and agricultural supply dealers.

Intravenous injection should be given slowly. At least 20 to 30 minutes should be allowed for treatment. Intraperitoneal injection may be given more rapidly.

If treatment is given during the first few hours after the development of the symptoms, recovery is usually fairly rapid and uneventful. The chance of recovery is slight if treatment is delayed 8 to 12 hours. No type of treatment has been found that will be successful in cases when treatment is delayed.

The removal of the cow from wheat pasture for a few days appears to speed complete recovery. It is unusual for an animal to have a second attack after recovery from the first one.

Grass tetany

Grass tetany is a disease that occurs most often within a few weeks after cattle are turned out to pasture that has been heavily fertilized. It is highly fatal. Symptoms are almost identical with those of wheat-pasture poisoning.

The malady is accompanied by lack of magnesium and calcium in the blood, but the exact cause of this is not known. There is said to be more involved than simple mineral deficiency.

Since death often occurs within an hour after first symptoms appear, prompt treatment is necessary. One recommended treatment consists in intravenous injections of a solution containing calcium chloride and magnesium chloride. Proper solutions of these salts are prepared by manufacturers with recommended dosages.

Selenium poisoning

Selenium poisoning is caused by eating plants that have taken up selenium from the soil. In regions where it occurs, it is commonly called "alkali disease," since it was formerly believed to be caused by drinking alkali water.

Symptoms of the disease are slow and uneven growth of the hoofs of horses, cattle and swine, loss of hair from tail and mane of horses, the switch of cattle and the loss of hair of swine. When hoofs are affected, animals are often lame for months and cannot get around properly for food and water.

When affected animals are fed selenium-free grains and forage they usually recover from the disease, provided it is not too severe. When animals have been badly affected, they suffer permanent injury and make little or no gain in weight even though given plenty of nutritious food. The amount of selenium in a ration is very critical—more than 10 parts per million is toxic or poisonous, but less than 2 ppm causes deficiency symptoms to appear.

How to collect semen from a bull

SEVERAL METHODS HAVE been devised for collecting semen from bulls. But collection by means of an artificial vagina has almost completely supplanted the others. Semen collection is largely a procedure for a specialist at an insemination ring or stud. The demands for sterility and temperature control are so exacting that they can be met only under conditions especially set up for them.

The artificial vagina consists of a heavy rubber cylinder, usually 14 or 16½ inches long and 2¾ inches in diameter, with a thin rubber lining. The cylinder has a valve or opening through which warm water can be poured into the space between the cylinder and the lining. The lining is a rubber tube which is folded over the ends of the cylinder and held in place with heavy rubber bands.

A funnel-shaped piece of rubber, called a director cone, is designed to carry the semen to a glass collecting tube, as shown in the picture on the opposite page. This tube is usually graduated, that is, it has markings etched into it that indicate the amount of fluid it contains.

Absolute cleanliness necessary

Sperm are readily killed by some microbes and chemicals. For this reason an artificial vagina must be thoroughly cleaned and sterilized before it is used. It can be cleaned with soap or a so-called detergent and water. It should then be thoroughly rinsed to remove all traces of the cleanser. Many semen producers use distilled water for rinsing.

The apparatus can be sterilized by boiling it in water for 10 minutes. However, rubber deteriorates with boiling. For this reason vaginas are often sterilized with a 70-percent solution of ethyl alcohol.

Never use denatured alcohol for cleaning an artificial vagina. The poison in the alcohol is often hard to remove and will kill sperm. Even the least trace of alcohol, denatured or otherwise, is harmful to sperm. The artificial vagina should be dry before it is prepared for use.

Preparing the artificial vagina for service

The amount of water used between the lining and cylinder of the vagina must be regulated in accordance with the size of the bull's penis. If too much water is used, the vagina may be too small for the bull and the collecting tube may be blown off the end of the director cone and the semen lost. Some operators vary the length of the vagina in accordance with the length of a bull's penis.

Filling the water space about one-half to two-thirds full is usually about right for most bulls. The temperature of the water to be added should be between 115 and 130 degrees F. After adding the warm water, close the valve, or if the vagina is not fitted with a valve, close the hole with a fold of the tube lining. Temperature on the inside of the vagina should be 105 to 118 degrees F., varying with the preference of the bull .

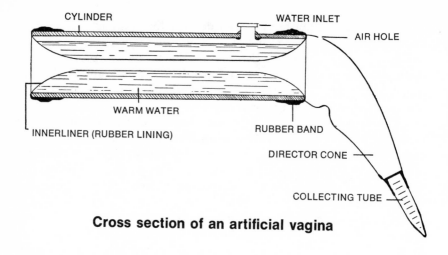

CYLINDER WATER INLET

AIR HOLE

WARM WATER

INNERLINER (RUBBER LINING)

RUBBER BAND

DIRECTOR CONE

COLLECTING TUBE

Cross section of an artificial vagina

The lining of the vagina should be smeared with a thin coat of lubricant such as sterile white vaseline, light mineral oil or a special lubricant made up of 3 grams of gum tragacanth, 5 cc. glycerine, and 50 cc. of distilled water, and allowed to jell. A prepared lubricating jelly containing tragacanth can be bought from supply houses.

Since mineral oil and vaseline are both injurious to rubber and are hard to wash off, the tragacanth lubricant is much preferred. The part of the lining near the collecting tube should not be lubricated. Do not use so much lubricant that it will contaminate the semen.

Just before the vagina is used, the temperature of the lining should be tested with a thermometer. It is highly important that this temperature should be between 105 and 115 degrees F., preferably close to 110, at the actual time of semen collection. Higher temperatures may kill the sperm and lower ones may slow down ejaculation or even make a bull incapable of ejaculation.

Quarters for collecting semen

The quarters or paddock for collecting semen should not be cramped and should, of course, be free from objects that might injure or frighten breeding animals. A smooth concrete floor should not be used since it might cause an animal to slip, especially when the floor is wet. Heavy large rubber mats are sometimes used to prevent slipping.

If possible the same quarters should be used each time for collecting semen. Males serve best in places that are familiar to them. An easy way to train a male to use an artificial vagina is to permit him to serve a cow in heat in a stall or breeding crate. Later, in the same place, you can substitute a cow not in heat, another bull or a dummy cow.

The use of a dummy

A dummy should be solidly made, and firmly anchored since it will, of course, weigh much less than a living animal. The framework may be of wood but metal is better. The top and sides of the dummy should be well padded and covered with skin, canvas or other durable material.

The dummy should be of proper height but need not closely resemble an animal. Space should be provided for insertion of an artificial vagina. Some bulls will not mount a dummy, especially those that were not trained to use one when they were young.

Collecting the semen

A bull should be conditioned, or teased, before the actual collection of semen. This is done by leading him up to the cow, dummy, or another bull, but not permitting him to mount. Such restraint results in a greater quantity and better quality of semen, since it permits the fluids that make up the semen to flow more freely.

After noticeable dripping occurs from the erected penis, the bull should be allowed to mount. If a dummy is used, the vagina is held between the dummy's hind legs; if a living animal is used, the vagina is held at the animal's side.

The vagina should be held with the open end tilted downward at an angle of about 45 degrees. This is the most favorable angle for collection of semen and also aids in ejaculation. The water collects in the lower part of the jacket and creates pressure that stimulates the ejaculatory nerves near the end of the penis.

As the bull mounts the cow or a substitute, the penis should be guided into the artificial vagina by means of a hand placed on the sheath. The penis itself should not be touched since this often causes a bull to dismount without ejaculation. The ejaculation which occurs at the end of the thrust of the penis, usually places the semen in the director cone from which it flows into the collecting tube.

After the bull dismounts, hold the vagina upright at once to make sure that all semen flows into the collecting tube. Then carry the vagina, tube and all, to the laborary for semen examination and dilution.

Sometimes two collections of semen are made with only a few minutes between them. The second ejaculate is larger and generally of much better quality than the first one. Collection of semen from a mature bull is usually limited to about once a week. If a bull is not doing his work properly, he should be given a rest period of three or four weeks.

Bulls differ widely in their ability to withstand service. A bull's sexual desire does not necessarily mean that he is a good producer of sperm.

Semen differs greatly in quality

Normal bull semen is a whitish, creamy fluid, resembling whole milk. The amount ejaculated at one time usually varies between two and six cubic centimeters ($\frac{1}{2}$ to $1\frac{1}{2}$ teaspoonfuls). Yearling bulls may yield only a few cc. while older ones may yield as much as 10 cc. A bull may yield different amounts at different times.

The number of sperm per cc. varies greatly. The most common number is about 800 million per cc. and the normal range is between 300 million and two billion. Thus, of two normal bulls, one may easily yield 25 times as many sperm per ejaculation as another.

The color of semen may give a clue to its quality. A yellowish color may indicate the presence of pus or urine, which can then often be detected by its smell. A pinkish or reddish color indicates the presence of fresh blood. A deeper red or brownish color probably indicates the presence of older blood from degenerating tissues. A sire from which abnormal semen is collected should not be used for insemination or other breeding purposes until the ailment is cleared up.

Sperm differ in their viability, that is, their ability to fertilize the eggs of females. The rate at which they swim and the percentage of normal, uncrippled sperm have a direct bearing on their fertility.

You can't look at semen and tell how good it is. If a bull is known to be fertile and his semen is not to be diluted very much, the chances are good that a high percentage of pregnancies can be obtained from the semen without laboratory tests.

Handling semen

In the handling of semen it should always be remembered that sperm are much more delicate than other cells of the body. They are killed by direct sunlight, undue shaking, soaps, antiseptics and substances that are either too acid or too alkaline. They are injured if their temperature is lowered too rapidly or is raised much above that of the body. They are killed at about 124 degrees F. They are injured if they come in contact with metal surfaces.

Sperm are not injured by certain antibiotics such as penicillin. Ordinarily they are killed when frozen but if frozen under certain conditions and kept at certain temperatures they will remain alive for at least a year and perhaps indefinitely, as explained further on.

It is seldom necessary to extend (dilute) semen when less than seven inseminations are to be made from one collection and semen is to be used within 48 hours.

If inseminations are to be made within half an hour after semen is collected, the semen may be kept at room temperature in a small clean bottle or vial.

If semen is to be used in from one-half hour to 48 hours, it should be immediately but gradually cooled, until it reaches 35 to 40 degrees above zero. This is ordinary refrigerator temperature.

How to cool semen

Gradual cooling of semen can be accomplished by wrapping the vial containing it in several layers of paper and placing it in the refrigerator. The vial may also be placed in a glass of water at room temperature and then refrigerated. Cooling the semen should take about one hour. It is not necessary to warm semen for insemination.

If semen is not to be used all at one time, it is better to divide it and store it in several vials. Frequent warming and cooling of semen sometimes causes so-called "temperature shock." The sperm lose their motility—their ability to swim.

Where practicable, vials should be filled to the top to exclude the air. A layer of neutral mineral oil (neither acid nor akaline) is often poured over the top of semen in vials. This excludes the air. Clean paraffin-treated corks should be used as stoppers for the vials.

In the field, a thermos bottle is often used to maintain temperature of semen. A hole can be bored through the cork of the thermos bottle to hold the vial of semen in place. The thermos bottle should then be filled about two-thirds full of water that is nearly ice cold. Ice may be added to the water. Where inseminating is to be done right along, it pays to buy a regular inseminating kit from an agricultural house. Or it may be advantageous to join an insemination ring and have a technician do the inseminating. This is usually done at a nominal charge for each cow.

The dilution of semen

The purpose of diluting semen is, of course, to extend its volume so that many cows can be bred from a single ejaculate. However, fluids used for diluting also prolong the life of sperm. Diluters provide energy for the sperm and one of the ingredients acts as a so-called "buffer." The purpose of the buffer is to keep the fluid at the degree of acidity necessary to preserve the life of the sperm.

Since microbes grow readily in semen, penicillin or streptomycin and sulfanilamide are usually added to halt this growth. For reasons that are not completely understood, the addition of these drugs also prolongs the life of sperm.

A number of good diluters have been developed. The principal ones are the egg yolk citrate diluter, the egg yolk phosphate diluter, and the milk diluter. Diluters, already mixed, are available at agricultural supply houses.

Bull semen is sometimes used in dilutions as high as 200 to 1. However, most members of the National Association of Artificial Breeders believe that 100 to 1 dilution should be the limit for general use. When dilutions are too high, conception rates are lowered. Dilutions should be made in accordance with the number of sperm in the semen. Authorities recommend a minimum of 5 to 10 million sperm per insemination.

Since only one sperm is necessary to fertilize an egg, it seems strange that so many sperm are required to bring a cow in calf. The reason for this has not been satisfactorily explained.

How to add diluters

If an ejaculate of semen is to be used for inseminating a large number of cows, the semen should be examined for quality, diluted and cooled as soon as possible. Even a few minutes delay in processing fresh semen has been known to make a difference of 5 percent in its conception rate.

To avoid damaging sperm, it is necessary that the temperature of semen be carefully regulated. The temperature of semen should be lowered gradually. In view of this, the diluter and all glassware used to hold semen should be about the same temperature as the semen when dilutions are made. However, bull sperm can withstand temperature changes much better when diluted than otherwise.

To avoid warming all of the diluter to the temperature of the semen, some technicians warm only a part of it and add it to the semen. When this mixture cools to the temperature of the remaining diluter, they add the rest of it. After semen is diluted, it should be cooled gradually as explained earlier in this chapter.

Good quality semen, properly diluted and cooled by ordinary methods, may be used for two or three days with practically as good results as on the day of collection. However, sperm rapidly lose their ability to fertilize eggs from the fourth day on.

A few successful inseminations have been made with sperm six days old with ordinary methods of processing semen, but the use of such old semen is not dependable. Most semen producers recommend that semen be used within 48 hours after collection.

Shipment of semen

Shipment of semen is made in small vials labeled with the date it was collected and the identity of the bull. Vials for shipment are generally placed in vacuum bottles with ice and water to maintain proper temperature. When shipments are made by mail, bus or express, bottles are packed to prevent breakage.

Frozen semen

As stated previously, when semen is diluted in the ordinary way and then frozen, the sperm are killed. The reason is that the water present forms ice crystals which puncture the thin membranes, or coverings, of the sperm. Upon thawing the diluted semen, the substance of the sperm leaks out and the sperm die.

However, if glycerol is used as one of the semen diluters and freezing is done in a certain way, ice crystals do not form. And if the temperature is lowered to 110 degrees F. below zero and kept there, the sperm will remain alive for years even though frozen. They become active immediately upon being thawed out. A temperature of minus 110 degrees F. is attained through use of frozen carbon dioxide (dry ice). With a more recently developed method, using liquid nitrogen, a temperature of minus 385 degrees F. can be maintained, thus greatly extending the life of the sperm.

Artificial insemination technique

SUCCESSFUL ARTIFICIAL breeding depends largely upon proper timing of the insemination and the care with which it is done.

For reasons explained in the chapter "What happens when a cow settles," the best time to inseminate a cow is just before the end of standing heat or just after that time. So-called standing heat is that part of the heat period when a cow permits other cows to "ride" her or she tries to ride other cows.

Before insemination, a cow should be properly restrained in a stanchion or tie stall. Her vulva and adjoining rear parts should be thoroughly cleaned and then rinsed to remove all traces of soap.

Two principal methods are used to inseminate cows. They are known as the speculum method and the deep cervical method. The speculum method requires less skill than the deep cervical method but is not quite so efficient.

The speculum method

A speculum is an instrument or device used by medical men and veterinarians to enlarge temporarily a body opening so you can see better what's inside. For artificial insemination, the speculum used is nearly always a tube of plastic, glass or metal, 12 to 14 inches long and of an outside diameter of about 1½ inches.

A speculum is lubricated before it is put to use. One end is then carefully inserted into the vagina until it is lodged near the cervix. The cervix can then be seen by shining a small flashlight into the speculum or by means of a headlight like those used by eye specialists.

Inseminating is done by means of plastic or glass tubes about 16 inches long and 3/16 of an inch in outside diameter. The tips of the

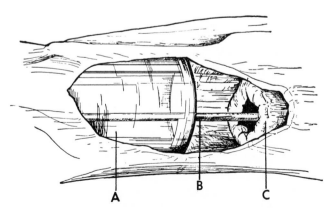

This cut-away section of a vagina illustrates the speculum method of insemination. It shows (A) the speculum, (B) the inseminating tube and (C) the cervix

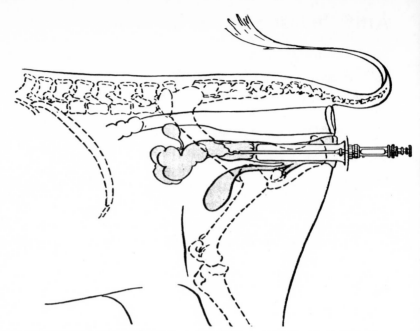

In the speculum method, a large glass tube is inserted into the vagina. A smaller tube is then used to inject the semen into the cervix

tubes are rounded so as not to injure animals. A small glass syringe, usually with a capacity of 2 cc., is attached to one end of the tube by means of a piece of rubber tubing or a specially made adapter.

Plastic inseminating tubes are much preferred to glass ones. They are less liable to injure an animal since the plastic will bend but not break. But their biggest advantage lies in the fact that they cost only a few cents apiece so can be used once and then thrown away.

After the speculum is in place and the opening to the cervix has been located, the semen is drawn into the tube by means of the syringe. The syringe is used only as a pump and does not come in contact with the semen.

Amount of semen to use

The amount of semen to be used depends upon its dilution. It varies between $1/2$ and $1^1/2$ cc. The number of sperm per insemination should not be less than five million and some authorities recommend as high as 15 million.

The free end of the inseminating tube should be carefully inserted into the opening of the cervix and the semen slowly expelled by pushing in the plunger of the attached syringe. The tube and speculum should then be slowly withdrawn.

The deep cervical method

The deep cervical method of insemination is the one used by practically all professional technicians. It is sometimes called the cervical fixation method, or the recto-vaginal method.

It is quicker than the speculum method, requires less equipment and results in a somewhat higher percentage of conceptions. However, it requires a little more training and is beset with certain dangers.

Before applying the deep cervical method, the excess manure should be removed from the rectum with the hand.

The method consists in reaching into the rectum and, through its lining, grasping the cervix lightly with gloved hand, while guiding the inseminating tube through the vagina and into the cervix with the other hand.

Untrained persons often have difficulty in locating the opening in the cervix, known technically as the os uteri. The best way to find this is to hold the cervix between the second and third fingers and then search for the opening with the thumb. After the opening has been located, hold the tip of the thumb above the opening and let it serve as a guide by which to insert the inseminating tube. This is the same kind of tube that is used in the speculum method and it is filled in the same way.

The cervix has a number of folds in it. This makes it necessary to manipulate the tube gently so as not to cause injury to the passage.

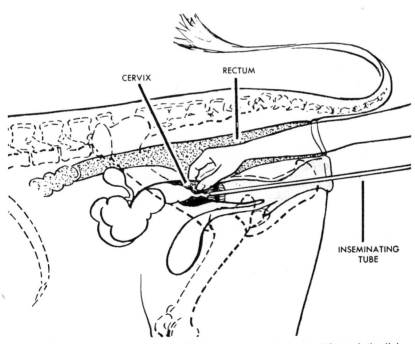

CERVIX

RECTUM

INSEMINATING
TUBE

In the deep cervical method of insemination the cervix is grasped through the lining of the rectum with one hand. At the same time the end of the inseminating tube is gently inserted through the vagina into the cervix with the other hand

Where should semen be deposited?

Opinions differ as to whether semen should be deposited in the middle of the cervix or in the uterus.

Insemination records of thousands of cows, both in England and in the United States, show that there is practically no difference in conception rates whether semen is deposited in middle of the cervix, the body of the uterus or in the horns of the uterus.

In view of this, most authorities now recommend that semen be deposited in the mid-cervix only. This is safer for two reasons: there is less danger of infecting the uterus and there is little danger of causing abortions in cases where pregnant cows are inseminated by mistake.

Although semen is deposited in the vagina when a cow is served by a bull, this site results in a very low conception rate when semen is diluted, as is the case in routine artificial breeding. The reason for this is that not enough sperm reach the opening in the cervix when diluted semen is used.

Portable pens cut calf losses

MANY DAIRYMEN are making astonishing cuts in calf losses by means of portable pens.

The portable-pen system is of greatest benefit in warm climates where all of the organisms that cause calf ailments are highly active the year around. But the system is also being used to cut calf losses in northern states. Calves in portable pens have withstood near zero temperatures with no apparent harmful effects.

On many farms, a new-born calf is placed in an old stall or pen which has been used for calves and cows for many years. Such a place usually abounds in parasites and in the organisms that cause white scours, coccidiosis and pneumonia.

In these surroundings, a calf can become infected with disease-producing microbes within 24 hours. As a result half the calves often die before they are six months old. And those that survive usually show the results of this mistreatment the rest of their lives.

How the system works

With the portable-pen system, the calf is dropped in a small clean pasture. It is removed from the dam within 24 hours after birth and placed in a portable pen by itself.

The pen, with the calf in it, is moved by two men to fresh, unsoiled ground once each week. The pen is not heavy since it has no floor, only half a roof, and its sides consist largely of woven wire. The calf, being nudged along, walks to the new location.

By moving the calf weekly, it is taken away from contaminated material before most of the coccidia have become infective. What's more, a week is too short a time for dangerous contamination by disease-producing microbes.

Calves are being raised by the portable pen system that are free from pneumonia, worm parasites, Johne's disease and coccidiosis. The animals, of course, do get some coccidia in their systems, but not enough to affect their health noticeably.

To raise such healthy calves, you must place them in portable pens within 24 hours after birth and move them every week, preferably at seven-day intervals.

Colostrum must be given calves preferably within the first six hours of life, and the earlier the better. Milk is given twice a day by means of the usual calf-feeding pail with a rubber nipple at the bottom. In addition, legume hay and grain are made available beginning when the calf is two weeks old. This is placed in a combination feeder (Fig. E).

The milk pail, water bucket, and feeder are hung on the side panels of the pen, high enough to prevent contamination by the calf (Figs. A and D). Each calf has its own feeding pail. A small block of iodized salt is kept in each feeder.

The calf is kept in the portable pen until it is four or five months old. Then it is placed with other calves of the same age in a clean pasture—one that has not been contaminated by cows or older calves.

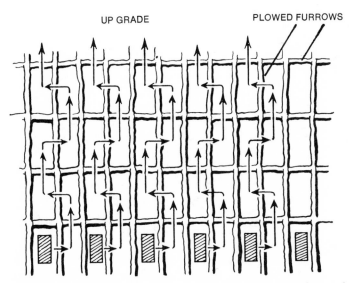

UP GRADE   PLOWED FURROWS

Each arrow indicates a weekly move of a pen. The small plots of ground are occupied only once a year

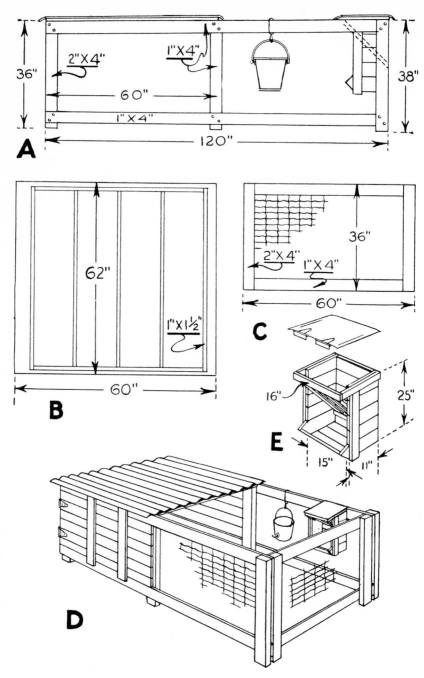

Details of construction of portable pen

At the regional laboratory, the pens with the new-born calves are first placed in a row at the foot of a wooded hillside, as shown in the sketch. A hillside is used so that the rain will not wash contaminated material over clean ground.

After one week the pens are moved one space to the right. At the end of the second week they are moved up hill one space. The next weekly move is made to the left, and so on, following a zig-zag course up the hill. A year is allowed to elapse before the same ground is used again.

The zig-zag course for the pens has two advantages. It permits full use of the plot of ground without having pens too close together, and the plot need be only half as deep as would be necessary if the pens were moved in a straight line. Other similar plans for movement of the pens can of course be devised for use on various-shaped plots of ground.

When a pen is moved, the ground that it occupied does not have to be cleaned. But unsightly bedding should be burned.

Specifications for portable pens

(All measurements are approximate)

The pen measures 5 x 10 feet. The sides and ends, Figs. A and C, require:

4 pieces 1 inch x 4 inches x 10 feet
4 pieces 1 inch x 4 inches x 5 feet
2 pieces 1 inch x 4 inches x 38 inches
8 pieces 2 inches x 4 inches x 38 inches
30 feet welded woven wire with 2 x 4-inch mesh, 36 inches high
4 pairs 3-inch loose-pin butt hinges for joining sides and ends

Removable side and end panels, Fig. D, are 60 x 31 inches and are made of one-inch materials. These panels are attached by wood screws.

Weight and cost can be reduced by making the pen without hinged joints and by using only one upright in each corner instead of two, as the diagram shows.

The removable top (60 inches x 62 inches) is made of $1 \times 1\frac{1}{2}$-inch material and corrugated-aluminum sheeting (Fig. B).

5 pieces 60 inches x 1 inch x $1\frac{1}{2}$ inches
2 pieces 62 inches x 1 inch x $1\frac{1}{2}$ inches
2 pieces 60 inches x 26 inches aluminum sheeting
1 piece 60 inches x 13 inches aluminum sheeting
Lead-headed or aluminum nails for nailing the sheeting to the wooden frame.

The combination grain and hay rack (Fig. E) is 25 inches high, 15 inches wide and 16 inches deep. The lid is an aluminum-covered frame which is hinged at the front.

Materials and design

The sheltered portion of the pen (Fig. D), is just big enough for one calf. The roof is made of corrugated-aluminum sheeting and is removable. The end and two sides are removable panels made of one-inch wood. These are hinged together and are removed in warm weather. Some dairymen use black waterproof building paper for these panels to reduce weight and cost. Burlap can be draped over the open end of the shelter in extremely cold weather.

The ground under the shelter should be raised a little so that water will run off, and dry bedding should be provided. A furrow should be plowed around each pen for drainage in rainy weather and to prevent cross-contamination.

You may want to omit the hay and grain rack (Figs. C and E) and substitute a lighter weight feed box to be used under the roof of the pen. Some farmers have complained about the weight of the feeder and said that it took as long to make as the rest of the pen.

Some farmers are making pens 4 x 8 ft. instead of 5 x 10 ft., especially for smaller breeds. They thus make more economical use of lumber and roofing materials. But of course they have to remove the calves earlier with smaller pens.

At the Regional Laboratory they are now using angle irons bolted together instead of wooden frames. They are lighter and last longer.

Hog cholera

PRIOR TO the early 1960's hog cholera was by far the most destructive disease of hogs. It occurred year after year. Since then, a strenuous eradication program has been carried on throughout the United States, with the result that most states are now free of the disease. Consequently, hog cholera virus and anti-hog-cholera serum may be used only by your veterinarian—and by him only under very special circumstances and only on specific authorization by his state veterinarian.

Therefore, much of what follows regarding hog cholera may not apply within the United States.

The disease is caused by a filtrable virus and is highly contagious. The blood, urine and other excretions all contain the infecting agent. It can be spread by man, dogs, cats, insects and even vehicles that have crossed infected premises.

The virus will live in meat as long as 90 days even if the meat is brine-cured or dry-salt cured. Sunshine kills the virus quickly and in warm weather it may lose its virulence in 24 hours even when not in the sun.

The virus usually gets into the body in feed. It quickly spreads to all organs where it causes hemorrhages and other changes.

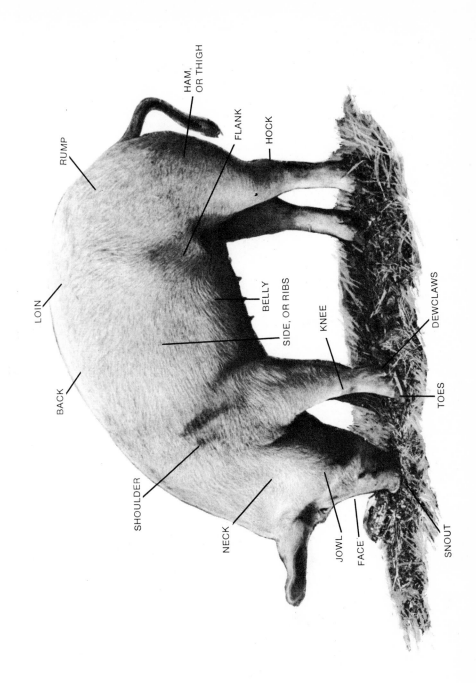

RUMP

HAM, OR THIGH

FLANK

HOCK

LOIN

BACK

BELLY

SIDE, OR RIBS

KNEE

DEWCLAWS

TOES

SHOULDER

NECK

JOWL

FACE

SNOUT

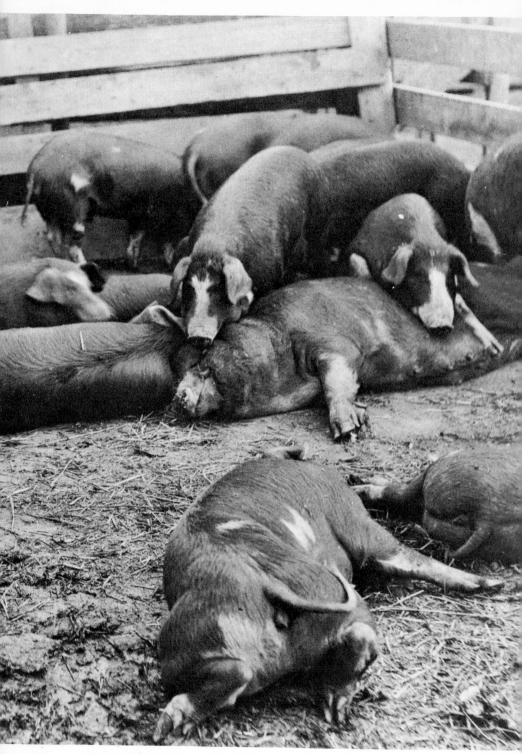

Hogs in advanced stage of hog cholera

USDA ph

Symptoms

First symptom of the disease is loss of appetite. Animals stay in their beds, scour and have high fever. When forced to move, they do so reluctantly and with great effort. Red blotches that do not turn white when pressed may appear on the abdomen and elsewhere. Convulsions may occur in advanced stages of the disease. Eyelids are stuck together with a discharge. Temperatures are usually 106 to 107 F.

Signs of weakness appear, particularly in the hind legs, which cross when the animal walks. This causes a peculiar wobbly gait.

Under usual conditions, one or two animals in a herd are stricken first. The rest of the herd is thus exposed to the disease, and a week or so later a number of animals may become sick at the same time. Hogs usually die within a week after symptoms appear. The death rate among animals contracting the disease is nearly 100 percent.

Diagnosis

Symptoms closely resemble those of a number of other diseases, including swine erysipelas and infectious necrotic enteritis.

Hog cholera has a more sudden onset than erysipelas. In hog cholera the eyelids become glued together whereas in erysipelas they do not. Erysipelas seems to be more painful than cholera and fever is higher. The red spots in hog cholera do not disappear when pressed whereas those of acute erysipelas do.

Hog cholera can be distinguished from infectious necrotic enteritis because cholera affects swine of all ages—not only the very young.

Highly accurate laboratory tests can be made to determine the presence of the disease. Such diagnosis should be made immediately if your veterinarian suspects hog cholera. When a positive diagnosis is made, the swine herd and the farm are placed under quarantine.

Prevention

There is no cure for hog cholera. At present the most widely used method for protection against the disease is the simultaneous injection of modified live virus vaccines and anti-hog-cholera serum. Injections should be made in accordance with instructions of manufacturers of these biologicals. Remember that this may be done only by a veterinarian and only on specific authorization by state and federal veterinarians.

The virus is often injected in the armpit, while the serum is injected under the skin of the flank. Some inject the serum into the abdominal cavity of small pigs and favor a spot behind the ear for large ones.

Because the weight of an animal determines the amount of a biological necessary to bring immunity, it is cheaper to vaccinate pigs against cholera when they are small. A large percentage of farmers vaccinate their new crop of pigs each year. Vaccination should be done either two weeks before or two weeks after pigs are weaned or castrated. A more solid immunity is conferred if vaccination is done after these procedures because the pigs are then a little older.

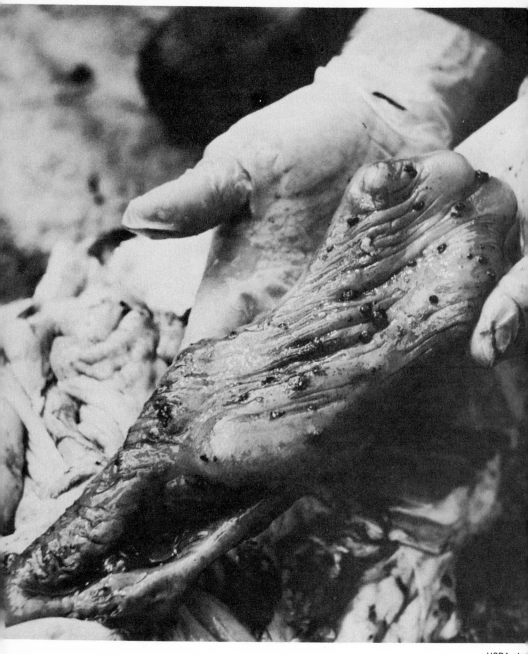

Button ulcers in the large intestine, a common sign of hog cholera. Each infected hog is a virus factory, multiplying chances for the disease to spread

Hog-cholera vaccines

Hog-cholera virus is prepared from the blood of pigs that are sick with hog cholera. Their blood is defibrinated and mixed with a preservative to make whole-blood virus.

Two types of vaccine have been developed, but neither one may be used in the U.S. except as stated previously.

Chemically treated vaccine does not produce cholera. It gives an immunity that is sufficient where exposure to the disease is not great.

The vaccine made by passing the virus through rabbits confers a more solid immunity. The virus is live but has been modified so that it does not produce cholera. As a precaution, however, the simultaneous use of antiserum is usually recommended.

The use of attenuated vaccines is subject to the same regulations as the unattenuated.

Hog cholera eradication program

A federal-state campaign to eradicate hog cholera from the United States got under way in 1962.

The law authorizes the Agricultural Research Service to prohibit interstate movement of virulent hog cholera virus, considered dangerous because it can help to spread the disease.

Close cooperation between swine producers, state and local agencies, and ARS enable best use of all the eradication tools. Here are the tools:

For swine owners

Isolation of replacement pigs until they are proved free of cholera.
Segregation of swine from visitors.
Sanitation of premises, vehicles, equipment, and workers' footwear, and the cooking of raw garbage fed to pigs.

For federal and state officials

Regulation of virus and of animal shipments within and across state lines, and inspection and quarantine where necessary.

Condemnation, destruction and proper disposal of infected and exposed animals, and payment of indemnities to owners with quarantine on the premises.

Information, to the swine industry, on campaign progress, requirement of prompt reporting of new hog cholera outbreaks, and training of specialists in eradication techniques.

Exploration through surveys, diagnosis, and traceback to infection sources, and research to improve eradication methods.

Hog cholera has been eradicated in the United States, Canada, Australia, England and perhaps a few other countries but is still prevalent in many parts of the world. Hence the danger of the disease is still here. The remnant of an imported pork sausage fed to a hog might lead to another epidemic.

Swine erysipelas

SWINE ERYSIPELAS is principally a disease of shotes between three and 12 months old, but also occurs among older and younger animals. Very young pigs seem to have great resistance to the malady.

The disease has become more widely distributed year by year and in some areas has become the most destructive malady of swine. It generally makes its appearance in warm weather, in the North from May to September, but it may occur at any time of year.

The disease is caused by *Erysipelothrix rhusiopathiae*, which can live in the soil for a long time. They do not form spores, but have a waxy covering that protects them. Once the infection appears on a farm it is likely to appear again.

The microbes are contained in the urine and dung of infected swine and may be carried in the bodies of healthy animals that have recovered from the disease. Man, cattle, horses, sheep, poultry and dogs are susceptible. The manner in which the disease is spread is not completely understood.

Symptoms

There are two forms of erysipelas, acute and chronic, both caused by the same microbe.

The acute type occurs most often. Symptoms so closely resemble those of hog cholera that it is difficult to tell them apart.

The onslaught of the disease is often rapid. Sometimes the first indications are the deaths of several animals that appeared to be in good health a few hours before.

Early stages of the disease are accompanied by high temperature, loss of appetite, stiffness of gait, occasional vomiting, arched back and the inclination of sick animals to withdraw from the herd. Sick hogs lie in their bedding, watching every move of an attendant even though they don't want to move themselves. If forced to move, they start with energy but squeal loudly as if in great pain.

Swine erysipelas is often called "diamond-skin disease" because irregular red patches, roughly diamond-shaped, appear on the lighter parts of the skin. These are not tender or swollen. Sometimes they appear in acute cases where animals die in a few days, but they are more often associated with milder cases. In the latter, swine recover within two weeks unless complications set in.

The affected areas of the skin later die and slough off. The ears and tail are often lost in this manner. Denuded areas may become the site for secondary infections.

In the chronic type, the infection localizes in the tissues or joints of the animal. No symptoms can be noticed when the disease settles in the heart valves, gall bladder or tonsils, but vegetative growths do appear on the heart valves and interfere with the free circulation of blood.

When the joints are affected, they become stiff and the bones become enlarged. The animal has a tendency to walk on its toes. The diamond-shaped blotches may be so faint that they are not readily noticeable. Death losses are low. But like the survivors from the acute type, the chronic animals are usually unprofitable.

The chronic type may appear following the acute type or it also may come without pronounced symptoms of illness.

Since man is susceptible to swine erysipelas, gloves should be worn when handling diseased animals. When localized skin infections do occur, they may be treated by applying anti-erysipelas serum under a loose bandage.

Specimens from suspected outbreaks of the disease should be sent to a laboratory for examination. Most states have such laboratories and there is no charge for examinations. Information may be obtained from veterinarians or livestock sanitary officials.

Treatment

Swine-erysipelas serum is a highly effective remedy if given when the disease starts. Sick animals, when treated, recover within 24 hours.

When an outbreak occurs, all animals in a herd should be given antiserum. The immunity conferred by this lasts only 10 to 20 days, but this affords time to carry out other control measures. What's more, if animals pick up live organisms during this period, they will be actively immune to the disease for six months. The serum is of no value against the chronic form of the disease.

Penicillin is quite effective in treatment of the disease.

Prevention

In heavily infected areas, simultaneous vaccination consisting of immune serum and live microbes is used. This can be done only by a veterinarian and under arrangements with state and federal officials. This form of vaccination has the drawback of possibly infecting areas which might otherwise be free of contamination.

Following an outbreak, infected houses, pens and feeding troughs should be thoroughly scrubbed and disinfected. A 2 percent lye solution is a good disinfectant, and when applied warm has the added advantage of being an excellent cleansing agent for walls, partitions, and floors.

Healthy animals should be removed to clean grounds where practicable, and grounds should be plowed up and planted with crops for a while.

Necrotic enteritis, or pig typhus

INFECTIOUS NECROTIC ENTERITIS is also called infectious gastro-enteritis, paratyphoid, pig typhus and "necro." It is caused by a microbe known as *Salmonella choleraesuis (suipestifer)*.

The microbe is peculiar in the way it acts. It may be present in the intestine of an animal for a long time without causing any trouble. Then suddenly, with a change in feed or in the presence of other infections such as hog cholera or swine influenza, it flares up and infects all the young pigs and shotes in a herd.

Symptoms

Usually necrotic enteritis starts with a fever, loss of appetite and diarrhea. The dung often contains fiber, pieces of dead tissue or blood. In the beginning "necro" may be confused with swine erysipelas or hog cholera. Here caution is necessary. If animals sick with the disease are treated with hog-cholera virus and anti-hog-cholera serum, deaths may occur in large numbers.

This type of Salmonellosis may appear not only as enteritis, but sometimes as a form of septicemia (blood poisoning), or it may involve the lungs. This has led to the suggestion that a second agent may sometimes be involved, and play a role in reducing resistance in certain organs.

The disease appears with suddenness in pigs from two to four months old. Younger pigs are sometimes affected. Hog cholera alone causes death in about 15 days, but if it appears with pig "necro," death comes in from five days to a week.

Post-mortem examinations reveal damage principally to the large intestines and cecum, but the small intestines and stomach may also show signs of the disease. The walls of these parts of the digestive tract are thickened and covered with a yellowish-gray layer of dead tissue. There is often a purplish discoloration of the tonsils and surrounding tissues.

Treatment

Many treatments have been tried over the years, copper sulfate, and oats soaked in an alkaline solution being among the more common. No drugs have been found that will completely rid an animal of Salmonella bacteria. Sulfaguanidine, Sulfathalidine, nitrofurazone, and some of the antiobiotics including Terramycin have been used in treating the disease but none have been outstandingly successful.

Prevention

Rigid sanitary methods are recommended for control of the disease. It is sound practice to have pigs farrowed in the early spring so that dams and litters can be turned into clean pastures when youngsters are 10 to 12 days old. In this way they have the benefit of green forage and sunshine. A so-called "A" house should be provided for each litter, and these houses should not be too close together.

Supplementary feed and drinking water should be provided in such a way that there is least danger of contamination. Over-feeding, especially from self-feeders, is reported to help bring on the disease. "Necro" thrives on farms that abound in filth and mud holes. When an outbreak occurs, sick pigs should at once be separated from healthy ones to help keep the disease from spreading.

The McLean County System of swine sanitation (see index) has been highly effective in preventing the disease.

Transmissible gastroenteritis (TGE)

THIS DISEASE is characterized by producing death in 90 percent to 100 percent of baby pigs less than 10 days old. The causative agent is a filtrable virus of the coronavirus class. TGE usually enters a herd with older animals, where it causes very little disturbance. But once it gets into the farrowing house it is devastating. The importance of bacterial secondary invaders is still being debated, but it is known that the virus can establish itself in the cells of the intestine without the presence of pathogenic or disease-producing bacteria.

Once the premises become infected and contaminated, the disease is likely to recur with succeeding farrowings. The incubation period may be only 16 to 18 hours, and diarrhea appears quickly, being followed by death in five to seven days. Because viruses multiply only in living cells, transmission from pig to pig must include very fresh bowel excrement. From this it readily invades the cells of stomach and intestines, and then spreads to widely separated tissues of the body.

The clinical signs of infection in older animals vary greatly, in fact a sow may lose all of her pigs from it but show no disturbance herself. In feeder pigs there may be a rapid decrease in rate of gain, but in young pigs diarrhea is always evident. The bowel discharge may be whitish, or yellowish, or greenish.

Diagnosis is usually made by observing the rapid spread of the disease, and the extremely high death rate. It may be confirmed by laboratory procedures.

No treatment has been found effective, although many have been tried with some degree of success. One program of immunization has also been tried. It consists of feeding the intestines and their contents from dead pigs to the pregnant sows at weekly intervals for the last three weeks of pregnancy. This appears to immunize the sow to the extent that the colostrum she produces will protect her pigs during the first days of life, and until they can build up their own immunity from contact.

In many instances, the outbreaks are "self-limiting" in that they disappear at the end of the farrowing period. However, the disease susally reappears at a subsequent farrowing period, because the infection persists in the bodies of older animals and in filth and litter protected from exposure to air and sunlight.

Vesicular exanthema, or "V.E." of swine

VESICULAR EXANTHEMA, commonly called "V.E.," attacks hogs of all ages and is highly contagious. It is caused by a virus.

The disease was first identified in California in 1932 but caused little damage. Then suddenly in 1951 it spread to the central part of the country and within ten months there were outbreaks in 40 states.

Vesicular exanthema is found almost exclusively on premises where hogs are fed garbage containing infected raw pork scraps. When the disease occurs on grain-feeding ranches, it can nearly always be traced to the addition of raw garbage. Once the disease gets started in a herd, up to 85 percent of the hogs may become infected.

Symptoms

Usually the first symptom noted by a herd owner is lameness of one or more animals. Close examination then reveals the presence of vesicles, or blisters, on or about the snout, on the lips, gums, tongue or other portions of the mouth of the infected animal. The blisters are whitish and contain varying amounts of clear fluid. Some of them are flat whereas others are raised to about the size of an almond. Fever reaches 104 to 107 degrees F. Appetite falls off.

In 24 to 48 hours, temperature becomes normal and at the same time blisters break and leave raw areas. At this time lameness appears, due to infection in the feet. Hoofs may slough off and the pain may cause hogs to walk on their knees and hocks. Symptoms are almost identical with those of foot and mouth disease. The big difference is that V.E. will not infect cattle or sheep.

In some cases, V.E. affects feet only. No blisters occur elsewhere.

The disease may occur on the same farm more than once with only short intervals between outbreaks. This may be because immunity to the disease is short-lived or due to another type of virus. Four distinct types of the virus that causes the disease have been established.

Sores caused by the disease may heal in five to seven days but healing can take two to three weeks.

Few death losses occur among older hogs but in some outbreaks mortality among pigs is high. Greatest losses lie in the abortion of sows in the late stages of pregnancy, breeding difficulties, and loss of weight from lack of appetite.

Control

There is no effective treatment known for V.E. However, the disease no longer has much significance. In the 1950's an eradication plan was put into effect by U.S.D.A., and the states which called for (1) inspection, (2) quarantine, (3) prompt disposal of infested swine, (4) thorough disinfection of all contaminated areas, and (5) laws forbidding the feeding of raw garbage to swine. These measures eradicated the disease in four years.

Leptospirosis in hogs

LEPTOSPIROSIS in hogs is caused by the same organism that causes it in cattle—*Leptospira pomona*, a parasite. In some other countries when man becomes infected with it, the ailment is known as swineherd's disease. It was first reported in the United States in 1952. The disease is spread through the urine of infected animals.

Symptoms

Symptoms among hogs may vary from mild jaundice and slow gains in weight to severe nervous and digestive troubles. There may be poor appetite, fever, frequent urination, mild inflammation of the eyelids, weakness of the hind legs, stiffness, blood tinged urine and drowsiness.

The disease may cause serious losses from abortions and pigs dead or weak at birth. Jaundice and anemia may lead to condemnation of slaughtered hogs. A more positive diagnosis of the disease can be made through laboratory tests.

So far as practicable, control measures as set forth in the chapter "Bovine leptospirosis" should be applied with hogs. Vaccination is common practice among good hog managers.

Sore mouth, or necrotic stomatitis

NECROTIC STOMATITIS, or sore mouth, is a form of necrotic rhinitis, and is caused by *Actinomyces necrophorus*.

Symptoms

Suckling pigs that are affected show signs of pain. Inflamed patches may be found on the gums, lips and palate. These later develop into what are known as necrotic ulcers. This means that skin and surface tissues die and then slough off. Pigs are unable to eat on account of the severe pain. A disagreeable odor is associated with the disease.

Treatment

Pigs seldom recover from sore mouth unless treatment is begun early in the course of the disease. Treatment consists of cleaning the mouth with mouthwashes such as potassium permanganate solution or applying a 5 percent silver nitrate solution.

Atrophic rhinitis

ATROPHIC RHINITIS was first reported in the United States in 1944. Since then it has become a major disease of hogs. Its cause is not definitely agreed upon, and may be a combination of infection and nutritional factors; and it is not known exactly how the disease is transmitted from one animal to another.

Symptoms

The disease is most prevalent in pigs two to five months old, and has a slow, mild onset when introduced into a herd so that it does not cause any great damage in the year following its introduction.

A few pigs in a litter begin to sneeze and sniffle, and later show evidence of chronic nose trouble. On examination, it is noted that the cartilagenous bones in the nostril (the turbinate bones) have been decreased in size, or have disappeared. This allows dust to reach the trachea and bronchi, and the lungs, thus interfering with growth to the extent that severely infected pigs may never attain normal market weight—or if they do, it is at a cost which leaves no profit.

But in the second year, gilts retained in the herd will produce litters that are seriously affected. Sneezing is frequent about three weeks after farrowing among all pigs of an infected litter. A clear sticky discharge comes from the nose. Often an affected pig will rub its nose vigorously against bedding or walls and shake its head as though it wanted to dislodge something in the nose. Pneumonia may develop within the first week or ten days of life.

Animals that survive are unthrifty, have a rough hair coat and suffer from diarrhea with consequent loss of weight. This disease does not kill outright but among litters of pigs from affected dams the death rate, after weaning, may be as high as 30 percent.

In its early stages, atrophic rhinitis may be confused with a cold, baby pig disease, various deficiencies or another infectious disease.

Of the pigs that survive an attack of the disease, about 20 percent are stunted for life. Their faces are twisted and have a typical dished-in appearance. This distortion interferes with breathing, causes frequent sneezing and nose bleeding.

Another group of surviving pigs will show no apparent ill effects but will take three weeks longer than normal to attain market weight. The remaining pigs may attain market weight in the usual time but may nevertheless remain carriers of the disease.

Control

There is no way known to treat the disease effectively or to vaccinate against it, but favorable results have sometimes been reported after using nasal sprays or nasal swabs in which various sulfonamides and antibiotics have been used.

According to the United States Department of Agriculture, the most satisfactory method of control is to keep the disease, out of a herd. Much can be accomplished by learning everything possible about conditions in the herd from which replacements are to be obtained.

A more drastic method is to dispose of the affected herd. Thorough cleaning and disinfection of the buildings and equipment should follow. It would be well to renovate the lots by filling in wallows and by providing drainage in the low, boggy areas. Replacements from disease-free herds can be made after several months.

A third method involves the selection within the herd of normal-appearing pigs for breeding purposes and the elimination of those that are obviously affected. Such a program could be improved by using the rhinoscope to aid in the selection and rejection of the pigs.

A rhinoscope is an instrument with an attached light that enables a person to examine the inner parts of the nose. When atrophic rhinitis has been present, the inner bony structure and the cartilage between the nostrils are wasted away.

Unfortunately the nasal structures cannot be seen completely; therefore there may be inaccuracies of diagnosis, particularly when the changes are not far advanced. This method is about 75 percent accurate.

Bull nose, or necrotic rhinitis

NECROTIC RHINITIS, also called bull nose, is a chronic disease that appears in the form of a swollen snout and face of pigs. It affects both the bones and the tissues. Pigs six to eight weeks old are the most susceptible.

The disease appears to be caused or spread by several groups of organisms, associated with insanitary conditions, abscesses and ulcers. They invade the body through wounds caused by fighting, blows from sharp sticks, pieces of barbed wire, and so on. Mud holes, filthy lots and old manure help to bring the disease on.

Symptoms

Among the first symptoms are loss of appetite and frequent sneezing. The discharge from the sneezing often contains blood. Swellings or lumps appear on the snout and surrounding area. These contain a cheese-like substance with a foul odor. Affected pigs have trouble eating because of the pain, sometimes becoming so weak from lack of food that they die.

Treatment

Treatment, to be of any use, must be started early. It consists in dipping the snouts of infected pigs into a creolin solution, which comes in standard strengths of 2 or 3 percent. The swellings should be opened and the pus removed before dipping. Painting the snouts with half-strength tincture of iodine is another standard remedy. In young pigs, sulfamethazine given as a drench has been found useful.

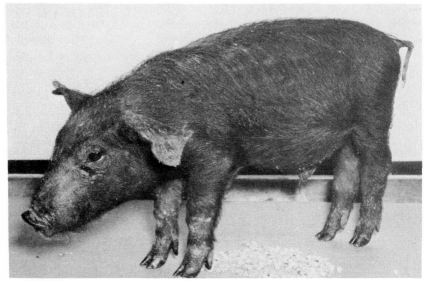

Pig shows the typical swollen snout of bull nose

Large roundworms of swine

LARGE ROUNDWORMS, or ascarids, are the most common hog worms and the ones that do the most damage. They cause digestive troubles and retard the growth of the animals, especially affecting young pigs.

When they first emerge from eggs, roundworms are too small to be seen with the naked eye. During this period they penetrate the intestines, enter the blood stream and migrate through the body, damaging the liver and lungs. After six to 10 days, many of them pass through the lung tissue into the windpipe and esophagus. Here they are swallowed with food and water and again resume life in the intestines. In about two months more they are fully grown and start laying eggs.

Roundworms cause a thumping cough while in the lungs, commonly known as "thumps." This may be followed by pneumonia. Hog men often blame the thumps on cold weather, an over-fat condition, or lack of exercise, but usually thumps are caused by roundworms. The larvae that migrate through the liver seldom cause immediate symptoms, but may cause a mild case of jaundice, and they leave spots of whitish scar tissue throughout the liver.

How roundworms are spread

When hogs get older, they become resistant to roundworms. But once infected, older hogs still harbor them and act as carriers. Each roundworm lays millions of eggs while in the intestines, and these are spread around the premises in the hog droppings.

Roundworm eggs do not always cause infection when swallowed. But if weather and other conditions are favorable, the tiny worms develop inside of the eggs. These are infective.

The eggs are resistant to cold weather, drought and most disinfectants. They have been known to live as long as five years under suitable conditions.

Treatment

Many drugs for treating roundworms have been used. Those that can be added to water or feed are the most popular. Among them are piperazine, dichlorvos, levamisole, sodium fluoride and cadmium compounds. The latter two are the least expensive but their use is hazardous since they are poisonous and may result in death if the animals get an overdose.

Prevention

A system that provides about 98-percent protection against roundworms and other parasitic diseases was developed a number of years ago in Illinois. It is known as the McLean County System of swine sanitation.

Since young pigs are more susceptible to roundworms than older ones, the system is based on the idea of keeping young animals from becoming infected. Here's the way it's done:

1. Clean farrowing pens thoroughly and then scrub them with scalding water and lye.

2. Clean the sows, particularly their udders, just before putting them in the clean beds to farrow.

3. When sows have farrowed, haul them and their litters—do not drive them—to a clean pasture. This pasture should consist of a forage crop sown on land that was cultivated for the purpose—not just an old pasture.

4. Keep the young pigs on this land until they are at least four months old. One further step would be to worm the sows before moving them to the farrowing pen.

Not only does this system provide almost 100-percent protection against roundworms, but pigs raised in this manner are ready for market several weeks sooner than those raised in muddy hog lots or on old contaminated pastures.

Swine kidney worms

SWINE KIDNEY WORMS (*Stephamurus dentatus*) are among the most injurious pests that prey upon livestock in the Southern states. The worms cause losses by damaging the kidneys, liver and other organs. Sometimes they even invade the loin and other muscles and thus may ruin a whole carcass. Under meat-inspection rules, infested meat and organs are condemned as unfit for use as food.

In addition, kidney worms make swine unthrifty. Infected kidneys and livers do not perform properly, so the animals cannot digest and assimilate their feed as they should.

Although the worms are most common in the South, they have been reported in the northern part of the country and even in Canada.

Kidney worms are black-and-white, and when fully grown are between one and two inches long and from 1/20 to 1/10 of an inch thick. Swine become infected with them by swallowing the larvae that are in contaminated soil. The larvae enter the blood stream through the intestines. They can also get into the blood by penetrating the skin. The larvae are so small that they cannot ordinarily be seen with the naked eye.

The larvae are carried by the blood to the liver, lungs and other organs. Those that lodge in the liver and nearby blood vessels grow to many times their original size in a period of four to five months. During this time, many of them burrow extensively through the tissue where they leave crooked bloody tracks. Others break through the outside wall of the liver and wander around until they reach the kidneys. Here they cause quite an extensive inflammation.

The time required for kidney worms to reach maturity seems to vary considerably in different pigs. According to one authority, the worms reach adulthood in from six to seven months after they enter the blood stream. In another investigation, the time was more than a year. They lay their eggs in the tissue of the kidneys and in the ureters, which are the tubes that lead from the kidneys to the bladder.

The eggs are discharged with the urine. One moderately infested hog has been known to pass as many as a million eggs in one day.

The eggs that fall on moist shaded soil hatch in 24 to 48 hours. In warm weather, the larvae develop rapidly and become infective in three to five days. In cooler weather, development may take a week or longer.

Neither eggs nor larvae can withstand sunlight, drying or freezing. Corncobs, cornhusks, pine needles, leaves and other litter often afford the shelter and moisture that keep them alive for several weeks.

How to eradicate swine kidney worms

Swine kidney worms can be eradicated from infested pastures in three farrowing seasons by using only first-litter gilts for breeding, then removing them after they weaned their pigs.

Kidney worms may require as long as a year to attain egg-laying maturity in swine. A gilt normally weans her pigs and can be disposed of before she starts passing kidney worm eggs in her urine.

This gilt-only method of removing kidney worms should cost farmers little or no more than the conventional practice of retaining older, frequently infested sows for breeding. After three or four farrowing seasons (about 2 years), hog lots will be free of the parasite so that older sows can be used more profitably.

Kidney worm control with drugs isn't satisfactory because none have been found effective in all areas of a pig's body where the parasite is active—liver, kidneys, kidney fat, loin muscles, central nervous system, and other organs.

Lungworms

LUNGWORMS cause general unthriftiness and are among the most injurious parasites occurring in swine. They are whitish, threadlke roundworms about one-half inch to two inches long and about one-fifteenth of an inch thick. They are technically called *Metastrongylus elongatus*.

Female worms in the lungs of infested pigs lay many eggs which are coughed up, swallowed and eliminated in the droppings. The eggs are swallowed by angleworms, and the larvae emerge when the eggs hatch. Pigs become infested with lungworms when they eat the angleworms. A single earthworm may harbor as many as 2000 larvae. The young lungworms penetrate the walls of the swine intestines and find their way into the lymph and blood streams. They are carried to the right side of the heart and to the lungs, where they complete their life cycle.

Prevention

Preventive measures consist in keeping pigs from rooting and keeping them on soil where angleworms are at a minimum.

Ringing the noses of pigs keeps them from rooting. Providing adequate rations tends to keep them from hunting feed in sheltered places where earthworms are numerous. Keeping pastures free from boards, logs and trash helps to keep earthworms underground.

Moist shelters with dirt floors, and the accumulation of humus and manure in permanent pastures favor an increase in earthworm population. On the other hand, temporary pastures are comparatively free from them. This is especially true where ground is plowed repeatedly. In short, the use of clean, well-drained temporary pastures and dry, clean shelters will do much to avoid or wipe out lungworm infestation.

Treatment

Effective treatments against lungworms are claimed, but they are not always efficient because they do not reach the smaller bronchioles where the worms are found.

Acute hypoglycemia—baby pig disease

THIRTY PIGS out of every hundred farrowed die before weaning. Many of these deaths are caused by "baby pig" disease, also known as acute hypoglycemia. This means "not enough sugar in the blood." The disease generally occurs from 24 to 72 hours after birth.

Hypoglycemia is not contagious. It may occur in any breed of swine. Small litters are just as susceptible as large ones. Animals farrowed in spring—whether early or late—seem to be more susceptible than those born at other times.

Symptoms

Pigs that get baby pig disease seem normal at birth. After 24 hours they appear listless. They shiver and have no desire to nurse. They tend to wander away from the dam, and may burrow into the bedding. When disturbed they emit squeals. Hair stands on end, skin is cold, and within 48 hours after symptoms appear, usually many, if not all sick pigs in a litter are dead.

Post-mortem examinations do not reveal any damage to the organs of animals other than a slightly yellowish or deep red color of the liver. There is generally no diarrhea except in cases where the course of the disease has been unusually prolonged.

Treatment and control

The exact cause of baby pig disease is not known and methods for its prevention have not been found. But it is known that the disease is associated with decreased milk flow of dams and lack of sugar in the blood of pigs. These facts have given rise to treatments that have greatly reduced losses.

The cause of hypoglycemia is lack of carbohydrates in the diet, which means "lack of milk." Why so many sows suffer from agalactia is not evident, but can be partly corrected by feeding a full ration right up to farrowing time.

Experiments conducted for a number of years by veterinarians at the University of Illinois show that baby pig disease can be greatly reduced if sows and gilts are fed a liberal ration throughout pregnancy. Contrary to common practice, grain rations should not be reduced during the last few weeks of the gestation period.

To stimulate the flow of milk, pregnant females should be fed $1\frac{1}{4}$ to 2 pounds of grain per hundred-weight per day, the smaller ration for big sows and the larger one for small gilts. The animals should also have free access to best-quality hay or other legumes.

Grain should be so placed that pregnant animals have to exercise to get it. Such animals should be well fed but not fat. They should be fed lightly just before farrowing time and not at all for 24 hours thereafter.

Pigs should be dried promptly after farrowing, and kept warm. They should be watched carefully for any indication of failure to nurse, any tendency to burrow into the bedding, lack of energy, or rough coat. These are all indications for a prompt examination of the sow to insure that she has milk for the pigs. If she does not, your veterinarian can give her a hormone (pituitrin) which will stimulate "letdown" of her milk.

A hover or brooder should be available to the pigs, and if this does not prevent or correct the situation, individual treatment is required. This can consist of feeding of corn syrup and fortified cow's milk. If the pig is too weak to swallow, when spoon-fed such materials, it may be advisable to inject a dextrose solution, either subcutaneously or intravenously.

For early hand feeding, corn syrup dissolved in an equal amount of water is recommended. Each pig should be given one or two tablespoonfuls every two or three hours. When appetite has returned, modified whole cow's milk can be used, adding the white of one egg, three ounces of cream and three ounces of limewater to every two quarts. This should be heated to body temperature on feeding. It may be advisable to return pigs to the sow after several feedings.

The exact amount of syrup given a pig depends upon its vigor, age and appetite. Too much will cause scours. Pigs need not be hand fed after they are four or five days old. They should then be given a mixture of whole and skim milk which they can drink from a pan.

Myoclonia congenita

THIS IS an inherited condition, called popularly by such names as dancing pigs, jumpy pig disease, shakes, shivers, and trembles. It usually affects litters instead of single pigs.

Distribution and total incidence of the condition are very sketchy. Minnesota has the best data, and reports more than 150 litters affected in 18 months.

Because information is vague, causes other than genetics have been blamed. These include hog cholera vaccination of pregnant sows, virus infection, and improper nutrition.

No treatment appears to be effective, but many pigs recover spontaneously and without treatment.

Rickets in swine

RICKETS is a disease of young animals caused by lack of the proper amounts of calcium and phosphorus or by failure of the body to absorb these substances properly. In the latter case the underlying cause is usually insufficient vitamin D.

Symptoms

The first symptoms of rickets are usually loss of appetite, bloating, weakness and perverse appetite—pigs eat filth and gnaw one another's tails and ears.

In the more advanced stages of the disease, animals are lame, their joints become enlarged and their legs bowed. Sometimes affected animals crawl on their knees or lie on one side, too weak to get up. Pigs with rickets lose weight and become runts unless the condition is corrected.

In slowly developing or chronic cases the enlargements at the growing ends of bones are particularly noticeable on the ribs, where they produce what has been called "The Rosary of Rickets."

Prevention

Rickets is very likely to develop when pigs are kept indoors and fed rations composed largely of cereal grains without any sun-cured roughage.

The cheapest source of vitamin D is direct sunlight. Since there is usually not enough sunshine in the North during the winter, other sources of vitamin D should be provided. One of the best sources is high-grade sun-cured hay, particularly alfalfa.

Other hays rich in vitamin D are soybean, lespedeza, sweet clover and red clover. These have the disadvantage of not being so palatable as alfalfa. The latter may be fed either free choice or at the rate of 5 to 10 percent of the total ration for fattening pigs and 10 to 15 percent for sows and boars.

A ration containing enough calcium and phosphorus is as important as supplying enough vitamin D. Buttermilk, skim milk, fish meal, tankage and meat scraps all contain a liberal amount of calcium and phosphorus. Legumes and hay are good calcium sources. Wheat bran and meals such as linseed and cottonseed are rich in phosphorus but low in calcium content. Commercially prepared swine feeds are frequently fortified with supplemental amounts of vitamin D.

Infectious arthritis, or navel ill, of swine

INFECTIOUS ARTHRITIS, commonly called navel ill or joint ill, is a disease of recently farrowed pigs. Generally it starts when the stump of the navel cord becomes infected with pus-producing germs before it has had time to dry up, but this can be prevented by dipping the navel in tincture of iodine as soon after birth as possible. These germs enter the blood stream. In other cases, infection occurs prior to birth. The germs were present in the blood or womb of the mother.

The disease may be caused by a number of different microbes, but streptococci are the most common. Upon entering the blood stream, the organisms settle in the joints and surrounding areas causing lameness, either with or without swelling.

Damp, unsanitary quarters and inadequate bedding are said to be important factors in bringing on the disease.

Symptoms

Infectious arthritis usually appears in the first week of life. The pigs don't want to suckle. They are at first dull and constipated and this may be followed by diarrhea. There is often a discharge of pus from the navel. Joints are hot and swollen and the little animals are lame. Failure to suckle brings on weakness and many of the sick pigs die. The disease may recur among those that recover.

Navel ill may be confused with other types of lameness such as that brought on by erysipelas or swine brucellosis. Infection of the navel is one symptom that helps to make a definite diagnosis.

Prevention and treatment

The most important prevention step is to provide clean quarters for sows about to farrow. Young pigs should be provided with clear bedding and not permitted to lie directly on concrete floors. As soon as possible after birth, dip the stump of the navel cord in the tincture of iodine.

Treatment of the navel is often unsatisfactory. If the navel shows signs of infection, infiltrate a solution of penicillin and Streptomycin. Since a variety of organisms may be involved, the so-called "broad spectrum" antibiotics are often more effective.

Anemia of suckling pigs

MODERN METHODS of raising pigs have cut down losses from parasitic and other diseases. But at the same time, losses from anemia have gone up. This is because so many pigs no longer have access to as much iron and copper as they did formerly.

Anemia among pigs occurs most often in the late fall, winter or early spring. Sow's milk is poor in iron and copper. Yet pigs need these elements for building the blood necessary for growth.

Pigs normally get their needed supply of iron and copper from soil and green feed. In winter proper feed is not so readily available and since modern pigpens have cement or tight wooden floors, pigs do not have access to soil.

Anemia appears most often among pigs from one to six weeks old, with the greatest number of cases occurring in about the third week of life. Anemic pigs are pale, lack vigor and fail to make normal gains in weight. The slightest exertion brings on labored breathing, commonly called the "thumps."

Symptoms

Young pigs may be severely anemic and yet look fairly well developed and fat. Some of them die suddenly. Others may later become thin and linger for several weeks before dying.

Watery blood, paleness of muscles, lungs and kidneys, and a grayish-yellow mottled liver are revealed by post-mortem examination. Digestive disturbances and pneumonia may also be present.

Methods of treatment

Injection of copper solution subcutaneously when the pigs are only a few days old is effective.

Several products are available commercially, and the directions of the manufacturer should be followed.

These have completely replaced the old procedures of putting sod in each pen, painting the sows' udders with iron solution, and giving iron tablets.

Iodine deficiency in pigs

IN THE so-called "goiter belt," comprising the north central and north-western states, losses among spring litters of pigs often occur as a result of iodine deficiency. The soil, water, and crops of this region lack iodine. The pigs are born hairless, or nearly so and they have enlarged thyroid glands (goiter). Such pigs are usually weak at birth and die within a few hours.

Iodine deficiency may be prevented by adding one or two grains of potassium or sodium iodide to the daily ration of the pregnant sow. Iodized salt will prevent the deficiency if made available to breeding animals.

Mastitis of sows

MASTITIS, also called garget, is an inflammation of the udder or mammary gland. Because the udder of a sow hangs close to the ground, it is often injured.

Mastitis is often a part of the MMA syndrome—mastitis-metritis-agalactia. A Streptococcus is often involved in this condition, but there is no general agreement as to the degree of relationship between mastitis and metritis, while the connection between mastitis and agalactia is readily understood.

In most instances a single segment of the gland is involved; in which case a single pig may be starved for milk and be forced to "rob" from adjoining segments of the udder.

Cuts and bruises are responsible for most cases of mastitis. The microbes that cause the disease gain entrance through such openings and multiply until the udder is inflamed and painful. Another source of infection is through the teat canal. Pus-producing microbes are principal offenders.

Symptoms

Mastitis is easily recognized. Mammary glands are hard, swollen and hot. Pain is often so great that a sow will not permit pigs to nurse.

Treatment

Mastitis can be prevented to a large extent by proper care, feeding and quarters. Farrowing quarters should be disinfected and properly bedded before farrowing time.

Inflammations should be treated with hot applications and massaged twice a day to reduce swelling. An udder ointment as used for cattle is used to advantage here. Or the affected section may be treated by injecting through the teat canal a penicillin or sulfa drug—or a combination.

Swine brucellosis

SWINE BRUCELLOSIS may occur wherever hogs are raised. It is not so serious as brucellosis of cattle because it can be wiped out of a herd with less financial loss. But if not controlled it may cost two or three pigs per litter between acute outbreaks and more during them.

The microbe that causes it is called *Brucella suis*. It is related to the microbes that bring on brucellosis in cattle and goats, and like them, it is a public health hazard since it causes undulant fever.

Symptoms

The most common symptom of swine brucellosis is abortion. This results in infection of the womb, and the birth of weak pigs, of which many die.

But the disease also attacks other organs of the body, usually only one or a few in the same animal. Lameness, abscesses, swelling of the testicles, and inflammation of the backbone (spondylitis) that sometimes results in paralysis are some of the more common symptoms. But the presence of such conditions is not always the result of brucellosis and swine may be infected without visible signs.

Post-mortem examinations show that the disease may lodge in the intestines, liver, gall bladder or urinary bladder. Sterility in both male and female frequently follows infection of the sex organs. A thin watery discharge often flows from the vagina of infected sows.

When brucellosis first invades a herd, the percentage of abortions is high, but thereafter the number falls off. Animals that have aborted once usually do not do so again. This does not mean that the disease is no longer present but merely that it has become chronic. Gilts and sows that apparently recover become carriers and infect any susceptible animals newly introduced in the herd.

Abortion that occurs early in pregnancy often escapes notice. The discharged fetus is trampled and becomes mixed with the dirt and litter. The thing that is noticed is that the sow or gilt again shows signs of heat although she was believed to be pregnant. Abortions that take place late in the second month of pregnancy or thereafter are readily observed.

How the disease is spread

Swine brucellosis is spread in many ways. Sucking pigs become carriers after drinking milk from an infected dam. Water and food become contaminated from urine, infected afterbirths and dung and discharges. If there is an infected animal in a herd it is practically impossible to keep brucellosis from spreading.

The disease is usually introduced into a herd by the addition of infected animals, but it may be brought in on infected feed bags or drainage from infected premises.

Swine should be purchased only from sources known to be free from the disease, that is, where every member of a herd is negative to a blood test. If animals are purchased from a herd where a single member is a reactor, there is danger of introducing the disease, even though the particular animals purchased are not reactors.

Abortion caused by brucellosis should not be confused with abortion due to other causes such as mechanical injuries, the presence of other infections, and vitamin or mineral deficiencies.

Diagnosis

Brucellosis of swine cannot be diagnosed by outward symptoms. The standard blood agglutination test as used in cattle is also used for testing swine, but is much less accurate for swine. Strangely, the antigen of cattle brucellosis works just as well with swine as that made from swine *Brucella.*

Many animals that have recovered from swine brucellosis show a negative test, even though they are carriers of the disease, and sometimes swine known to be non-infected show positive reactions. However, the blood agglutination test is practical in determining herd infection. If titers of 1:100 or over are found in any of the animals, all swine in the herd should be considered as possible carriers.

Control measures

There is no effective drug for treatment of swine brucellosis. But the disease can be wiped out with very little loss since the value of a gilt for slaughter is about the same as the cost of replacement. This of course does not apply to valuable blood lines.

Where brucellosis occurs in swine maintained for producing pork, elimination of the disease is not difficult. It does not spread from such groups to others and tends to die out because the animals become immune.

The breeding herd is responsible for keeping the disease alive. If the sale of infected pigs from such herds were stopped, the problem of swine brucellosis would disappear.

Swine brucellosis eradication plan

"Validated Brucellosis-Free Herd" is the term used in the intensified swine brucellosis eradication effort begun by the states and U.S.D.A. in 1961. Here's how the program works:

Individual herds are validated brucellosis-free for one year, using all procedures recommended by the U. S. Livestock Sanitary Association and approved by U.S.D.A. and cooperating states. In brief, these procedures consist of two consecutive negative blood tests of each adult animal in a herd. When a herd qualifies, the owner is supplied with an appropriate sign bearing the symbol of validation—identifying his herd as a source of brucellosis-free hogs.

Eventual eradication of the disease in all swine herds is the goal of the program. However, major emphasis first will be on validation of purebred herds. These are the source of most breeding boars—and swine brucellosis is primarily spread by infected boars.

So a producer's *best* plan is to validate his herd, then purchase boars and replacement breeding stock from other validated herds *only*. Programs for establishing brucellosis-free swine herds now exist in 30 states. In addition, herds in the SPF (Specific Pathogen-Free) program qualify as Validated Brucellosis-Free Herds.

If a herd blood test reveals infection, a producer has three alternate methods of eradicating the disease. Information on these methods—and on the Validated Brucellosis-Free Herd program—is available from state or federal disease control officials and county agents.

Swine dysentery

SWINE DYSENTERY is also known as infectious hemorrhagic enteritis, bloody diarrhea, black scours, and by several other names. It is an acute, highly fatal inflammation of the large intestines. *Salmonella choleraesuis* is usually a primary infective agent.

The disease occurs most often in the swine-producing states of the Middle West. Nearly all outbreaks can be traced to swine purchased from sales barns or public stockyards. Within a week or 10 days after infected animals are added to a herd, the disease appears.

Losses among them are between 10 and 90 percent. In feeder hogs mortality is from 10 to 20 percent, while in brood sows losses are from 2 to 5 percent.

Swine dysentery is often associated with a diet of corn and frequently follows vaccination against hog cholera. It seems to be spread through contaminated food but there is no evidence that it is carried from one farm to another except by transfer of sick animals. The microbe that causes the disease is given off in the bowel discharge from infected animals.

Symptoms

The principal symptom of swine dysentery is a profuse bloody diarrhea. The discharge contains shreds of tissue and a varying amount of blood.

At first only a few animals are sick. Then, within a week or so, the whole herd comes down with the disease. Some animals go off their feed, but others show no loss of appetite. The pigs show a rise in temperature to as high as 106 degrees Fahrenheit from the fourth to the seventh day following the onset of the disease.

Diarrhea appears about the sixth day and the elimination of blood a day or two later. In severe attacks, some animals become weak and gaunt. The dung is usually red and is mixed with blood and mucus. In older animals it is a darker color that has given rise to the term "black scours" that is sometimes applied to the disease.

Some pigs die suddenly after a few days of illness while other linger two weeks or more. Those that recover are usually unthrifty.

Treatment

Aureomycin, bacitracin, streptomycin and drugs containing arsenic have been found effective in reducing death losses. Symptoms often reappear after first treatment, making a second treatment necessary. Soluble streptomycin and the arsenicals are most convenient to give since a herd can be treated by adding them to the drinking water.

Care should be taken not to overdose with arsenic. Two arsenic compounds are commonly used. They differ in strength, and each must be used in strict accordance with the directions of the manufacturer.

Control measures

There are no vaccines or other biological products known that will protect animals against the disease. Sanitary measures consist in keeping sick animals away from the others and providing both groups with clean well-drained quarters. Wholesome feed should be given in clean troughs or on concrete floors. Mud, manure and other sources of infection should not be allowed to accumulate.

In many cases the best way to handle an outbreak is to sell the herd for slaughter and start over on fresh grounds with healthy animals and strict methods of sanitation. The purpose of good diet is not only to put on weight but to build up resistance against disease.

Trichinosis

TRICHINOSIS is a disease caused by small roundworms that become embedded in the muscles of human beings, swine, dogs, rats, mice and many other animals. It is spread principally by eating infected pork that has not been sufficiently cooked or otherwise treated so as to kill the worm, called *Trichinella spiralis*, or commonly, trichina.

Symptoms

The disease is seldom diagnosed in living swine or other animals. The reason is that infected animals do not often become visibly sick. When they do, trichinosis is hard to identify because the symptoms are so much like those of other diseases.

Trichinae can be seen under a microscope by examining a thin layer of infected meat, but this method is not completely dependable.

In man, symptoms appear within nine or 10 days after trichinous meat has been eaten. Severity of the disease varies with the number of trichinae that have entered the intestines.

In mild cases symptoms may hardly be noticeable. In severe cases, there are pronounced pains in the muscles, particularly in the arms and legs. Eyeballs become inflamed. There is difficulty in chewing and swallowing because the muscles of the tongue are involved. In the fourth and fifth weeks after infected meat has been eaten, profuse sweating occurs, there are asthmatic attacks and the sick person has difficulty in breathing. In the sixth week the face, legs, forearms and abdomen become swollen.

In adults, fever is present throughout the course of the disease. Death usually occurs between the fourth and sixth weeks.

Prevention

There is no effective treatment for the disease in humans or animals once symptoms have apeared. But prevention is comparatively simple. Trichinae in pork are killed when the meat is thoroughly cured, or heated to 131 degrees Fahrenheit, or refrigerated at a temperature of not over 5 degrees continuously for not less than 20 days.

Trichinosis is prevented in both hogs and humans if the pork they eat is thoroughly cooked before it is eaten. The disease occurs five times as often among garbage-fed hogs as it does among grain-fed hogs. For this reason the feeding of uncooked garbage to hogs should be avoided. The feeding of raw garbage is prohibited by federal regulations, but still goes on in a small way in the feeding of family garbage. Another preventive measure is to get rid of rats, since they are often infected with the parasites. Moreover, never throw dead rats or mice into hog pens.

Swine influenza, or "hog flu"

SWINE INFLUENZA, also called "hog flu," is a highly contagious disease caused by the combined infection of a virus and microbe, *Hemophilus influenzae suis*. It occurs principally in the Middle West in the fall and early winter, and is associated with exposure to cold and dampness.

Symptoms

The disease comes on with suddenness and often affects practically every animal in a herd. The incubation period is between two and seven days.

Principal symptoms are loss of appetite, listlessness, coughing and a discharge from the nose. The eyes may be red, swollen and weepy. Breathing is labored and jerky. Fever runs from 104 to 107 degrees Fahrenheit. Owing to soreness of muscles, swine often squeal when handled.

After five or six days of sickness, animals recover quickly. Deaths usually run from 1 to 4 percent, but may reach 10 percent in severe epidemics. Losses are caused mainly by pneumonia and other secondary infections rather than by the "flu" virus itself. Some authorities say that animals affected with the disease are immune to it for the rest of the season; the experience of others indicates that swine may have several attacks during a year.

Treatment

There is no effective vaccine or serum for the disease. Present treatment consists entirely in providing warm, clean, well-ventilated quarters with plenty of fresh drinking water. Secondary complications are most frequent where bad sanitary conditions prevail such as in garbage feeding lots.

The virus that is partly responsible for the disease is carried by the swine lungworm, which in turn spends part of its life in the earthworm. If rooting of swine is prevented, an important source of infection is eliminated. A further preventative measure consists in keeping in quarantine for 30 days all new additions to the herd and all animals returning from shows.

Hemorrhagic septicemia or swine plague

HEMORRHAGIC SEPTICEMIA of swine, sometimes called pasteurellosis, or swine plague, is caused by an organism called *Pasteurella multocida*. This is ordinarily a harmless microbe that is present all the time in the air passages and intestines of healthy swine. But when animals get run down physically, the organism becomes active and sometimes causes heavy losses. Stresses such as exposure to cold, weaning, poor shelter and improper feed often bring on swine plague.

Symptoms

Symptoms of the disease are the usual ones that are noticed in very sick pigs such as fever, coughing, loss of appetite, discharges from the nose and mouth and constipation, sometimes followed by diarrhea. "Thumps" are often present. Onset of the malady is fairly sudden. With such symptoms, animals rapidly become weak and thin. Post-mortem examinations reveal lungs full of pus, as in pneumonia.

Diagnosis of swine plague is difficult. The disease often accompanies others, particularly hog cholera. The outward effects of the two maladies are so much alike that it is impossible to tell one from the other except by laboratory examinations. The pneumonia caused by swine plague and other forms of pneumonia are also hard to tell apart.

Treatment

No completely satisfactory treatment is known. Serums, bacterins, and aggressins are available, but are chiefly useful in preventing the disease rather than treating it. Sulfamethazine, sulfamerazine, and dihydrostreptomycin have been successful in some experimental cases, but are not dependable in naturally-occurring outbreaks.

Swine pneumonia

PNEUMONIA in swine is usually a secondary disease, that is, it affects animals after some malady has lowered their body resistance. Cholera and influenza are often accompanied by pneumonia.

In cases where pneumonia does not occur with other ailments, it nearly always stems from some sort of irritation of the lung tissue. Severe temperature changes, improper drenching so that medicines find their way into the lungs, and inhaling of foreign materials are common causes.

Symptoms

Fever, chills and rapid breathing attend pneumonia. When the disease appears alone, usually only one or a few members of a heard are affected and temperatures are not over 104 degrees Fahrenheit. But when pneumonia appears with some other disease, many animals generally will be affected and temperatures will be several degrees higher.

There are no medicines or biological products whose use is practicable in the treatment of swine pneumonia.

Prevention

Pneumonia as a primary disease can be largely avoided by proper care of animals. Keeping them from getting chilled will help a lot. Allowing them to burrow into straw until they are overheated and then getting them out in the cold for feed is particularly bad. When associated with or following another disease, the primary conditions should first be corrected.

To be healthy, swine require clean, dry, roomy shelter, free from drafts. And they should not be vaccinated when sick.

Swine pox

SWINE POX affects principally suckling pigs. Animals over six months old seldom get it. The disease occurs most often in the Middle West.

Two types of virus are responsible for swine pox. Pigs that recover from the disease caused by one type are thereafter immune to that one but may be infected with the other one. From a practical standpoint the only difference in the two infections is that in one case the course of the disease is more rapid than in the other. Death losses from either kind are generally small.

Swine pox does not usually spread directly from sick pigs to healthy ones. It is transmitted by the hog louse and possibly by flies and other insects. In cold climates, even when lice are not present, the disease sometimes occurs in summer but not in the winter. This indicates that insects other than lice are sometimes to blame.

Symptoms

The first signs of the disease are small red spots that appear over a large part of the body, mostly on the face and ears, in the armpits, on the abdomen and inner surface of the upper hind legs. The spots grow rapidly to the size of a dime or larger.

After a few days, small firm blisters or pustules appear in the centers of these spots. The blisters cause itching and animals break many of them by rubbing against rigid objects. At first the blisters contain a clear fluid, but later this becomes cloudy or puslike. A few days thereafter, the blisters dry up and are replaced by dark-brown scabs. When these fall off, they leave depressions in the skin.

Severe cases of the disease are often accompanied by fever, chills, weakness and loss of appetite. In mild cases, symptoms may hardly be noticeable.

At first the disease may be confused with erysipelas or hog cholera, in which there are also skin lesions. But later, skin depressions, or pock-marks, make it easy to tell the difference. The course of the disease is from 12 to 14 days.

Treatment and prevention

The only way known to ward off swine pox is to keep swine free from lice. No specific treatment for the disease is known. So far as possible, affected pigs should be kept away from others and should be given the care that is usually given sick animals, such as warm quarters, palatable feed and an abundance of fresh water. Hot lye solution is a good disinfectant to apply to infected premises.

Animals sick with swine pox should not be vaccinated, otherwise heavy losses may occur.

Swine mange

SWINE are affected by two kinds of mange—sarcoptic and demodectic. Sarcoptic or common mange is a contagious skin disease of major importance. It is most prevalent in the Corn Belt area where the swine population is greatest and is caused by *Sarcoptes scabeae.*

Mange stunts the growth of young pigs, causing an estimated loss of $2 a head in infected herds. What's more, mangy hogs sell at a discount of 50 cents to $1.50 per hundredweight. The marks of mange on the skin of hams and bacon make them unsalable to the public, so the skin has to be removed.

Cause

The disease is caused by small white or yellowish mites that resemble insects. Adults are about one-fiftieth of an inch long and have four pairs of legs. They can be seen with the naked eye, especially if placed on a black background, and kept warm to encourage them to move. But they are studied more effectively with a low-power magnifying lens or a simple microscope.

The mites burrow into the skin where each female makes a separate gallery in which she lays from 10 to 25 eggs. Cone-shaped swellings appear, accompanied by inflammation and intense itching. The eggs hatch in three to 10 days. Mites begin laying eggs when they are 10 to 12 days old. The disease progresses most rapidly among swine that are in crowded quarters. That is why it increases during the winter.

Symptoms

In its early stages, common swine mange is not always easy to see, particularly among vigorous well-fed animals. That is why it is often overlooked until it is well established in a herd.

At first, the mange usually appears around the eyes, ears and nose, but the mites also take up residence inside of the ears. Many of them are covered with a brown scurf. When this is removed, inflamed areas are revealed where they have dug in.

From the head the infection spreads over the neck, shoulders and back, and along the sides. If animals are not treated, the entire body becomes involved.

The itching of sarcoptic mange makes swine restless and causes them to rub themselves. This rubbing often injures the skin. Large scabs form and when these are scuffed off, the skin is often red or yellowish with blood or serum. In bad cases there is an offensive odor. The thick wrinkled skin of mange is unmistakable.

Sarcoptic mange is spread from animal to animal mostly by contact. Mites that drop to the ground don't live long in sunshine, in dry places or in freezing weather. But they may survive four weeks or longer in moist shady places.

Treatment

Formerly, a number of insecticides such as crude petroleum, crank case oil, lime and sulphur, and arsenical solutions were used to control swine mange. Methods for applying the insecticides included self-oilers, homemade rubbing posts, spraying, dipping, or medicated wallows.

Regardless of the methods employed, eradication was difficult, once the disease became firmly established in a herd. Repeated treatments were often necessary because many of these insecticides kill only the mites— not the eggs.

Better insecticides have virtually replaced the old ones for treatment of mange. Among these are benzene hexachloride, chlordane and lindane. These products kill both mites and eggs in one application and often in a few hours. Their use is simple and economical.

Benzene hexachloride, commonly called BHC, is sold as a wettable powder. The potent part of the substance—the part that indicates how strong it is—is called its "gamma isomer."

BHC should be used in accordance with the instructions of manufacturers. The substance is poisonous, particularly to young animals, if concentrations are too high. It can be applied as a spray, dip or wash. For its most effective use, some precautions are given by those experienced in its application.

The solution should be applied to all parts of the body, including the insides of the ears. Dipping is the most efficient way to treat small pigs but is more trouble than spraying.

Sprayers equipped with agitators give best results. Pressures of 50 to 250 pounds per square inch are recommended, using a half gallon to a gallon on each hog.

BHC has one drawback. It has a persistent musty odor that lingers for days on the bodies of animals and for three or four weeks in barns or on the clothing of operators. It is even noticeable in the fat of treated animals. For this reason do not treat hogs with BHC within 30 days before they are to be sold.

Lindane is the trade name for a product which contains 99 percent or more of the gamma isomer of BHC. It has practically none of the disagreeable odor of BHC so does not have the disadvantage of the latter product. During cold weather when dipping and spraying are not feasible, dust hogs and their bedding with lindane or BHC dust.

Demodectic, or follicular mange

Demodectic or follicular mange in hogs is caused by *Demodex folliculorum*, a wormlike mite so small it can be seen only under a microscope. Unless present in large numbers, the mites seem to cause no lesions or discomfort whatsoever.

The disease may spread rapidly on a hog but spreads very slowly from one animal to another. The lesions appear as small pimples around the eyes and snout but may grow as big as hazelnuts. They usually contain a thick white substance. In severe cases the nodules break and discharge their contents.

There is no practical cure for all cases of demodectic mange though some respond to treatment with lindane or BHC. Fortunately the disease is self-limiting.

Hog lice

THE HOG LOUSE, *Hematopinus suis*, is the largest of the lice that attack domestic animals. The female is about a quarter of an inch long when fully grown and the male is slightly shorter. Both sexes are grayish in color but look darker when on dark-skinned hogs.

The lice attack hogs and spend their entire lives on their hosts. The female lays from one to 20 eggs on a hog bristle, usually locating behind the ears, on the shoulders or flanks. These hatch in 12 to 20 days. When separated from an animal, the pests live two or three days.

Symptoms

Hog lice feed by puncturing the skin and sucking blood, seeking a new place each time. The itching causes hogs to rub and scratch themselves. The open sores that follow often become infested with screw-worms.

The pests are most active in the winter—in fact may seem to disappear completely in warm weather. But unless animals are treated, the lice come back stronger than ever when cold weather sets in.

Treatment

Hog oilers, devices using crude petroleum or crankcase oil, are in common use. Hogs oil themselves by rubbing against these devices.

Two other simple methods for controlling lice consist in dipping hogs in vats containing crude petroleum or applying kerosene emulsion by hand. A solution containing 5 percent lime-sulphur suspension and $1\frac{1}{2}$ percent DDT is very effective. Spraying both hogs and hog houses with this mixture once a month keeps lice under control.

Sprays and powders that are newer and in some ways better than those mentioned above contain Lindane, Chlordane, Toxaphene or Methoxychlor, Co-Ral, ronnel, malathion, rotenone or synergized pyrethrins.

Pantothenic acid deficiency

This deficiency disease is interesting and puzzling, but has not been of great economic importance. It results in "goose-stepping" and other incoordination. It may be corrected by supplementing the feed with this amino acid.

Parakeratosis

A further nutritional problem is the skin ailment called parakeratosis, elephant hide, or scaly skin disease. It is due to a deficiency of zinc, which is often related to an excess of calcium. The skin gets dry and crusty, and may resemble dandruff. Increasing the zinc, or decreasing the calcium, in the ration often corrects the condition very promptly.

Pseudorabies or mad itch

These names are applied to a disease officially known as Aujesky's Disease. It is caused by *Herpesvirus suis,* and it has assumed increasing importance in the swine-producing states of the Middle West in recent years, although it was recognized as early as 1813. No reason for this increase has been reported.

The disease may often exist in older animals with no outward signs, but young pigs exposed to such "carrier animals" may develop paralysis, have a high fever, fall into a coma, and die—all within 24 hours. The condition is transmissible to cattle and sheep as well as to dogs and cats.

There is no recognized treatment, outbreaks being comparatively rare and affecting only young animals. Mortality may be high in pigs, but those that recover appear to have a solid immunity.

Virus pneumonia (of pigs) (VPP)

THIS DISEASE, also known as Enzootic pneumonia may be the world's most disastrous swine disease. Losses in the United States annually run into millions of dollars, some years more than $100 million.

The cause is not fully established beyond the point that *Mycoplasma suipneumoniae* is a primary infection and is frequently triggered by or followed by viruses and/or other bacteria. But, it should not be confused with swine influenza, pasteurellosis, or other types of pneumonia.

Herd treatment is only partially effective, if started very early in an outbreak. Tylosin or one of the tetracyclines checks the secondary invaders. The best way to establish a VPP-free herd is to begin with specific pathogen-free (SPF) pigs and follow very strict procedures of management and replacement purchases.

Cervical abscesses or jowl abscesses

BEING CAUSED by a Streptococcus, this condition is more accurately called Streptococcal Lymphadenitis. The bacteria first localize in the tonsils, then in the lymph nodes of the neck.

Infected pigs usually appear thrifty, but have small abscesses scattered along the lymph channels of the neck. These completely destroy the lymph nodes and lymph glands in three weeks. If only the deep lymph glands are infected, the condition may not be diagnosed in the living hog. However, at slaughter various tissues will be condemned, and this may mean the whole head.

For heavily infected herds, a vaccine is available, and a number of antibiotics may be added to the feed and/or water to reduce the number and the virulence of the Streptococcus.

Porcine stress syndrome (PSS)

A CONDITION loosely termed the porcine stress syndrome has assumed an increasing degree of importance, although it has been recognized for at least 30 years.

The importance lies in the fact that the condition occurs chiefly in market hogs at the time of marketing—when they represent the greatest loss.

The total syndrome is estimated to cost more than $300 million annually. The increase of this loss during recent years is probably related to the fact that swine selection and breeding has progressively emphasized the muscling of the loin and the hams, because it is most prevalent in hogs which show this tendency most strongly. Also, *reducing* the back fat and the fat cover appears to *increase* the incidence. This process, of course, emphasizes the meat/fat and the meat/bone ratios at time of slaughter.

The problem becomes serious during the period of stress which accompanies the sorting and loading of hogs for market. And the further stress of movement by truck aggravates the situation still more, so that 3 percent to 5 percent of the hogs may die on the way to market.

At the time of slaughter, the muscles are pale and soft, and exudative called PSE, with fibers that are coarse and open-textured. The relationship of the carcass changes and the stress has been clearly demonstrated. The muscle changes occur in the living animal, but are seen only in the carcass.

Evidence of the stress syndrome is found at first as a tremor of the muscles, usually beginning at the tail and progressing to the rear limbs. Breathing becomes difficult, the animal collapses, and dies. Muscle biopsy and blood sampling technics help in diagnosis, but do not prevent losses.

Attempts are being made, and with considerable success, to recognize stress susceptibility in the breeding herd. The selection is based on the total syndrome, not on any single symptom. Differences in individuals within a breed are greater than the differences between breeds.

It is expected that careful selection of breeding stock will help to rapidly establish the best balance between production of muscle meat and losses from mortality and inspection condemnation.

Edema disease

THIS CONDITION is also called gut edema, gastric edema, and edema of the bowel. It is not known to occur in any other species.

Edema disease is quite widespread over the world and over the United States, being especially prevalent where hog population is heavy. The exact cause is not known, and may not always be the same, but is generally recognized as a toxemia of some type.

The disease may progress so rapidly that animals die without having been seen sick. When observed they may refuse to eat, may tend to walk in circles, and seem weak and wobbly. Paralysis develops rapidly.

As the various names indicate, there is an extra amount of fluid in the walls of the stomach and/or the intestines, but also in the mesentery. Sometimes the eyelids, ears, and jowls are swollen.

Because no specific cause has been found, treatment has included practically all types of medication; but results have been disappointing with all. Therefore, no prevention or correction procedures can be recommended.

Poisoning

THREE TYPES of toxemia or poisoning are of economic concern.

Salt poisoning

Salt or brine poisoning is mentioned most frequently, but is a problem only when the excessive intake can not be balanced with a readily available and abundant supply of fresh, clean water.

It is characterized by epileptiform seizures, and by bunching the feet under the body—like a horse backing up a heavy load.

Treatment consists of providing water plentifully, and the best is prevention or very early watering.

Cocklebur poisoning

Another type of poisoning occurs most frequently in the spring when young pigs are in an old hog lot and they eat the young shoots of the cocklebur—because these are the only green plants available. The pigs rapidly become depressed, weak, and unsteady on their feet. There may be spasms of the neck muscles, and death can occur within a very few hours after the first symptoms are observed.

Pitch or tar poisoning

A baffling toxemia is that caused by the pitch or tar in clay pigeons, and can only occur when pigs are pastured in an area used for skeet or trap shooting.

Frequently, the first evidence of trouble is a dead pig. Examination of the carcass shows a characteristic engorgement and mottling of the liver. There is no treatment, but pigs should be removed immediately from that pasture.

Internal parasites of sheep

SHEEP HAVE LESS SICKNESS than other farm animals. They have no devastating diseases such as brucellosis of cattle or cholera of hogs. The most serious losses of sheep are caused by internal parasites. This is especially true of farm flocks.

Some 40 internal parasites prey upon sheep. Among the principal ones are stomach worms, nodular worms and lungworms. Tapeworms and head grubs also commonly infest sheep, but these parasites do relatively less harm.

Comparatively few sheep are killed by internal parasites. Nearly all the damage is done because the infested animals become unthrifty, and therefore less valuable for marketing or breeding.

Some of the symptoms of worm infestation are loss of weight, diarrhea, paleness of skin around the mouth and eyes, potbellies and soft swellings under the jaw. The last symptom is called bottle jaw, or poverty jaw. Often a lot of damage is done by internal parasites even when infestation is not great enough to cause pronounced symptoms. Many lightly infested animals just don't thrive the way they should.

Stomach worms

Common stomach worms, *Haemonchus contortus*, of sheep are about three-fourths to one and one-half inches long and about as thick as a pin. The body appears to have a twisted or "barber pole" appearance because the ovary is white and it twists around the digestive tract which usually contains blood that has been sucked from the host.

They hatch from eggs laid by mature females in the fourth stomach of sheep. The eggs pass out with the droppings. The larvae which emerge from them pass through several stages of development before they become infective. Then, if there is rain or dew, they crawl up blades of grass where they are swallowed by grazing animals.

The larvae soon reach the fourth stomach. They mature and start laying eggs in two or three weeks. With proper weather conditions it is possible to have a new generation of the parasites every 30 days.

The principal symptom of infestation by common stomach worms is severe anemia. If animals are not treated, this condition sometimes causes death.

The old treatment of copper-nicotine sulfate has been replaced with thiabendazole or levamisole. Thiabendazole has a wider range of safety and is therefor preferred.

Nodular worms

Nodular worms, *Oesophagostomum columbianum*, are white, fairly large and about five-eighths of an inch long. Usually their heads are bent to form a hook. Adults are found principally in the cecum and large intestines. Their life cycle is similar to that of stomach worms, and sheep become infested with them in the same way.

The worms are called "nodular" because they cause nodules, or lumps, often as large as peas, in the digestive tract. These nodules not only impair the health of infested animals but render the intestines unfit for the manufacture of surgical sutures and sausage casings. The nodules contain worms and a green, cheesy material or a brown, gritty mass. Sometimes the worms break out of the nodules and germs enter the cavities and cause ulcers.

The worms irritate the large intestine, making it red and thick. Sheep harboring only small numbers of the worms may not show symptoms. But with heavy infestation, the dung becomes soft, and the animal loses weight. Later chronic diarrhea develops, which greatly soils the wool. Passing of the dung becomes painful and the straining that results causes the animal to assume a characteristic hunched-up appearance. Affected animals become dull, inactive and weak.

Despite the severity of the disease, animals nearly always survive and the marked symptoms gradually disappear. However, affected sheep continue to suffer from the effects of thickened, nodule-studded intestines.

Thiabendazole is an effective treatment, and has a good range of safety.

Lungworms

The common lungworm, *Dictyocaulus filaria*, is common in the temperate zone, but requires moisture and it prefers swampy pastures.

Lungworms are whitish in color and grow to four inches in length. The eggs hatch in the lungs. When an infected animal coughs, the eggs are expelled. They either leave the mouth directly or are swallowed and pass out with the droppings.

Upon being swallowed by sheep, lungworms bore through the walls of the intestines and reach the lungs by way of the lymph stream. They break through the walls into the larger passages. Worms reach maturity in the lungs. Eggs may be produced in 26 to 35 days after infection.

The worms, eggs and larvae set up an irritation in the lungs which causes a cough that is usually harsh in light infections but may be mild or even absent in heavy infections. In severe cases the air passages in the lungs become clogged and a large portion of the lung tissue becomes useless. This makes the animals short of breath and may lead to death if much of the lung tissue is involved.

Heavily infected animals become weak and listless. Bronchitis may be brought on through irritation of the bronchial tubes, and collapsed portions of the lung may lead to pneumonia.

Treatment is not entirely satisfactory but methyridine and tetramisole are helpful if the flock can be moved to clean pasture immediately after treatment, and can also be fed supplementarily.

Tapeworms

Several kinds of tapeworms infest sheep, both as mature worms and as larvae. Two common tapeworms—*Moneizia expansa* and *Thysanosoma atinoides*—infest the small intestine, but are of minor economic importance. Treatment with niclosamide is effective against both types, and has largely replaced the older treatment with lead arsenate and phenothiazine.

Treatment for worms

Several drugs have been found that are effective in the treatment of lungworms. Two principal kinds of treatment are used against worms other than lungworms. They are a mixture of copper-sulphate and nicotine-sulphate, often called Cu-Nic, and the phenothiazine treatment. The Agricultural Extension Service of the University of Illinois has issued the following summary of the treatments:

Treatments in most cases should be given before placing sheep on fresh pasture in the spring, once a month while on pasture, and in the early winter after the flock is taken off pasture. Be sure of the diagnosis before giving these treatments.

Copper-sulphate-nicotine treatment. One-percent copper sulphate is prepared by mixing one and one-third ounces of copper sulphate and one ounce of 40-percent nicotine sulphate (Blackleaf 40) in one gallon of soft water. Before giving the drench withhold feed for at least 32 hours. Use in the following doses: for yearlings and full-grown sheep, four ounces; for 75-pound lambs, three ounces; for 50-pound lambs, two ounces; and for 25-pound lambs, one ounce.

Phenothiazine treatment. Phenothiazine has proved an effective treatment both for nodular worms and for stomach worms. The dose for a ewe is about one ounce and for a lamb one-half ounce. Avoid treating ewes in the late stages of pregnancy.

The breeding flock should be treated for nodular worms in early winter after it is taken off pasture and in spring before going on pasture. Nodular-worm larvae infesting the pasture are generally killed by freezing during the winter. If treatment of the ewes has removed most of the nodular worms, the pastures will not be rapidly reinfested in spring and the lambs will remain relatively free from them.

Only lambs kept over for breeding stock need be treated the following winter and spring, but occasionally it may be advisable to treat all lambs. Different methods of administering phenothiazine, which does not mix with water alone, have been successfully employed.

Individual drenching is the surest way to know that each ewe and lamb receives the prescribed dosage. For 16 sheep thoroughly mix one pound of phenothiazine with six or seven ounces of blackstrap molasses, then add enough water to make one quart. Two ounces of the mixture may be given to each adult sheep and one ounce to lambs. The mixture should be thoroughly shaken before using, as it tends to separate on standing.

Whole milk can be used with phenothiazine instead of molasses and water. With a paper funnel place one-half pound of phenothiazine (enough for eight sheep) in a gallon jug or bottle, add one-half gallon of milk, and shake until thoroughly mixed. Then pour eight ounces (one dose) into a measuring cup and from the cup through a funnel into a 12-ounce pop bottle. Hold the sheep between the legs and tilt its head slightly upward, keeping one hand over the side of its mouth to prevent slobbering. Pour the dose into the sheep's mouth by inserting the neck of the bottle in the back part of the mouth between the animals cheek and teeth.

A mixture consisting of one part phenothiazine to 14 parts of salt has also given good results. It is substituted for the usual salt supplement necessary for sheep and is kept before the sheep continuously for a month or longer. The sheep may then be given salt alone in the usual way for a period of several days before being placed on the salt-phenothiazine mixture again. (Note: The U.S. Department of Agriculture recommends a stronger dose—one part of phenothiazine to nine parts salt.)

For tapeworms, lead arsenate—0.5 to 1.0 Gm.—is probably the drug of choice. It may be used with phenothiazine solution. These treatments have been widely replaced with thiabendizole and levamisole.

Head grubs, or sheep nose bots

Head grubs, or sheep nose bots, are the larvae of sheep nasal flies, *Oestrus ovis*. They cause sheep great discomfort but little actual damage.

The flies bring on a condition commonly called grub-in-the-head, so called because they deposit tiny grubs or maggots around the nostrils of sheep. The grubs fiind their way into the nasal passages of the animals and after a while enter the frontal sinuses, or hollows in the bone of the forehead.

After a period of development, the grubs re-enter the nostrils, drop to the ground and burrow into the soil where they become pupae. After a period of from three weeks to two months, depending upon soil and weather conditions, they emerge from their pupal cases as flies.

The flies are a little larger than common horse flies, are dull yellowish in color and have hairs on their bodies. They annoy sheep greatly in their efforts to deposit grubs in the nostrils of the animals. The sheep stop feeding and try to protect their noses from the flies, often huddling together for protection.

Animals are molested by flies mainly during the heat of the day. The flies become inactive when it is cooler.

While the grubs are in the nose and sinuses, they irritate the tissue so that the nose runs as though the animal had a bad head cold. At first the discharge is thin and clear, but later it thickens and becomes dark in color. Affected animals sneeze often and breathe with difficulty.

Treatment

Head grubs can be controlled through the use of two comparatively new drugs. Ronnel, a systemic insecticide, kills the larvae in their first stage. It is given once a month for three or four months, after fly activity has ceased. Slaughter of treated animals for food should not take place within 60 days of treatment.

Dimethoate, also a systemic, kills larvae in all stages. Its use produces immediate response and permits slaughter two weeks after treatment.

Anthrax

The disease is very similar to that described for cattle. Control and immunization are as described there.

Blackleg

This disease has often been confused with anthrax and with malignant edema. Symptoms in sheep closely resemble those in cattle, and control and immunization procedure follow the same pattern.

Bladder worms or sheep measles

These are the larval forms of tapeworms which mature in other species of animals. The dog tapeworm cysts or bladders are found on the peritoneum and are seldom economically important.

Another type may be seen in the muscles. They, too, are rarely significant, and are controlled by treating the dogs more often.

A third type is called Gid, and develops in the brain. It was of some interest early in the century, but has disappeared.

Scrapie

SCRAPIE is a nervous disease of sheep and probably goats which commonly occurs in sheep more than two years old. Symptoms are seldom seen in animals under 18 months old because of the long incubation period —18 months to three years or even longer.

The disease has been known in Britain, France and Germany for 200 years but appeared in Canada for the first time in 1938 and in the United States in 1952. It is caused by a virus. It is spread by means of contaminated pasture but lambs can also acquire it before birth from their mothers and from infected rams.

Symptoms

Symptoms of the disease develop slowly. An infected sheep at first becomes more excitable than usual. Fine tremors, or quiverings, extend over the head and neck and produce slight rapid nodding movements. Itching starts in the region of the rump and finally extends over the whole body. Often the itching becomes so intense that an affected animal cannot rest or feed normally. As an animal rubs itself, it makes licking movements with its tongue and grinds its teeth. There is no rash present.

Temperature remains normal. Despite a good appetite, weakness and loss of condition progress to the extent that in the later stages of the disease a victim can no longer stand. Previous to that stage, the animal may have an abnormal gait. When made to trot, it has a high-stepping action of the forelegs and galloping movements of the hind legs. Convulsions may occur as may paralysis of the hindquarters.

The symptoms usually last from six weeks to six months. Generally the animal dies. There have been instances, however, of complete recovery.

Scrapie may attack 20 to 30 percent of the animals in a newly infected herd. The disease may become progressively more severe in an area and infect as many as 50 percent or there may be only occasional cases over a period of years.

Control

There is no way known to prevent the disease or to cure it. Control is exceptionally difficult because of the long period of incubation. Infection may incubate many months in a flock without the owner knowing it. The only means of control found thus far is to slaughter and burry or burn animals showing symptoms, slaughter exposed animals for meat, clean and disinfect the premises, establish a clear history of the flock, and make long-term inspections of flocks that may have been affected by the disease.

Recommended disinfectant solutions for use on infected premises and conveyances are: a 2-percent solution of sodium hydroxide (lye), made by adding a 13-ounce can to 5 gallons of water; a 4-percent solution of sodium carbonate (soda ash), made by adding 1 pound to 3 gallons of water; a 4-percent solution of sodium carbonate (sal soda), made by adding a 13^1/$_2$-ounce can to 1 gallon of water.

Campaign against scrapie

The U. S. Department of Agriculture has set up a 6-point program to eradicate scrapie. It embraces: (1) Immediate reporting of suspicious cases. (2) Diagnosis of the disease. (3) Quarantine. (4) Indemnity for losses. (5) Disposal of infected and exposed animals. (6) Flock history and inspections.

Indemnities are paid on a basis similar to that employed in the brucellosis eradication program.

Bluetongue

BLUETONGUE is an infectious disease of sheep caused by a virus. It was identified for the first time in the United States. Prior to that the ailment was known in South Africa and Palestine. It has been causing heavy losses in Africa for many years.

Bluetongue is spread by biting insects. It can also be spread through inoculation but not by direct contact.

Symptoms

First symptoms of the disease are loss of appetite, depression and fever of 107 degrees F. Within a few days the mouth parts, including the tongue, and the inside of the nose become inflamed and there is a flow of saliva and froth from the mouth.

In some cases there is labored breathing. The mouth parts and tongue may become blue which gives the disease its name. There is often a discharge from the nose that forms a crust on the upper lip.

After the fever disappears, reddening and pain often become evident around the coronary bands of the feet, accompanied with lameness. The acute stage of the disease lasts five to ten days. It takes an animal several weeks to fully recover. About ten percent of affected sheep die.

Prevention

No medical treatment has proved of any value. Affected sheep should be separated from healthy ones so far as possible.

Sheep can be vaccinated for protection against the disease.

Contagious ecthyma or sore mouth

SORE MOUTH, a highly contagious disease of sheep and goats, is caused by a virus. The technical name of the malady is contagious ecthyma. It occurs often among lambs in feed lots, in fact is believed to be present to some extent wherever lambs are fattened for market. It also sometimes occurs in range and farm flocks. It seldom affects animals over one year old.

Symptoms

When lambs shipped to feed lots get the disease, symptoms generally appear between a week and 10 days after the animals arrive. The first symptom is a reddening and swelling of the lips, gums or tongue, together with small vesicles, or blisters, on these mouth parts.

Later the vesicles break and leave raw sores that bleed easily and become covered with thick grayish-brown scabs.

Animals recover from sore mouth within three or four weeks. The scabs fall off and leave no scars. Death from the disease is rare but sometimes secondary ailments cause losses. These are brought on when other disease-causing organisms enter the body through the open sores. In some parts of the country, screwworms infest sore-mouth wounds.

Sore mouth is expensive to sheep owners because it brings about loss of condition. Affected animals do not eat properly. On account of the painful sores, lambs and kids nurse with difficulty, and older animals do not graze normally. Affected animals don't even like to eat from troughs.

Among ewes, other possible results of the disease are caked udder and mastitis, or blue bag. These may be brought on when the virus attacks the udders, making them so sore that dams will not permit lambs to nurse. In such cases the young also suffer from lack of milk.

Prevention

Almost complete protection against sore mouth can be obtained by vaccination. The vaccine is applied by scratching the skin in a manner similar to that used in vaccinating against smallpox. The scratches are usually made on the underside of the tail or on the inside surface of the thigh.

In range areas where the disease prevails, lambs are commonly vaccinated at the time they are castrated, docked and earmarked. Immunity lasts anywhere from several months to two years or even longer.

Sheep that are to be sent to feed lots should be vaccinated at least 10 days before they are shipped. The scab that appears after vaccination contains the virus, just as do the scabs caused by the disease itself. By waiting until the scabs fall off and complete healing occurs before making shipments, there is no danger of spreading the disease to susceptible animals that may be encountered en route or in feed lots.

Enterotoxemia or pulpy kidney disease

THIS IS an acute disease occurring chiefly in feedlots when lambs are being fed a highly nutrition ration. The causative agent is *Clostridium perfringens*, which is widely distributed in soils and is abundant in feedlots. Six types are recognized, each producing a specific toxin which differs from the others. Type D is most prevalent in the United States, and it also produces the condition known as "over-eating disease".

Its presence is commonly recognized by finding animals that have died suddenly, often with evidence of convulsions, but while in apparently excellent condition. The findings on autopsy include edema of the lungs, the rumen, and the true stomach. The digestive tract contains ample feed, while the kidneys are pulpy due to rapid decomposition after death.

Control can be had by reducing feed, but this is often not economically advisable. Therefore, preventive vaccination with a toxoid is common.

Bacillary hemglobinuria or red water disease

THIS ACUTE DISEASE is caused by *Clostridium hemolyticum,* an anaerobic microbe. The organism apparently multiplies only in the animal body, but may live for long periods in soil or in the bones of animals dead of the disease.

The most striking evidence of the condition is a port-wine colored urine, which foams freely when voided. Mortality in untreated lambs is about 95 percent, and can be prevented only by early and vigorous treatment with penicillin or other antibiotics. Blood transfusions may be resorted to in valuable animals. When the disease appears repeatedly, vaccination with a bacterin offers preventive protection.

Pregnancy disease, or ketosis, of ewes

PREGNANCY DISEASE, or ketosis, of ewes is a noncontagious malady that occurs before lambing, especially among animals that are carrying twins or triplets. The disease is most common among ewes between three and six years old. It occurs more often in small flocks than in bands on the range.

Usually animals are affected when they are in the fourth or fifth (last) month of pregnancy. The ailment affects ewes the world over.

The exact cause of the malady is not known but it is believed to be brought on by faulty metabolism. Affected animals do not have enough sugar in their blood and develop an acid condition in their bodies. Some authorities say that the added burden on ewes in having more than one lamb is beyond their normal endurance.

Symptoms

Ewes with pregnancy disease often lag behind the flock when driven, or stand off by themselves when at rest. They nearly always grind their teeth. They become dull and weak and urinate often. They tremble when exercised.

Later, affected animals refuse to eat, their breath comes fast, they drink hardly any water, urinate very litle, become stupid or excited and may appear blind. Finally they become so weak they can no longer stand. They lie on their breastbones, heads to one side. They may lie in this position for days. There is no fever.

The course of the disease is from one to 10 days. Ninety percent of affected animals die. However, if lambing occurs in the early stages of the ailment, the animals usually recover. Lambs born in such cases are usually weak and many of them die.

Treatment and prevention

Treatment of animals sick with pregnancy disease is generally not satisfactory and rarely successful in advanced cases. Some success has been reported with the injection of certain sugar solutions into the blood stream.

Exercise and proper feeding will largely prevent the disease. If pregnant ewes are not on green pasture, they should be fed a liberal amount of good-quality legume roughage such as clover or alfalfa hay. In addition they should get one-fourth of a pound of good grain daily during the eighth to the sixth week before lambing and one pound daily during the fourth to second weeks. Ewes in good condition may not require more than a half pound daily during the last few weeks.

Small amounts of molasses, corn syrup, brown sugar or dextrose may be given with the grain. Salt should be made available, and it is best to avoid sudden changes in the quantity or kind of feed.

A moderate amount of exercise is necessary. Animals should not be driven rapidly but should be forced to walk about a quarter to a half mile a day. A convenient way to accomplish this is to feed the ewes at some distance from where they are kept at night. Pregnant ewes should be kept in good thrifty condition, neither too thin nor too fat.

Liver flukes and black disease

THESE PARASITES cause failure to gain, or loss of weight, and sometimes death. The condition is called fascioliasis because it is caused by *Fasciola hepatica*, a flattened oval worm having a sucker on the bottom.

Flukes infest the sheep when the tiny larvae enter the digestive tract with contaminated water or grass to which the larvae cling at the water's edge. In the duodenum, the young fluke bores through the wall and enters the periotoneum. It easily migrates to the liver, where it bores its way into the bile ducts. This whole migration may take 10 to 12 weeks, during which time great damage may be done in the liver by the growing and burrowing flukes.

For many years, treatment consisted of administering carbon tetrachloride, but more effective drugs have been synthesized, and some are effective against developing flukes as well as those which are mature.

It is necessary for the flukes to pass a part of their life cycle in the snail, so that the best approach to prevention and control is by providing good drainage, and sometimes taking additional steps to reduce the number of snails. Also, fencing off the snail-infested areas is helpful, but not fully effective because rabbits and deer grazing the same area are also susceptible and can infest and reinfest sheep by persistent contamination of the pastures.

Circling disease, or listerellosis

CIRCLING DISEASE, also known as listerellosis and encephalitis of sheep, is a highly fatal malady that affects sheep, goats, cattle and sometimes swine. It is caused by a germ called *Listerella monocytogenes* which attacks the brain. It is not known how the microbes are spread.

The disease occurs most often in the Middle West and in eastern states where it usually appears year after year on certain farms. Most cases occur in the late fall and winter but cases have been noted in New York state as late as July. In sheep it is seen most often among adults but it may attack spring lambs that are only six weeks old.

Symptoms

First symptoms of the disease are dullness and an inclination of affected animals to wander off by themselves and become indifferent to feed. An affected sheep may keep some hay in its mouth for hours. The head is often held to one side, held low or pulled in towards the body. If the head is pushed into its normal position, it will return to the former one when released.

In most cases animals with the disease will walk in a circle, either to the right or the left, but always in the same direction. If they run into a fence or other obstruction, they will not turn to go in another but will stand indefinitely with their heads pressed against the obstacle. Often the lower lip or an ear is paralyzed. Complete paralysis usually precedes death.

A cow with circling disease has symptoms that resemble those of acetonemia—a wild or anxious facial expression and insane behavior. Two differences between the diseases are that a cow with acetonemia does not usually move in circles, nor does a cow with circling disease have the odor of acetone on her breath.

Circling disease among ewes is sometimes mistaken for pregnancy disease. Here, also there are differencses. In both diseases, the head of a victim may be turned to the side, but in pregnancy disease the head will not return to the distorted position if straightened out. Paralysis of an ear or the lower lip is not present in pregnancy disease.

Symptoms of circling disease in swine are trembling, stilted movements of the forelegs and dragging of hind legs. Among affected animals, the greatest number of deaths occur in suckling pigs.

Treatment

The disease is generally regarded as almost 100 percent fatal though there have been some reports of recoveries following treatment with sulfanilamide, aureomycin and penicillin. To be effective, drugs must be given early in the course of the disease.

Wool maggot and sheep tick remedies

WOOL MAGGOTS, the larvae of certain kinds of blowflies, cause serious losses of sheep in some parts of this country. They can be successfully controlled by using formula EQ 335, a remedy developed by the United States Department of Agriculture. One part of EQ 335 should be diluted with nine parts of water and the liquid applied to infested portions of the sheep. (See index for formula for EQ 335.)

For treatment of sheep ticks, two remedies are lindane and toxaphene. (See index.)

Sheep scab, or mange

FIVE KINDS OF MITES cause scab, or mange, in sheep. They are known as psoroptic, sarcoptic, chorioptic, demodectic and psorergatic. Each kind has habits whereby it can be identified.

Psoroptic mites live on top of the skin, usually on the back, withers, rump and sides. Sarcoptic mites burrow into the skin, generally where there is little wool, such as on the head and face. Chorioptic mites live on the skin and are usually found on the legs. Demodectic mites are found in hair follicles and in glands of the skin. They are the smallest of the five and resemble worms. Their presence is indicated by small hard pimples or nodules. Psorergatic mites cause a mild irritation and itchiness like that caused by lice. The sheep scratch and bite the parts most easily reached. The mites are about one-third as big as the common scab mite.

Psoroptic or common scab is the most widespread form of scabies and does the most damage to sheep. The disease is highly contagious and spreads rapidly through a flock once it gets a start.

The mites of common scab are white or yellowish and can be seen with the unaided eye. Their entire life is spent on the body of the host. The mites irritate animals, causing unthriftiness and loss of weight. A loss of wool also results from the disease. Where weather conditions are bad and animals are undernourished, death sometimes results.

Each female lays between 15 and 24 eggs in her lifetime. These hatch in about four to seven days after they are laid. Young mites become mature, mate and the females start laying eggs in from 10 to 12 days after hatching.

Symptoms of common scab

Common scab mites prick the skin of sheep to obtain food. Since this causes itching and slight inflammation, it is believed that poisonous saliva of the mites is introduced into the wounds.

As the mites multiply, itching becomes intense and blood serum oozes to the surface. This becomes mixed with dirt and the oil from the skin and soon hardens into crusts or scabs. At first these are yellowish, but later they become dark in color.

Areas of skin affected by scab become hard and thick. The itching makes sheep restless. This is particularly noticeable when animals are warm with exercise. They scratch and bite themselves. They rub themselves against rigid objects that may be at hand.

As the disease progresses, fleece becomes matted in affected areas and the animals pull out masses of it with their mouths. This leaves denuded patches of skin that resemble parchment. Blood sometimes appears in the cracks as in severely chapped hands.

The parasites are most numerous at the outer edges of the infected areas. Here the surface of the skin is greasy, bright and glistening. On the other hand, in the centers of the patches where the mites have been destroyed or are no longer active, the region appears dull and dry.

Mites can be found by scraping crusts from a victim's skin with a knife and dislodging the mites that are attached to the crusts. They can be more easily seen if placed on a warm black cloth or other surface. They are most active at body temperature or in warm sunshine.

Treatment of common scab

The best way to get rid of common sheep mange is to dip the animals in a solution that will kill the parasites and their eggs. This was formerly done with dips containing lime and sulphur, or nicotine. These substances, however, have been replaced by the better benzene hexachloride (BHC), and lindane.

When BHC is used, animals should not be slaughtered within three weeks after dipping since the substance has a disagreeable odor. Lindane does not have this drawback. Both products should be applied in accordance with recommendations of their manufacturers.

When dipping is impracticable because of cold weather or for other reasons, the animals can be treated by hand. This consists in soaking the affected parts in warm dip. In both dipping and hand treating, any hard scabs that the animals may have should first be dressed by rubbing them with warm dip and then breaking the scabs with a stick or with a stiff brush, taking care not to cause bleeding.

Treatment for other forms of scab

Sarcoptic mange does not occur often in the United States. It can be eradicated by dipping affected animals in warm lime-and-sulphur solution every five or six days for period of a month to six weeks.

Chorioptic scab can be wiped out by using the same method employed in eradicating common scab. During cold weather, wading tanks can be used instead of dipping vats, since the disease does not affect the upper part of the body except in severe cases.

Demodectic scab seldom occurs in the United States. Since there is no known way to cure it, the only practical way to eradicate demodetic scab from flocks is to sell affected animals for slaughter. The laws of some states prohibit the shipment of afflicted animals, however.

There is no specific treatment for psorergatic mites. Attempts to control them with BHC have shown some promise, but the condition seldom progresses to a point where it has economic significance.

White muscle disease of lambs and calves

WHITE MUSCLE DISEASE of lambs and calves occurs principally across the northern half of the United States. It is most serious in some of the fertile irrigated districts of the western inter-mountain area. In sheep flocks it is often called stiff-lamb disease.

Losses range from a few individuals to a high percentage of young in affected flocks and herds. Among lambs it occurs most often between the ages of three and four weeks and in calves between the ages of four and six weeks.

Cause of the disease is not known but is closely associated with lack of vitamin E, and its interaction with selenium and possibly sulfur.

Symptoms

The disease brings on muscular deterioration. An early sign in a lamb is a slight difficulty in rising and following the ewe. This is followed in three or four days by stiffness of the legs and finally by paralysis. A paralyzed lamb will take milk if raised in position to suckle. But paralysis is usually followed by death. The lambs that recover from the disease are often permanently stunted.

Affected calves are weak. They walk slowly and with difficulty. Most calves are strong enough to rise and nurse but they show no inclination to run and play.

Injury to the leg muscles occurs most often among lambs whereas heart muscles are injured more often among calves. When the heart is affected there is labored breathing and death may occur a few hours after symptoms appear. When calves die in this way, a blood-tinged foam is often discharged from the nostrils just before death. Muscles of the diaphragm, between the ribs and in the tongue are often affected.

Damaged muscles of animals that have died from the disease have areas where the normal coloring is gone. The color may be slightly lighter than normal or muscles may be bleached with white streaks.

The lining of a lamb's heart may contain patches that look like white enamel. Where there has been heart damage and labored breathing for some time before death, the lungs are congested with blood. This is sometimes mistaken for a sign of pneumonia.

Prevention

White muscle disease is not generally a problem where animals have access to range in the winter. Although investigations indicate that the disease is caused by faulty nutrition or metabolism associated with lack of vitamin E, the problem is not so simple as it appears.

The disease can be prevented by adding an inexpensive chemical containing selenium (Na_2SeO_3) to the ration of ewes during pregnancy or drenching them with a dilute solution of the substance. (See package for directions.) Where ewes have not received such supplements, the disease will not occur in the lambs if they are given the drug as prescribed.

Docking and castrating

DOCKING keeps sheep clean and thus reduces danger of disease. Tails on ewes sometimes interfere with breeding and result in losses to owners.

Docking is easy when done with a knife or orchard-pruning shears. Pull the skin of the tail towards the body and clip off so as to leave a stub about one inch long. When you let go of the tail, the skin will go back in place and cover the stub. To prevent bleeding, pinch the skin between the thumb and forefingers for about half a minute. This will close the arteries.

Always disinfect instruments and hands before you dock.

Another good way to dock lambs is with a hot docking chisel or pincers. When they are heated only to a cherry-red color there is no danger of losing blood. The wound is seared over. If the irons are too hot, profuse bleeding may occur. The method is particularly good for docking older lambs, since these animals are much more apt to bleed heavily.

Castration

Male lambs that are not to be used for breeding should be castrated when they are between seven and 14 days old. This will make the rams more desirable for market. To save time, lambs are usually castrated and docked at the same time, although they can be docked without injury when only three days old.

Castrating should be done on a bright day, never when the weather is damp, chilly or rainy. It is easy to do with a pair of castration shears or a knife. First cut off one-third of the scrotum, or bag. Then force the testicles out and hold them with a firm grip, pulling them out with the attached cords. This should be done with a steady pull. The cords should then be cut and the wound treated with tincture of iodine or some other standard disinfectant.

One method of castration preferred by many is done with the so-called Burdizzo forceps, or emasculatome. If properly done it does not cause a wound in the external tissues.

The jaws of the instrument are placed over the cords leading to the testicles, one at a time. When the handles of the emasculatome are pressed together, the jaws do not quite meet. In this way the cords are severed without injuring the bag. Following the operation, the testicles gradually shrink and waste away.

Elastration

A method of castration and docking that has come into use to some extent, principally since World War II, is called elastration. It consists in applying a rubber band around the scrotum or high up on a lamb's tail. This cuts off the supply of blood to these parts and in a short time they shrivel up and drop off. A special instrument, called an elastrator, is used to apply the rubber bands. The method is "bloodless." However, soreness and swelling occur.

Footrot

THIS IS ONE of the oldest and most costly diseases of sheep. When it appears it usually affects a large percentage of the flock or band, and commonly involves more than one foot of each animal. Losses are seldom due to death, but rather to excessive loss of weight as a result of lameness and pain, which usually lasts for a number of weeks.

The causative agent is *Bacillus necrophorus*, which may also be involved in lip and leg ulceration.

At the onset, infection gets under the sole, often because the wall of the hoof has grown too long and has curled under the sole. This provides space for pebbles and filth to accumulate, and the curled-under wall places excessive pressure on this material and on the sole.

Treatment must begin with the trimming of the hoof so that walking can be normal. When the feet have been trimmed, the sheep must be placed on soft soil or in well-bedded pens. Because of the number of animals involved, it is necessary to build a trough through which all sheep will walk at least twice a day. This trough must contain a solution of copper sulfate (30 percent), sometimes with formalin (5 percent) added. Because of the materials carried in on the feet of the sheep, the treatment solution should be renewed regularly, and it must be kept at a depth of two inches or more to cover the entire hoof up to and including the coronary band.

A good preventive procedure is to examine the flock before the rainy season, or before it is placed on wet pasture. Regular exercise through the winter will assure wearing of the walls of the hoof so that it will not curl under the sole.

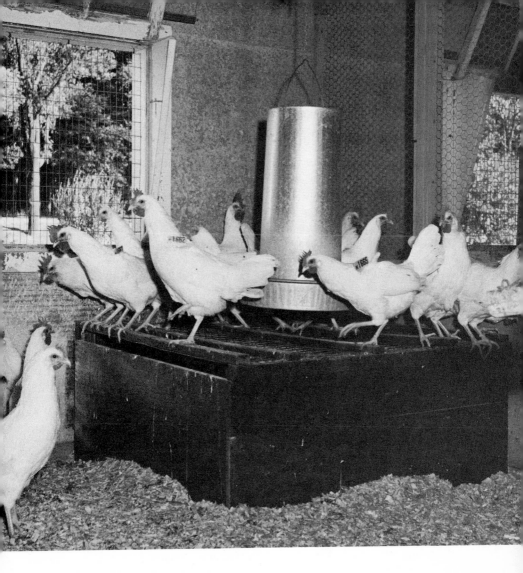

The small poultry flock

(Reprint of Extension Bulletin 773, Farm Science Series, Michigan State University, East Lansing, MI 48824*)

SUCCESS IN RAISING poultry depends on many things. The three most important are: proper feeding, sound management and good sanitation. Of course, genetically well-bred birds capable of high production are a prerequisite to good management.

*The authors are: Professor, Extension Specialist, and Associate Professor in the Department of Poultry Science, and Extension Agricultural Agent, Lapeer, Michigan, respectively.

Selecting chicks for egg production

Buy from a reputable hatchery. Your County Agent or perhaps a neighbor can tell you where to buy chicks from a U.S. Pullorum-Typhoid Clean hatchery.

If possible, work closely with the person from whom you buy the chicks. If you are new in the poultry business, the hatcheryman can help you.

Select the breed or strain for the purpose intended. There is no really good dual purpose chicken. There are broiler strains and egg-laying strains of chickens.

Almost all of the egg-laying strains of birds lay white eggs (they are Leghorn-type birds). Brown egg-laying strains are available. However, there is no difference between white and brown shelled eggs—except for the shell color.

Getting ready for new chicks

Remove all equipment possible, such as: feeders, waterers, brooders, etc., from the hen house.

Wash all equipment with a soap or detergent and rinse thoroughly. If possible, place in the sun to dry. This will help disinfect the equipment.

Remove used litter and rubbish from the house, such as: bags, paper, tools, buckets, etc.

Clean the building thoroughly—sweep ceilings, walls, remove and wash windows, remove any caked material on the floor.

Use a high pressure sprayer to completely wash down the building interior or soak caked materials to loosen them. Apply an approved insecticide in buildings where lice, mites, beetles or other insects have been a problem.

Use a good rodent control program inside and outside of the building.

Rinse equipment with a disinfectant. Quarternary ammonium and chlorine bleaching agents are good disinfectants. Follow instructions on the container.

Put clean, dry litter in the building after it has been cleaned and disinfected and dried. Chopped straw, wood shavings or crushed or coarsely ground corn cobs make good litter.

Brooder stoves for chicks

You must provide heat for the baby chicks. Brooder stoves are available that use gas and oil. These stoves have hovers that contain or retain the heat close to the floor. Electric heat lamps (without hovers) are also used to brood chicks.

Start the brooder stove at least 24 hours before the chicks arrive to properly adjust the stove and dry out the house.

Provide a temperature of 90-95° F at chick level. Use only new or cleaned chick guards at least 3-4 feet from edge of brooder hover for first 7 days. Use solid chick guards in cold houses. A chick guard is a paper, cardboard or a fine wire mesh ring around the heat source (brooder stove) that confines the birds to the warmed area.

Reduce temperature under the hover gradually over a period of weeks. It is good to have heat under the hover and have the rest of the pen or house cool. Chicks will gradually learn to regulate their location in the temperature zone most comfortable for them.

Over a period of several weeks (outside temperature will make a difference) gradually raise the brooder hover or heat lamps. Birds should gradually become accustomed to the idea that the heat source is not necessary. Remember, the brooder has been a foster mother to them.

Chicks indicate when they are too cold or too warm. When too cold, they chirp—complain a lot; when too hot, they will lie down or try to pile up in corners. When comfortable, young chicks form a ring on the floor under the heat source.

Litter

The purpose of litter is to provide comfort, and to absorb droppings and excess moisture.

Use clean, dry, dustless litter 2-3 inches deep on concrete or wood floors. Dirt floors are not to be used as it is impossible to clean and disinfect them.

Remove wet and caked spots in the litter immediately; replace with dry litter.

Day-old (and up to a week old) chicks may eat the litter instead of the feed. Cover the litter with paper or egg filler flats to prevent litter eating. When the birds are eating the feed well, remove the paper (slippery paper may cause leg problems).

Feeding chicks

Use freshly-made feed; do not buy more than a month's supply of any feed, as feeds tend to deteriorate with age.

Start chicks on a commercial chick starter purchased from a local elevator or feed dealer. Follow the feed manufacturer's recommendations closely as to length of time each feed should be fed.

Usually four different rations are fed to egg-type chickens. A 21% protein starter ration is fed for the first 8 weeks. An 18% protein grower ration is fed from 8-14 weeks of age. A 14% protein maintenance ration is fed from 15-20 weeks of age. A laying mash is fed to pullets after 20 weeks of age.

Grit may be provided in a small box in the house. Gravel—take out the large stones—will provide all of the grit needed for birds of any age. Grit helps grind coarse feed in the gizzard of poultry.

Poultry housing for all ages

A well-constructed brooding and/or laying house should be well-insulated, and well-ventilated to remove ammonia odors, excess moisture and airborne disease organisms. A small fan with a thermostat is useful for small houses; for large houses, request the poultry housing bulletin listed on the last page of this publication for information.

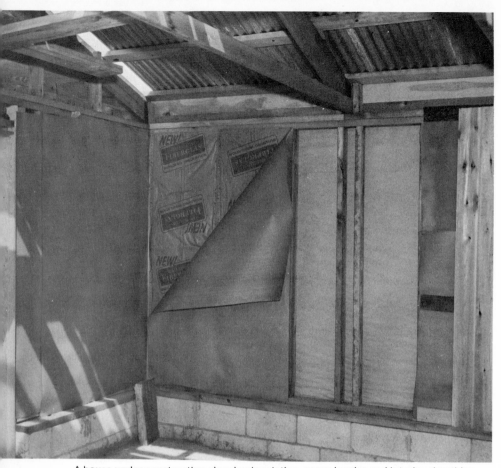
A house under construction showing insulation, vapor barrier and interior sheathing

Do not protect the birds too much—they are usually comfortable at cool to cold temperatures. Adult birds do well in temperatures that range from 0° to 80° F. Avoid freezing the water and rapidly and widely fluctuating temperatures.

Birds (baby chicks to adult birds) do not like drafts.

Insulation

To maintain a warm (above freezing) house in winter and a cool house in summer, you must use insulation.

Two to 3½ inches of fiber glass batts, or equivalent, in the walls and ceilings will provide adequate insulation under most conditions.

Birds produce heat. The purpose of the insulation is to confine this heat to the house during the cold weather. Large egg production units of 10,000 birds or more can maintain a minimum temperature of 60° F during the coldest Michigan winter months. A flock of 25 birds will not provide enough body heat to maintain this house temperature. Electric heat tapes

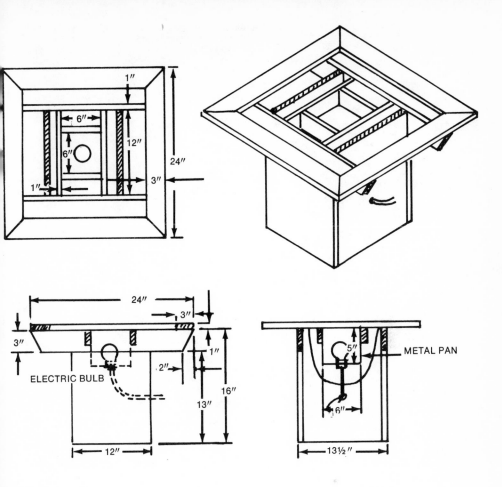

A simple plan for a water stand with light bulb to prevent water from freezing

on the water pipes and a heat bulb over the waterers may be needed to keep water from freezing in houses with small flocks.

Space and equipment requirements

Allow ½ square foot of floor space per chick to 3 weeks of age, 1½ square feet to 14 weeks of age and 1½-2 square feet per hen in well-ventilated and well-insulated houses.

Allow 40 linear feet of feeder space per 100 hens. You should have enough feeder space so all birds (of any age) can eat at the same time. Feeders and waterers should be raised as the birds get older. The top of the feeder side should be raised to at least the level of the bird's back as it stands (in a normal position) on the floor. The birds should have to reach up and over the edge of the feeder. This will help prevent feed wastage.

Allow three ½-gallon water founts per 100 chicks at one day of age. After a week or so, use larger founts so that water intake is unrestricted. Clean founts every day.

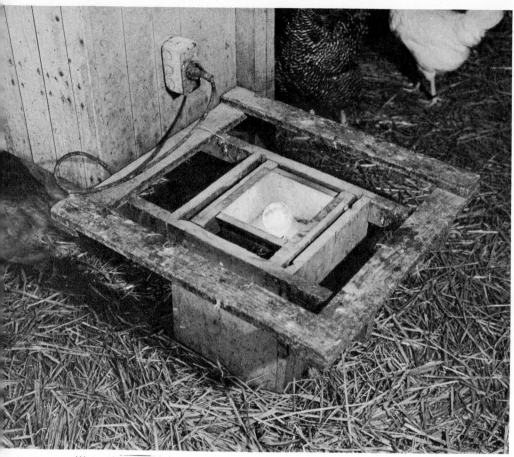

Water should be unrestricted. Here is a heated water stand

Allow one 5 gallon water fountain or 4 linear feet of watering trough for each 100 hens. Water is the cheapest nutrient; keep it clean, fresh and always available.

Egg Production

You may want to keep a few hens for egg production. Many producers buy 20-week-old started pullets for the laying house. Producers who wish to have a small flock might consider this approach to getting started with some birds.

Other producers might want to contact a commercial egg producer who is selling off his flock of old hens. A few of these hens will do a fine job of laying eggs. You should expect to molt these birds (allow them to replace their feathers—take a rest for 8-10 weeks). They should then come back into production with nice, large eggs.

Management for egg production

Put new birds in a clean, dry, well-insulated and well-ventilated house.

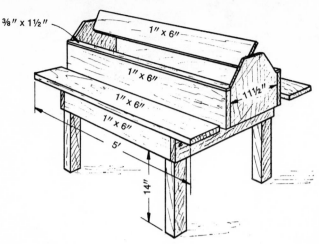

Here is an easy-to-construct dry mash feeder. The revolving board on top prevents contamination of the feed

Provide plenty of clean, fresh water. Clean water founts daily.

Provide fresh feed with adequate space for all birds to eat. Do not store feed for long periods of time. Keep feed in a cool, dry place until fed to the birds. A feed designed for layers should be fed. A 16-18% protein laying mash is desirable.

Keep poultry house clean and well-supplied with clean, dry litter. Used litter that looks dirty (with manure) is clean if it is dry!

Control rodents.

Cull non-laying hens. Laying hens have 3-4 inches distance between the pubic bones at the base of the tail (the vent) and the keel bone. They have more than 1 inch of space between the pubic bones (one on each side of the vent). The vent is oval and moist. (Non-layers have much less distance between the pubic bones and the vent is round and dry.)

Do not allow feed wastage; feeders must be placed at proper height and filled not over half-full.

Feed according to age and purpose of birds!

Provide one nest for each 4-5 laying hens. A 2x4 foot community nest will take care of 40 laying hens.

Light is essential for laying hens. It stimulates egg production and hens will not lay well if kept under conditions of declining light-day length (this occurs from late June until late December).

Pullets (young female chickens) become sexually mature (will lay eggs) at approximately 20 weeks of age. They should be given 16 hours of light (daylight plus electric) per day. Our longest day in Michigan is about 15½ hours. If you give the layers 16 hours of light, you will not be in danger of shortening their day length.

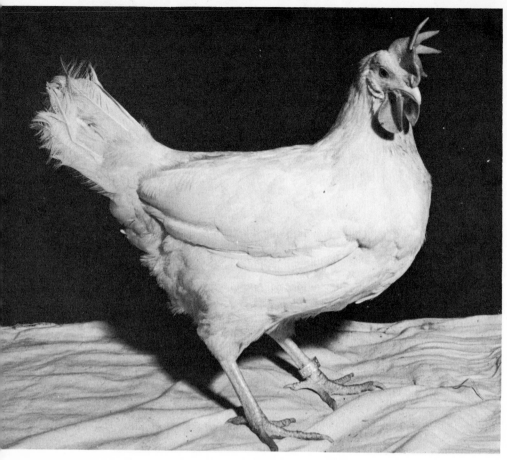

Here is a fine laying hen. Note the large comb and wattles

The amount of light needed is not great. One foot candle of light at bird level in the dark part of the house is adequate. A 40-watt bulb each 100 square feet of floor space is more than adequate.

Cannibalism

Cannibalism (picking) among chickens is always (at all ages) a distinct possibility. The best way to control this problem is to prevent its start. The actual cause of this problem is not really known. We suspect that too much of something is the cause; too much heat, too much light, crowding and starvation have been blamed.

Control is based on making the birds comfortable. Vary temperatures and light within the house when possible. Allow the birds some light and dark areas in the house. Space requirements are discussed in another part of this publication. Some small flock owners allow the birds to run free; this is good for cannibalism control.

Debeaking is the control (and preventative if done before the birds start) measure that is used if cannabalism gets started. To debeak the bird, remove one-half to two-thirds (when measuring from the nostril hole to the tip of the beak) of the upper beak and the tip of the lower beak. A pocket knife or small (very sharp) tin snips will do the job. If bleeding occurs sear the tip of the beak with a red hot soldering iron to stop the bleeding. Caution: do not burn the bird's tongue!

What to do when disease strikes

When excessive mortality or morbidity occurs, consult a veterinarian immediately.

Young birds (4 to 10 weeks old) are highly susceptible to coccidiosis. Coccidiosis is a disease of the intestinal tract and is usually transferred through the litter to susceptible birds. Outbreaks can be controlled, if caught early, by cleaning the house every 3 to 4 days—this removes most of the disease-producing organisms before they become mature, infective agents. Another common method of control is to feed rations that contain a coccidiostat until the birds develop immunity at 12-14 weeks of age.

Need for vaccination

In Michigan and some other states, it is imperative that all chickens—breeding and laying flocks—be protected against infectious bronchitis, Newcastle disease, epidemic tremor, fowl pox and Marek's disease. Failure to protect laying hens against these diseases invites disaster in all poultry enterprises. These diseases cause economic loss from mortality, inefficient growth, reduced egg production and low egg quality. Vaccines offer protection against these diseases.

Vaccine program (see Table 1)

Chicks, at the time of hatching, carry parental (passive) immunity against infectious bronchitis, epidemic tremor and Newcastle disease; this immunity is derived from the egg from which they hatched. Vaccinating chicks during the first week in the brooder house or cage does not stimulate maximum immunity to these three diseases. It is preferable to withhold vaccination until the parental immunity has subsided. However, day-old chicks must be vaccinated against Marek's disease using the turkey herpes virus vaccine.

Vaccination, whenever administered, causes a reaction (stress) in the birds because the vaccine produces a mild form of the disease. It is recommended that the several vaccines be administered separately, rather than in combination to reduce the reaction observed 5 to 7 days following administration.

Table 1.   Recommended vaccination program for Michigan

Age of birds	Vaccine	Method of administration
1 day old	Marek's disease	Individual hypodermic injection
7-10 days	Infectious bronchitis*	Drinking water or dust
17-21 days	Newcastle disease*	Drinking water, dust or spray
8-14 weeks	Fowl pox	Individual wing-web
10-16 weeks	Epidemic tremor	Drinking water
4 months	Newcastle disease	Drinking water, dust or spray
Booster every 3 months in egg production	Newcastle disease	Drinking water, dust or spray

*These two vaccines are often administered simultaneously at 10-14 days of age.

Six virus diseases

These can be controlled by the use of available, attenuated virus vaccines: 1) infectious bronchitis; 2) Newcastle disease; 3) epidemic tremor; 4) Fowl pox; 5) laryngotracheitis; and, 6) Marek's disease.

Dangers

Vaccines, except for the killed-type of Newcastle disease vaccine, contain living viruses intended to cause a mild form of the disease, thus, developing immunity to field strains of the respective viruses. Actually, the vaccines do cause a systemic reaction. The reaction will be mild if:

1. the birds are healthy at the time of vaccination;
2. the bird's environment is clean and dry;
3. there are no sudden changes in management practices;
4. the brooder temperature is maintained (the temperature may be raised 3° to 5° F for a few days after vaccination);
5. the instructions accompanying the vaccine are followed;
6. booster vaccinations are from the same manufacturer as the original vaccine; and
7. you follow instructions on the label.

To assure adequate protection from these diseases, it is important that the birds be in good health when vaccinated!

Broilers

You may want to keep a few broilers for meat production. Broiler chicks differ from egg production chicks. They grow rapidly if cared for properly. Broiler chicks will weigh 4-6 pounds in 8 weeks if they are really a broiler strain (bred to grow fast) and are fed a broiler ration. Since World War II a very large industry has developed in broilers. The U.S. raises approximately 3½ billion broilers a year.

Cultural practices for broilers

Follow the same cultural practices in caring for broilers discussed in the baby chicks for egg production portion of this bulletin. Broiler chicks will grow faster and eat more—in a shorter time, than egg production chicks.

Feeding broilers

A good broiler starting ration should contain 24% protein. If you feed anything less than this, you are not realizing the potential that the broiler is bred to produce. At 5 weeks of age drop back to a broiler finisher feed containing approximately 21% protein. Order the feed well in advance of when you need it as most feed dealers do not carry a stock of broiler feed. Table 2 will give you an idea of how broilers will eat, drink and grow if cared for properly.

Management check-list for chicks

1. *Litter*—Provide 2-3 inches deep of a mold-free absorbent litter.
2. *Chick guard*—Place 12-18 inch high chick guard (a ring of netting, paper, cardboard, etc.) around the heat source.
3. *Temperature*—Regulate the brooder temperature to the comfort of the chicks.
4. *Floor space*—Allow 0.5 square feet of floor space per bird the first 3 weeks, and 1 square foot of floor space per bird for the remainder of the growing period.
5. *Ventilation*—There should be enough draft-free ventilation to remove ammonia fumes and keep the litter dry.
6. *Vaccination*—All birds should be vaccinated.
7. *Feeder space*—Allow 250-300 linear inches (2- to 6-foot 3½ inch deep trough or use 4 tube-type feeders) per 100 birds.
8. *Water space*—Start with three ½ gallon water fountains per 100 chicks.
9. *Light*—Allow the birds a minimum of 12 hours of light per day with a minimum light intensity of 1 foot candle.
10. *Debeaking*—Remove upper beak ⅔ of the distance from tip to nostril openings and detip the lower beak.

Table 2. Average feed consumption, water consumption and growth rate of broilers

Age in Weeks	Avg. Wgt.	Feed Con- version	Feed Consumption/100 Birds			Water Consumption/ 100 Birds		
			Daily	Weekly	Cumu- lative	Daily	Weekly	Cumu- lative
			pounds			gallons		
1	0.23	0.70	2.3	16	16	0.5	3.5	3.5
2	0.47	1.11	5.0	35	51	1.2	8.4	11.9
3	0.82	1.37	8.5	60	111	2.0	14.4	26.3
4	1.23	1.58	11.7	82	193	2.8	19.6	45.9
5	1.72	1.72	14.4	101	294	3.5	24.5	70.4
6	2.29	1.85	18.3	128	423	4.4	30.8	101.2
7	2.92	1.94	20.5	144	567	4.9	34.3	135.5
8	3.52	2.08	23.8	167	734	5.7	39.9	175.4
9	4.13	2.20	25.4	178	912	6.1	42.7	218.1

11. *Feed program for broiler-type chicks:*

Age	Protein	Calories/lb	Ca	P
0- 5 weeks	24%	1425-1550	1.0%	0.6%
6- 9 weeks	20%	1425-1550	1.0%	0.6%

Feed program for egg-type chicks:

Age	Protein	Calories/lb	Ca	P
0- 5 weeks	20%	1250-1400	1.0%	0.6%
6-14 weeks	17%	1250-1400	1.0%	0.6%
15-20 weeks	14%	1200-1400	1.0%	0.6%

12. *Coccidiostats*—Be sure your chick starter contains a coccidiostat, for example, Amprol or Zoaline at the 0.0125% active drug level.

13. *House preparation*—Remove all litter and manure. Then scrape, scrub and disinfect the house and equipment.

14. *Brooder space*—Each chick should be allowed a minimum of 7 square inches of brooder space under the hover. For electrical brooders, 10 inches should be provided.

Suggested bulletins

The following bulletins are sometimes available at your local county extension office (through county agricultural agents), or the Superintendent of Documents, U.S. Printing Office, Washington, D.C. 20402 (price 20¢), Stock number 0100-2431.

Farm Poultry Management, Farmers' Bulletin No. 2197, U.S. Department of Agriculture.

Raising Livestock on Small Farms, Farmers' Bulletin No. 2224, U.S. Department of Agriculture.

The Chicken Broiler Industry, Report No. 930, U.S. Department of Agriculture.

Practical poultry feed formulas[1]—(*1000 lb. mix*)

Ingredients		Calculated analysis			
		Starter	Grower		Layer
		20% protein	17% protein	14% protein	17% protein
Crude protein	%	20.0	17.0	14.0	17.0
Crude fat	%	3.0	3.3	3.6	3.1
Crude fiber	%	4.8	4.8	6.5	4.2
Productive energy	Cal/lb	875.0	875.0	835.0	890.0
Calcium	%	1.2	1.1	0.9	3.25
Phosphorus (total)	%	0.7	0.6	0.6	0.8
Salt	%	0.3	0.3	0.3	0.5
Manganese (supp.)	mg/lb	28.0	28.0	28.0	28.0
Approximately					
Vitamin A	I.U./lb	3300.0	3100.0	2800.0	3400.0
Vitamin D$_3$	I.C.U./lb	700.0	700.0	700.0	700.0
Vitamin E	I.U./lb	4.0	4.4	4.9	4.3
Vitamin B$_{12}$	mcgb/lb	4.7	4.5	4.7	3.5
Riboflavin	mg/lb	2.6	2.5	2.3	2.1
Niacin	mg/lb	20.0	23.0	24.0	20.6
Pantothenic acid	mg/lb	6.6	6.7	6.6	5.7
Choline	mg/lb	650.0	575.0	520.0	540.0

Mention of commercial products or companies is for informational purposes only and does not imply their endorsement or prejudice against others not mentioned.

Practical poultry feed formulas[1]—(*1000 lb. mix*)

Ingredients	All-mash feeding			Layer
	Starter	Grower		
	20% protein	17% protein	14% protein	17% protein
Corn, yellow finely ground	542	—	—	—
Corn, yellow medium ground	—	547	422	570
Alfalfa meal, dehyd. 17% protein	25	20	20	25
Soybean meal, dehulled, 50% protein	—	—	—	—
Soybean meal, solv. 45% protein	255	160	45	195
Wheat middlings, standard	50	150	200	90
Oats, ground	50	50	250	—
Oat hulls, ground (or fine ground corn cobs)	—	—	—	—
Meat and bone scraps, 50% protein	25	25	25	20
Whey, dried	10	10	—	—
Fishmeal 60% protein	15	10	15	10
Salt	3	3	3	5
Dicalcium phosphate	5	5	5	15
Limestone, ground[5]	15	15	10	65
Vitamin-trace mineral premix[2]	5	5	5	5
Coccidiostat[3]	+	+	+	+

[1] **Modification of formulas:** Ground wheat or 39-40 lbs./bu. oats may replace corn if price is favorable. Light fish meals containing (or adjusted to) 60% protein may replace menhaden fish meal. Bone meal or defluorinated phosphate may replace dicalcium phosphate to provide equivalent amounts of calcium and phosphorus.

[2] **Vitamin-trace mineral premixes:** All starter or grower mashes can use Nopcosol M-5, layer mashes and layer mash supplement can use Nopcosol M-3, breeder mashes or breeder mash supplement can use Nopcosol M-4 available from the Nopco Chemical Co., Harrison, N.J. (Check manufacturer's recommendations, since Nopco proposed vitamin mixes may be the double potency which will be required at 2½ lbs. per 1000 pound mix.)

(or)

Dawe's Vitafac No. 1 can be used for all starter, grower, and layer mashes and layer mash supplement. Vitafac No. 2 can be used for all breeder mashes and the breeder mash supplement. These premixes are available from Dawe's Laboratories, Inc., 4800 S. Richmond St., Chicago, Illinois 60632.

Similar-type products may be purchased from these and other manufacturers: Peter Hand Co., 1000 North Avenue, Chicago, Ill.; Merck and Co., Rahway, N.J.; Chas. Pfizer and Co., Inc., Terre Haute, Indiana; Specificide Inc., 55263, Indianapolis, Indiana.

[3] Coccidiostat employed should permit development of immunity in starting chicks and developing pullets. Do not use coccidiostats in breeder-type rations unless manufacturer guarantees safety for breeding birds.

[4] Provide adequate coccidiostat to compensate for the grain portion of the ration.

[5] **To supply extra calcium in the mash:**
   A. An additional 30 lbs. of whole oyster shell should be added to each 1000 lbs. of all 15% and 17% protein layer and breeder mashes to supply adequate calcium for building normal egg shell strength.
   B. An additional 60 lbs. of whole oyster shell should be added to each 1000 lbs. of the 22% layer or breeder mash to be fed 1:1 with grain.
   C. An additional 120 lbs. of whole oyster shell should be added to each 1000 lbs. of 40% layer or breeder supplement to be fed 1:3 with grain.

To supply extra calcium free-choice:
   Limestone may be added in separate hoppers kept before the layers at all times.

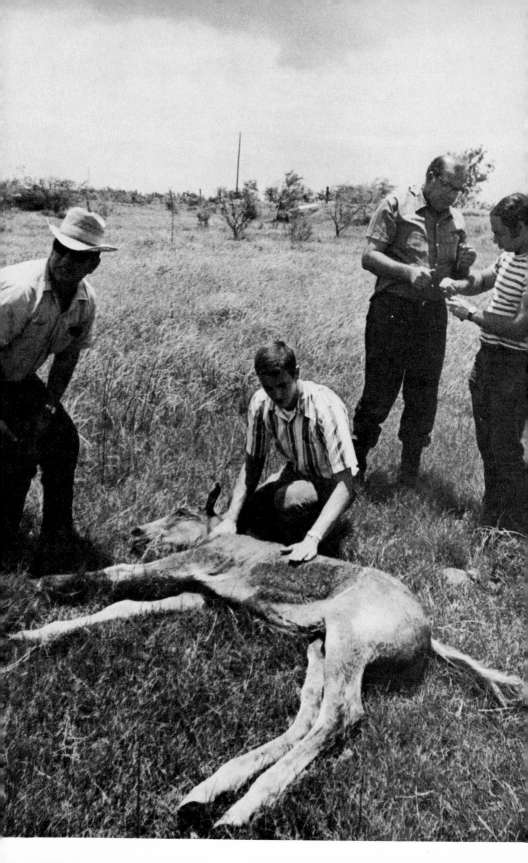

Encephalomyelitis

EQUINE ENCEPHALOMYELITIS, commonly known as sleeping sickness and brain fever, is caused by a virus that attacks the brain and spinal cord. There are three types of the disease, the Eastern, the Western, and the Venezuelan. They are identical in their effects, except for the severity, which varies with the strain of virus and the degree of exposure. They differ, in that immunity against one will not confer protection against either of the others.

The exact ways in which the malady is transmitted from animal to animal are not known. But experiments have proved that mosquitoes can act as carriers, and it is believed that other insects may also transmit the disease.

The malady is seasonal. It usually appears in April or May, reaches a peak in midsummer, and disappears after the first killing frost. It occurs principally among pastured animals, only rarely among those that are stabled. The eastern type virus is found on the Atlantic seaboard and in the Gulf coast states. The Western type predominates west of the Mississippi River, while the Venezuelan seems to be less selective, being more prominent in the lower Mississippi Valley, but overlapping both Eastern and Western types.

Sleeping sickness attacks equines of any age, breed or sex. During an outbreak, about 10 percent of the horses and mules in an area show signs of the sickness.

Symptoms

First symptoms of the disease are fever, sleepiness, grinding of teeth, uncertain gait and difficulty in chewing and eating. The animal may recover at this point and thereafter be resistant to the type of virus that caused the symptoms. On the other hand, symptoms may become more severe, with involvement of the brain and spinal cord.

In cases where the disease progresses, affected animals become dejected and then lapse into a stupor. Such "sleepers" must be aroused in order to give them food and drink. They often fall asleep while food is in their mouths. There are usually a watery discharge from the nostrils and a foul breath.

One in every four or five animals affected with the western type and nine out of every 10 having the eastern type become weaker and weaker and finally collapse. Nearly all of these that go down finally die. Mortality from the Venezuelan type virus is variable, but usually ranges between that of the Eastern type and the Western type.

Treatment and prevention

The use of medicine for the disease is of no value, but good care and treatment contribute to recovery. Anti-encephalomyelitis serum is often

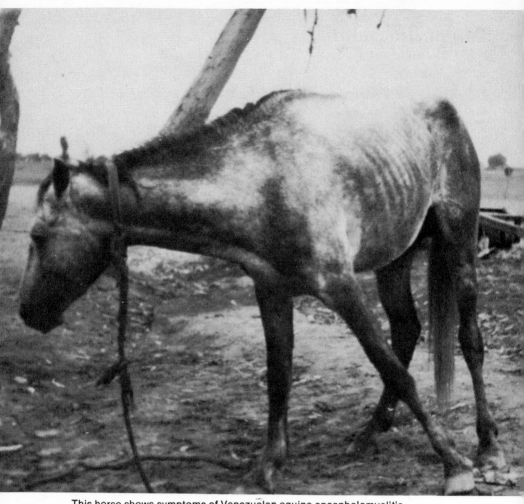

This horse shows symptoms of Venezuelan equine encephalomyelitis

given early in the course of the malady by veterinarians. If given later, it it not effective.

Protection against sleeping sickness is afforded by vaccination.

The vaccines available protect against specific types of virus used in their preparation, but none are cross-immunizing. Two doses of vaccine injected at seven to 10-day intervals, give protection for that year. Vaccination should be completed before the danger season begins.

Periodic ophthalmia of equines

PERIODIC OPHTHALMIA, or moon blindness, is a disease of the eyes of horses, mules and asses. The cause of it is unknown, even though for many years scientists have conducted every manner of research to find out what brings it on.

The malady seems to be infectious, since it flares up in specific areas. Sometimes an outbreak affects only a few farms. Then again it may affect from 5 to 30 percent of the animals in a region. The disease may run its course in a short time or may extend over a period of several years. On some farms the malady may affect new animals that are introduced year after year. These and similar contradictory occurrences add to the mystery of the ailment.

There is evidence that periodic ophthalmia is a symptom of leptospirosis, and other indications that limited intake of riboflavin may contribute to the severity of the problem.

Symptoms

The first symptom of periodic ophthalmia is an inflammation that may affect one or both eyes. Eyelids are swollen and the affected eye or eyes are kept closed. A watery discharge is present.

The symptoms appear suddenly. They are usually noticed in the morning in animals that showed no signs of the disease the night before. Affected animals have a slight fever and show other signs of illness.

After a week or 10 days the inflammation disappears. The eye or eyes may return to normal or may have turned chalky white and sightless. Another attack of the disease may occur in a week or perhaps in several months. There may be as many as 20 attacks occurring over a period of years. The disease may affect one eye and then the other or both at the same time.

Usually animals are not affected until they are three or four years old. Sometimes it does not develop until they are 15 or 20. No sure way has been discovered to prevent or cure the disease.

Treatment

Some success in warding off the disease has been attained by adding rather large quantities of riboflavin (vitamin B_2) to the rations of horses. The amount is 40 mg. per day and it can be given at a reasonable cost through the use of brewers' yeast. Riboflavin is of no value in treating established cases.

The daily intravenous injection of 400 mg. of ascorbic acid (vitamin C) during the acute stages of the disease has in many cases resulted in disappearance of symptoms. Streptomycin administered subcutaneously in doses of 5 gm. has also brought relief.

A dark stall while symptoms are present adds to an affected animal's comfort. In some animals, acute symptoms have been controlled by ophthalmic ointments containing cortisone, with or without antibiotics. Atropine should be used promptly to keep pupils dilated and prevent adhesion of the eye parts.

Azoturia, or monday morning disease

AZOTURIA is a disease of horses, usually of vigorous draft animals in good condition. It generally appears shortly after work is begun, following a day or more of idleness. This is why it is often called Monday morning disease.

The symptoms appear suddenly. They include heavy sweating, dark-colored urine and paralysis of the muscles, usually of the hind legs. The exact cause of the malady is unknown.

To prevent azoturia, the diet of animals should be regulated when they are not at work. Feed should be cut to a minimum and the ration should include a laxative feed such as bran. On off days, if possible, animals should be allowed to exercise of their own free will in a paddock.

Horses resuming work after a lay-off should be watched carefully. If symptoms appear, immediate rest is necessary. Animals should not even be moved from the field to the barn. If possible, immediate veterinary service should be procured. No irritating laxatives should be given. However, mineral oil helps to relieve the condition. Sedatives and alkalizing drugs may be necessary.

Among animals that have been stricken for some time, a large percentage die even when professional treatment is given.

Founder, or laminitis

FOUNDER is a serious ailment of the feet of horses. It commonly results from overfeeding, chiefly on grains, although gorging on other feeds will also bring it on. Other occasional causes of the disease are inflammation of the uterus in recently foaled mares, heavy work on hard footing and poisoning.

The chief symptoms of the malady are extreme pain and fever. Usually all four feet are affected, but the pain may be greater in the forefeet. In this case, the animal extends its forefeet in front of its body so as to throw the weight on the heels. If the hind feet only are involved, the legs are bunched under the body so as to throw the weight on the forefeet and the heels of the hind feet. Animals with founder have a crouching gait. They tremble, don't like to move and have an anxious manner.

Treatment

When the condition is caused by gorging, horses should be given a purgative. Feet should be placed in cold water, with ice, if possible. With prompt treatment, the symptoms usually subside in a few days.

Chronic laminitis often results in deformed feet. Little can be done to relieve it except suitable shoeing.

Malignant edema

MALIGNANT EDEMA is a highly fatal disease that affects horses, swine, sheep and cattle. It is also known as gas phlegmon, and sometimes as braxy when it occurs in sheep.

The disease attacks animals of all ages. It usually occurs in the spring, summer and fall.

The microbe that causes it is called *Clostridium septicum* and it gains entrance into the body through wounds. In horses, such wounds are likely to be made by nails or splinters. In sheep infection may follow castration, docking or shearing. In cattle the disease may follow castration or result from other wounds. Gas phlegmon of swine occurs now and then when vaccination against hog cholera is done under insanitary conditions.

Symptoms

The disease starts suddenly with symptoms that resemble those of blackleg. In a few hours to a few days after the injury, gas swellings appear in muscles and a thin dirty reddish fluid seeps from the original wound. The gas swellings crackle when pressed, like those of blackleg, but they are usually not so extensive as in blackleg. Other symptoms of the malignant edema are loss of appetite, dullness and fever that usually reaches 106 to 108 degrees Fahrenheit.

When infection starts with a wound on the face of a horse, the whole head of the victim soon becomes swollen and death follows in from one to two days.

The death rate of infected animals is almost 100 percent.

Prevention

There is no effective treatment for the disease. Protection is given by vaccination with a bacterin.

Infectious anemia, or swamp fever

INFECTIOUS ANEMIA, also known as mountain fever, swamp fever, malarial fever and slow fever, is one of the most serious diseases of the horse. It is caused by a virus.

The disease occurs most often in poorly drained, low-lying sections, but has been found on marshy pastures at high altitudes and in wooded sections. There are more cases of it during wet years and when biting insects are numerous.

Infectious anemia appears in May and June and reaches its height in midsummer, usually disappearing in late fall. Chronic cases are, of course, present the year around. It is especially prevalent among horses and mules in the Mississippi Delta region.

Animals are more susceptible to the disease when their resistance is lowered by such things as overexertion, extreme heat, improper feed and infestation with intestinal parasites. It is not exactly known how the malady is transmitted, but outbreaks often follow the introduction of an infected animal into a territory. Biting insects are suspected of being carriers.

Symptoms

Infectious anemia occurs both as a rapidly fatal and as a chronic malady. The virus may also be present in the blood stream of an animal all the time without causing any visible symptoms.

In the acute form of the disease, the onset is sudden and accompanied by a fever that reaches 105 degrees Fahrenheit. Breathing is rapid, the animal is dejected, the head hangs low, leg weakness appears, body weight is shifted from one leg to another, frequently hind feet are placed well forward, feed is refused and there is loss of weight. Attacks usually last from three to five days. The animal either dies or the disease becomes chronic.

In the chronic form of the malady, attacks follow at intervals of a few days, weeks or months. When the time between attacks is short, the victim seldom lives more than a few weeks to a month.

The attacks are accompanied by a heavy destruction of red blood corpuscles. Accurate diagnosis is difficult because the body changes brought about by the disease are so much like those of other maladies.

No cure or preventive measures known

So far as is known, there is no cure for the disease, nor have any methods been developed for its prevention. In areas where the disease is known to exist, the maintenance of good sanitary conditions and general health of animals, together with control of insects, helps to hold the damaging effects of the malady at a minimum. Since the disease may be present in the inactive form, great care should be taken not to transmit it when using hypodermic needles and other instruments.

Navel ill of foals, calves and lambs

NAVEL ILL, also called joint ill, is a disease of newborn or very young foals, calves, lambs and pigs. (See index for navel of pigs.)

It may be caused by any number of different microbes which gain entrance to the body by way of the navel. From there, the infection spreads throughout the body, settling in the joints and other parts.

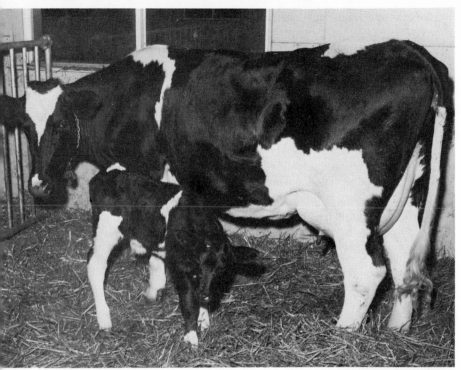

Maternity pen:—clean, well bedded, providing protection for the newborn calf from severe weather exposure

Authorities disagree as to whether the young animals get the disease while still in the mother's womb or whether the navel or umbilical cord becomes infected after the animal is born. Evidence indicates that infection may come about in either way.

Symptoms

Because the disease may be caused by various kinds of microbes, symptoms are of wide variety. The most common symptoms are the swelling of one or more joints which become hot and tender. The victim is lame or refuses to walk at all, does not want to suckle, has a high fever, fast pulse, fast breathing, and pus—often foul-smelling—runs from the navel. Animals with these symptoms seldom recover and when they do they are usually unthrifty.

In the acute form among foals—where the disease appears a few hours after birth—the death rate is 90 to 100 percent.

In lambs, there are two principal forms of the disease. In the acute form the lamb dies when about one week old. In the chronic form, which occurs among older lambs, victims may be lame, stiff or may become paralyzed. They may linger for some time before dying or they may recover.

Prevention and treatment

Where the disease might be acquired before birth, it is reasonable to suppose that the dam's blood contains antibodies against the microbes that cause the ailment. In view of this, injections of the dam's blood are sometimes given foals immediately after birth.

Bacterins are available for injection containing the killed microbes generally associated with the disease. Sulfanilamide has been reported to be of some value in the treatment of sheep and sulfamethazine in treating swine and foals. Streptomycin, either alone or in combination with penicillin, is effective in treating septicemia in new born foals.

To prevent navel ill before birth, only healthy animals should be bred. Buildings and bedding of maternity stalls should be kept as sanitary as possible. This applies to cattle as well as to horses.

To prevent the disease from being contracted after birth, umbilical stumps of susceptible animals should be immersed in some good antiseptic solution, such as tincture of iodine, immediately after birth.

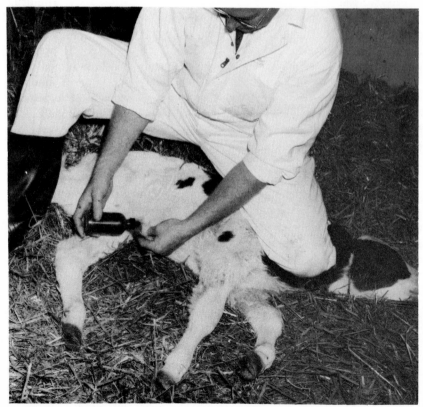

Apply tincture of iodine to the navel to prevent infections

Michigan State University

Horse strongyles

STRONGYLES are the commonest and most injurious parasites of horses. There are some 40 different kinds, of which about 15 do most of the damage. Most of them are less than an inch long, although a few of them attain a length of as much as two inches. The large strongyles are commonly known as palisade worms, redworms and bloodworms.

Strongyles have a complicated life cycle. When in the larval state, they crawl to the upper portion of grass blades and are swallowed by grazing horses. They do the most damage by attaching themselves to the lining of the intestines and sucking the blood of infested animals.

Symptoms of strongylosis are anemia, loss of appetite and falling off in weight. Strongyles are also sometimes responsible for diarrhea.

Treatment and prevention

Phenothiazine is regarded as the best drug for removing the worms. It must be given with care, however, since a small percentage of animals are injured by it.

A dosage of 25 to 30 grams (about one ounce) per 1,000 pounds of body weight is used and has generally proved satisfactory. The drug may be given in capsules, as a drench, or in ground feed. However, divided doses, for example, five grams daily in the feed for about a week, may be safer for anemic or heavily parasatized animals, for pregnant mares, for emaciated animals and for particularly valuable animals.

Some horses and foals will voluntarily consume sufficient amounts of a mixture of 40 parts of salt and one part of phenothiazine to provide reasonably effective control of strongyles. The mixture is provided as a salt lick which, for reasons of economy, must be protected from the weather. The animals are encouraged to take the medicated salt by adding a few handfuls of grain to it from time to time.

To use phenothiazine most advantageously as a preventive of strongylosis, full doses about twice a year are probably advisable. These should be given before, and again at the end of, the grazing season. Animals from about six months to five years of age may require additional medication midway in the grazing season, and animals over 10 years of age may do well on one treatment a year.

Tetanus

TETANUS is a disease that affects nearly all animals, including man. Horses, mules and asses are particularly subject to the kind of injuries likely to result in this disease.

The organism that causes the malady—*Clostridium tetani*—is commonly present in the soil. Heavily manured lands, swamps and some truck gardens usually contain large numbers of the bacteria and their spores. They infect punctures, cuts and wounds, forming a powerful toxin, or poison, that enters the blood stream.

Symptoms

Symptoms of the disease usually appear within one or two weeks after infection, although they may be delayed for months. In younger animals they often appear in less than a week.

The first signs of tetanus usually appear around the head. Chewing becomes less forceful; swallowing is slow and awkward. The so-called inner or third eyelid protrudes over the surface of the eyeball. Muscles become rigid, this condition affecting one group after another. Eating is greatly impaired, or is stopped altogether. This symptom gives rise to the word "lockjaw." Ears are held rigidly erect, tail is elevated and stiff and legs are spread and stiffened. This gives the animal a sawhorse appearance. Death is usually due to exhaustion, paralysis of internal organs or pneumonia.

Prevention and treatment

The disease can be largely prevented by removing objects that are apt to cause wounds, such as protruding nails, splintered boards, and farm machinery with projecting parts on which animals may injure themselves.

When slight, fresh cuts and wounds should be treated with tincture of iodine or other suitable antiseptic. Tetanus toxoid, a chemically treated toxin, brings on lasting immunity when properly administered.

Treatment of seriously injured animals consists in cleaning and draining wounds and applying antiseptics and suitable dressings to affected parts. Huge doses of tetanus antitoxin are sometimes given, particularly to valuable animals.

Horse botflies

HORSE BOTFLIES attack horses, mules and asses, but will not molest any other farm animals. Three kinds of them are common in the United States.

The nose botfly attaches its eggs to the hairs on a horse's lips. The tiny bots that hatch from the eggs enter the horse's mouth and burrow into the lining. After a month, they pass to the stomach and intestines where they remain for eight to 11 months, meanwhile growing to about three-fourths of an inch long. The bots do a lot of damage to the walls of these organs before they are finally ejected with the manure. On or in the ground they become pupae and later emerge as flies.

Throat botflies attach their eggs to the underjaw of a horse. The young bots, on hatching, enter the mouth and dig into the gums. Afterward, their life cycle is similar to that of the nose botfly.

The common horse botfly lays its eggs on a horse's body or legs, usually in back of the knee. Horses lick the eggs, causing the bots to emerge and stick to the horse's tongue. The bots burrow into the tongue and lips and complete their life cycle in a manner similar to that of the nose botfly.

How to control botflies

Adult botflies have no mouth parts. Since they do not eat, they cannot be lured into traps or to poisoned bait. Nor is there any practicable way to kill the eggs.

The treatment recommended by the Bureau of Animal Industry for removal of bots from the digestive tract is as follows:

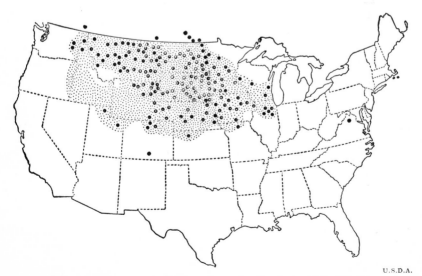

U.S.D.A.

This map shows the distribution of nose botflies in the United States

Fast the animal from noon of the day preceding treatment until 6 or 7 o'clock of the next morning. At this time the animal is given carbon disulphide by stomach tube or in flexible gelatin capsules, the capsules being given by hand or by means of a balling gun. The dose for a horse weighing about 1,000 pounds is one dose of six drams, or two doses of four drams each with a two-hour interval between doses, or three doses of three drams each with an hour interval between doses. Do not feed or water for three hours after treatment.

As a rule the single-dose treatment is most satisfactory, but if there is any question as to the animal's ability to tolerate the dose, divided doses may be given and the treatment suspended if bad effects follow a partial treatment. The dose should be diminished for smaller animals, and yearling colts should not receive over half the quantities given above. Very old or weak horses, or those suffering from febrile or debilitating diseases, are sometimes poor risks for treatment.

The carbon disulphide should not be followed by a purgative, and oil is especially undesirable. Preliminary purgation the evening before treatment is advisable only in the case of a constipated animal. The bots may continue to pass out for a month or more after treatment.

In view of the fact that carbon disulphide is a poison, intended to poison the bots, and a chemical which may cause unpleasant results or even death if given unskillfully or administered to animals having disease conditions which make the treatment unsafe, it is always advisable to have the treatment given by a competent veterinarian whenever possible. Serious consequences have resulted when poorly trained men used make-shift balling guns. When a capsule breaks in a horse's mouth and the carbon disulphide gets into the lungs, the horse may die.

A very important consideration in obtaining the best results is the matter of time of treatment. Carbon disulphide will remove many bots when administered at any time of the year, but the greatest efficiency can be obtained by treatment in winter months, preferably December or January. If treated before the botflies are killed by freezing weather, the horses may become reinfested.

Soon after February 1 some of the nose-fly bots begin to pass backward into the rectum where they cannot be reached with the internal treatment. In the South, January is the best month for treatment, as botflies may appear and lay eggs on horses in December. Another reason for early-winter treatment is that horses freed from the parasites will winter better.

Large roundworms of horses

LARGE INTESTINAL ROUNDWORMS, or ascarids, are more common among young equines than older ones. Roundworms are the largest parasites of horses and mules. Female worms are from six to 15 inches long, while males are somewhat smaller. Their life history is similar to that of roundworms of swine.

In heavy infestations, the larvae do a great deal of damage to the lungs and liver. Treatment is the same as for horse botflies, that is, with carbon disulphide.

Influenza of horses

INFLUENZA, also called shipping fever and pink eye, is one of the most common diseases of horses and mules. Death losses from the disease are usually low. Most of the financial loss is caused by the inability of affected animals to work. The ailment is caused principally by a virus, with complications resulting from other microbes.

Horses and mules coming through sales stables and other establishments where animals are assembled from scattered sources are most often affected with it. Excessive work and undue exposure make animals more susceptible to it.

Symptoms

Symptoms resemble those of the "flu" that affects people. These include loss of appetite, fever, weakness, rapid breathing, coughing and nose and eye discharges. In addition the lining of the eyelids becomes yellowish-pink in color, giving rise to the name "pink eye." This disease is not to be confused with "pink eye" in pigs, which is keratitis, or the shipping fever of cattle.

Where no complications occur, animals recover in about a week. A second rise in temperature takes place where the disease is followed by secondary disturbances such as pneumonia and various maladies of the digestive tract.

Treatment

Treatment consists in giving sick animals absolute rest in well-bedded, draft-free stalls, with small amounts of nutritious feed and a constant supply of fresh water. Animals should not be returned to work until their strength is regained—usually some days after fever has disappeared.

To prevent influenza, newly purchased horses and mules should be held in rigid quarantine, if possible with separate stable attendants, for three weeks before being permitted to mingle with other susceptible animals. Horses and mules acquire protection against secondary infections by repeated injection of specific bacterins. Such treatments should be completed before animals leave for their destinations.

Fistula of the withers

FISTULA of the withers is a general term applied to an inflammation of the withers. It is usually accompanied by infection.

Authorities disagree as to the cause of the ailment. Some believe that friction from a collar or other injuries bring it on.

First treatment usually consists in shaving the affected areas and applying tincture of iodine. In stubborn cases, the fistula, which is like the opening of a deep-seated boil, is cut open and allowed to drain. This of course is done only after proper sterilization of the affected areas and the necessary instruments.

Strangles, or equine distemper

STRANGLES, or equine distemper, is a germ disease of horses, mules and asses. It occurs mainly where these animals are brought together, such as at stockyards, sales stables, race tracks and remount depots.

In the days when horses were the principal mode of transportation, strangles was a common ailment. It is caused by a species of *Streptococcus*, an organism that is easily spread through such means as public water troughs and mangers. Young animals are more susceptible.

The early symptoms of strangles—fever, loss of appetite, discharge from the nose and so on—resemble those of influenza. In one to three days, however, the discharge becomes thick and is expelled in large quantities by snorting and coughing. Usually there are also swellings of the glands under the jaw and in the throat. These often become abscessed and a yellow, creamy pus forms.

These abscesses often interfere with breathing to such an extent that it is necessary to run a tube into the windpipe to keep the animals from suffocating. Pneumonia and blood poisoning sometimes follow.

Most animals recover from the disease and are thereafter resistant to it. Treatment and preventive measures are the same as for influenza. No patent medicines or home-compounded remedies are of any value in treating the disease. Bacterins are sometimes used as preventive measures.

Index

swine, 235-236
winter, 157

E

Ecthyma, contagious, 30-31, 255
Edema disease, 247
Edema, malignant, 26-27, 142, 283
Egg production, 270-272
   selecting chicks for, 266
Elastration
   in castration, 90, 263
   in dehorning, 95
   in docking, 263
Elephant hide, 244
Emasculatome, 88, 90, 263
Emasculator, 87-88
Encephalitis, sheep, 24-25,
   258-259
Encephalomyelitis, equine, 30-31,
   279-280
End-incision method of bull
   castration, 88, 89
Endometritis, 81-82
Enteritis
   chronic specific, *see* Johne's
      disease
   infectious hemorrhagic, 235
   infectious necrotic, 28-29,
      216-217
   vibrionic, 157
Enterotoxemia, 256
EQ-335, 161
Equine distemper, 292
Equine encephalomyelitis, 30-31,
   279-280
Erysipelas, swine, 32-33, 214-215
   similarity to hog cholera, 211
   similarity to necrotic enteritis,
      216
Eversion
   of vagina in cattle, 85
   of womb in cattle, 82-84
Eyes
   in diagnosis of disease, 16
   in hog cholera, 211
   in infectious keratitis, 173-174
   in periodic ophthalmia, 281
   pupil response, 16
   tearing in X-disease, 177
   in tetanus, 288
   in trichinosis, 237

Exanthema, vesicular, 34-35, 218-
   219
Extractors, calf, 73

F

False cowpox, 175-176
Farrowing, sanitation and,
   223-224
Feeding
   in baby pig disease, 227-228
   of cattle during shipping, 136
   chicks, 267
   in enterotoxemia, 256
   nutritional deficiencies, 187-
      194
   poultry feed formulas, 276-277
   to prevent azoturia, 282
   to prevent bloat, 125-126
   and reproduction in cattle, 66,
      67
   salt, 192
   and trichinosis, 237
   and urinary calculi, 171-172
   and vesicular exanthema, 218
Fertility, of cattle, 63-69, 112-115
Fetus
   determining age in cattle,
      59-62, 63
   malpresentation in cattle, 75-81
   mummified, 65
   normal position in cattle, 70-72
Fever
   as disease symptom, 16-17,
      22-35
   signs of, 17
Fistula
   of teat, 115
   of withers, 292
Flies
   blowflies, 160-162
   heel, 162-164
   horn, 165
   horse botflies, 289-290
   sheep nasal, 251-252
Flukes, 11
   liver, 258
Foals, navel ill, 284-286
Follicular mange, 243
Foot rot, 128-130, 264
   symptoms, 12
Foot-and-mouth disease, 147-149

rabies, 151
red water disease, 143
shipping fever, 135
sore mouth, 255
swine erysipelas, 215
transmissible gastroenteritis, 217
Impaction, gastric, 122-123
Incubation period of disease, 7
Indigestion, 122-123
in ketosis, 121
symptoms, 15
Infections, secondary, with virus diseases, 11
Influenza
in horses, 291
swine, 32-33, 238
symptoms in shipping fever, 134
Injections, 36-42
epidural, 83-84
filling syringe, 40
hypodermic, 36-37
intradermal, 37, 38
intramuscular, 41
intraperitoneal, 42
subcutaneous, 36-37
and tourniquets, 39-40
Insemination, artificial, 201-204
collecting bull semen, 195-200
Intestinal worms, 169-170, 249, 250-251
Intradermal injection, 37, 38
Intramuscular injection, 41
Intraperitoneal injection, 42
Intravenous injection, 38-41
Iodine deficiency, 190-191, 232
Iron deficiency, 191, 231

J

Jaw spreader, 127
Johne's disease, 24-25, 139-140
Johnin test, 139
Joint ill, 26-27, 230, 284-286
Jowl abscesses, 245-246
Jumpy pig disease, 228

K

Keratitis, infectious, 28-29, 173-174
Ketonuria, 28-29

Ketosis, 26-27, 120-122, 256-257
Kidney stones, see Urinary calculi
Kidney worms, 224-225
Knotting sutures, 46, 50

L

Labor
in abortion, 73
signs in cattle, 70
Lake shore disease, 191
Lambs
castrating, 263
docking, 263
enterotoxemia, 256
and ketosis, 257
navel ill, 284-286
vaccination, 255, 256
white muscle disease, 262
Lameness
in navel ill, 230
in poultry, 152
in vesicular exanthema, 218
Laminitis, 282
Laryngitis, necrotic, 24-25, 118-119
Lateral-incision method of bull castration, 87-88, 89
Lead poisoning, 186
Leaking teats, 115
Leptospirosis, 26-27, 110-111, 219
Lice
cattle, 166
hog, 243-244
and swine pox, 240-241
Ligature, of vein, 47
Lindane, 159-160, 161, 242-243, 261
Listerellosis, 24-25, 258-259
Liver flukes, 258
Lockjaw, 32-33, 45, 288
Locoweed poisoning, 184
Lumpy jaw, 132-134
Lungworm disease, 166-168
Lungworms, 226, 249-250
and swine influenza, 238

M

Mad itch, 172, 245
Magnesium deficiency, 190
Malarial fever, 283-284

and swine influenza, 238
    tapeworms, 250, 251, 252
    trichina, 237
Parasites, external, 11, 14-15
    blowflies, 160-162
    cattle grubs, 162-164
    cattle lice, 166
    heel flies, 162-164
    hog lice, 240-241
    horn flies, 165
    mange mites, 158-160, 260-261
    screwworms, 160-162
    sheep ticks, 259
    wool maggots, 259
Paratuberculosis, 24-25, 139-140
Paresis, parturient, see Milk fever
Pasteur treatment, 151
Pasteurellosis, 239
    pneumatic, 134-136
Pathogens, 7
Pens, portable calf, 204-208
Pericarditis, traumatic, 131
Pest control
    blowflies, 161-162
    cattle lice, 166
    heel flies, 164
    hog lice, 244
    horn flies, 165
    mange mites, 159-160, 242-243
Phagocytes, 8
Phosphorus deficiency, 187-188,
    190
Pig typhus, 28-29, 216-217
Pigs, baby
    acute hypoglycemia, 227-228
    anemia, 231
    atrophic rhinitis, 220-221
    as brucellosis carriers, 234
    goiter, 232
    jumpy pig disease, 228
    McClean County System of
        Swine Sanitation, 223-224
    milk requirements, 227-228
    navel ill, 230
    necrotic enteritis, 216-217
    sore mouth, 220
    swine pox, 240-241
    transmissible gastroenteritis,
        217-218
    vaccination for hog cholera,
        211-212

Pink eye
    in cattle, 28-29, 173-174
    in horses, 291
Pitch poisoning, 248
Placenta, retention in cattle, 81-82
Plague, swine, 239
Plants, poisonous, 178-184
    cocklebur, 247
    table of, 180-183
Pneumatic pasteurellosis, 134-136
Pneumonia, 28-29
    calf, 119-120
    in roundworm infestation, 223
    as secondary infection in
        coccidiosis, 155
    stockyards, see Shipping
        disease
    swine, 239-240, 245
    virus, 245
Poisoning
    algae, 184
    alkaloid, 179
    cocklebur, 247
    hydrocyanic acid, 178-179
    lead, 186
    locoweed, 184
    oxalic acid, 179
    pitch, 248
    resinoid, 179
    salt, 247
    saponin, 179
    selenium, 194
    from substances used on farm,
        186-187
    sweet clover, 185
    symptoms, 180-183
    tremetol, 184
    wheat-pasture, 193-194
Porcine stress syndrome, 246
Post-mortem, see Autopsy
Poultry, 265-277
Pregnancy
    detecting in cattle, 58-62, 63
    eversion of vagina, 85
Pregnancy disease, 28-29, 256-257
    similarity to listerellosis, 259
Probang, 127-128
Prolapse
    of vagina in cattle, 85
    of womb in cattle, 82-84
Protozoa, 11

in swine erysipelas, 214
in X-disease, 177
Sleeping sickness, 30-31, 279-280
Slow fever, 283-284
Snails, and liver flukes, 258
Soil contamination
  in anthrax, 145
  in blackleg, 141, 142
  in swine erysipelas, 215
Sore mouth, 30-31, 220, 255
  see also Diphtheria, calf
Speculum method of artificial
    insemination, 201-202
Speculum, mouth, 127
Sperm, bull, 53
Spinal anesthetic, 83-84
Splenic fever, see Anthrax
Spores, microbe, 10
Stance as disease symptom, 14
Sterility, in cattle, 63-69
Sterilizing instruments, 36
Stomach worms, 169-170,
    248-249, 250
Stomatitis
  gangrenous, 24-25, 118-119
  malignant, 24-25
  necrotic, 24-25, 118-119, 220
  ulcerative, 118-119
  vesicular, 111-112
Strangles, 32-33, 292
Strongyles, horse, 287
Subcutaneous injection, 36-37
Sulfa drugs, 43
Suture knots, 46, 50
Suturing, 46, 48-49, 50
Swallowing, in tetanus, 288
Swamp fever, 283-284
Swelling of skin, 15
Swine
  gestation period, 62
  McClean County System of
    Swine Sanitation, 223-224
  useful facts (table), 21
  vital signs (table), 21
Swine dysentery, 235-236
Swine erysipelas, 32-33, 214-215
  similarity to hog cholera, 211
  similarity to necrotic enteritis,
    216
Swine influenza, 32-33, 238
Swine plague, 239

Swine pneumonia, 239-240
Swine pox, 240-241
Symptoms, interpreting, 12-13
Syringe, filling, 40

T

Tapeworms, 250, 251, 252
Tar poisoning, 248
Teats
  injuries, 115
  leaking, 115
  removing extra, 85
Teeth, of cattle, 96
Temperature
  normal rectal (table), 21
  taking, 18-19
Testing
  acetonemia, 121
  bovine vibriosis, 112
  brucellosis, 107-108, 234
  hog cholera, 211
  in Johne's disease, 139
  ketosis, 121
  leptospirosis, 110
  mastitis, 98-99
  tuberculosis, 153
Tetanus, 32-33, 45, 288
Tetany, grass, 14, 194
TGE, see Gastroenteritis,
    transmissible
Torsion
  of artery, 47
  of womb in cattle, 74-75
Tourniquet
  in hemorrhage, 47
  and injections, 39-40
Trichinosis, 237
Trichomoniasis, bovine, 34-35
Triplets in cattle, 57-58
Trocar, 124
Tuberculosis, 152-154
Twins in cattle, 57-58, 65-66, 70,
    76-77
Tympanites, 123-126
Typhus, pig, 28-29, 216-217

U

Udder
  inflammation, 97-102, 232-233
  leaking teats, 115
  removing extra teat, 85

in sore mouth, 255
Ulcerative stomatitis, 118-119
Urinary calculi, 171-172
Urolithiasis, 171-172
Uterus
    prolapse in cattle, 82-84
    twisting in cattle, 74-75

V

Vaccination, 37
    for anthrax, 145-146
    for blackleg, 142
    for bluetongue, 254
    for bovine virus diarrhea, 109
    for brucellosis, 108
    in chickens, 273-274
    for encephalomyelitis, 279-280
    for enterotoxemia, 256
    for hemoglobinuria, 256
    for hog cholera, 211-212
    for leptospirosis, 111, 219
    for rabies, 151
    for sore mouth, 255
    for swine erysipelas, 215
Vaccines, 9
    hog cholera, 211-212
    temperature effects on, 41
Vagina
    artificial, 195-196
    prolapse in cattle, 85
Vaginitis
    nodular, 68
    symptoms in cattle, 14
Veins, stopping hemorrhage, 47
Venereal disease in cattle, 68,
    112-115
Vesicular exanthema, 34-35
Vesicular stomatitis, 111-112
Vibrionic abortion, 112-113
Vibrionic enteritis, 157
Viruses, 10-11
Vital signs, normal, 21
Vitamin A deficiency, 67, 178,
    192-193
Vitamin D deficiency, 178, 193,
    229
Vitamin E deficiency, 262

W

Warbles, 162-164
Warts, 175

Weight of dairy cow, determining,
    91-92
Weight loss
    in acetonemia, 121
    as disease symptom, 14
    in tuberculosis, 152
Wheat-pasture poisoning,
    193-194
White heifer disease, 67
White muscle disease, 262
White scours, 34-35, 116-117
Winter dysentery, 157
Withers, fistula of, 292
Wooden tongue, 132-133
Wool maggots, 259
Womb
    prolapse in cattle, 82-84
    twisting in cattle, 74-75
Worms
    bladder, 252
    horse strongyles, 287
    kidney, 224-225
    lungworms, 166-168, 249-250
    nodular, 249, 250-251
    roundworms, 223, 291
    stomach and intestinal,
        169-170, 248-249, 250
    and swine influenza, 238
    tapeworms, 250, 251, 252
    trichina, 237
Wounds
    and blackleg, 141
    and blowflies, 160, 161
    major, 45-49
    minor, 45
    punctures, 45
    stopping hemorrhage, 46-47
    suturing, 46, 48-49
    tetanus and, 45

X

X-disease, 34-35, 177

Y

Yellow body, 57
    persistent, 64-65

Z

Zinc deficiency, 244